Gynecology
for the
Primary Care
Provider

Scott B. Ransom, D.O., F.A.C.O.G., F.A.C.S., C.H.E.
Assistant Professor
Division of Gynecology
Wayne State University School of Medicine/Hutzel Hospital
Chief, Section of Gynecology
Veterans Administration Medical Center
Detroit, Michigan

S. Gene McNeeley, Jr., M.D., F.A.C.O.G.
Associate Professor and Director
Division of Gynecology
Wayne State University School of Medicine/Hutzel Hospital
Chief, Department of Gynecology
Detroit Receiving Hospital
Detroit, Michigan

W.B. SAUNDERS COMPANY
A Division of Harcourt Brace & Company

Philadelphia London Toronto Montreal Sydney Tokyo

W.B. SAUNDERS COMPANY

A Division of Harcourt Brace & Company

The Curtis Center
Independence Square West
Philadelphia, Pennsylvania 19106

Library of Congress Cataloging-in-Publication Data

Gynecology for the primary care provider / [edited by] Scott Ransom,
   S. Gene McNeeley.—1st ed.
        p.   cm.
      Includes bibliographical references and index.
      ISBN 0-7216-6433-4
      1. Gynecology.   2. Generative organs, Female—Diseases.
   3. Primary care (Medicine)   I. Ransom, Scott.   II. McNeeley, S. Gene.
      [DNLM: 1. Genital Diseases, Female.   2. Primary Health Care.
   WP 140 G9976 1997]
   RG101.G943   1997
   618.1—dc21
   DNLM/DLC   96-37235

GYNECOLOGY FOR THE PRIMARY CARE PROVIDER   ISBN 0-7216-6433-4

Printed in the United States of America

Last digit is the print number: 9   8   7   6   5   4   3   2

Contributors

Michael A. Allon, M.D.
Clinical Instructor
Division of Reproductive Endocrinology
   and Infertility
Department of Obstetrics and Gynecology
Wayne State University School of
   Medicine/Hutzel Hospital
Detroit, Michigan

Lisa J. Bazzett, M.D.
Department of Obstetrics and Gynecology
Wayne State University School of
   Medicine/Hutzel Hospital
Detroit, Michigan

Charla M. Blacker, M.D.
Assistant Professor
Division of Reproductive Endocrinology
   and Infertility
Department of Obstetrics and Gynecology
Wayne State University School of
   Medicine/Hutzel Hospital
Detroit, Michigan

John O.L. DeLancey, M.D.
Associate Professor
Department of Obstetrics and Gynecology
University of Michigan Medical Center
Ann Arbor, Michigan

Michael P. Diamond, M.D.
Professor of Obstetrics and Gynecology
   and Physiology
Director, Division of Reproductive
Endocrinology and Infertility
Wayne State University School of
   Medicine/Hutzel Hospital
Detroit, Michigan

Thomas Elkins, M.D.
Professor
Department of Obstetrics and Gynecology
Louisiana State University Medical Center
New Orleans, Louisiana

Kenneth A. Ginsburg, M.D.
Associate Professor
Division of Reproductive Endocrinology
   and Infertility
Department of Obstetrics and Gynecology
Wayne State University School of
   Medicine/Hutzel Hospital
Detroit, Michigan

Deborah Hamby, M.D.
Department of Obstetrics and Gynecology
Wayne State University School of
   Medicine/Hutzel Hospital
Detroit, Michigan

Susan L. Hendrix, D.O.
Assistant Professor
Department of Obstetrics and Gynecology
Wayne State University School of
   Medicine/Hutzel Hospital
Detroit, Michigan

Carolyn Johnston, M.D.
Assistant Professor
Division of Gynecologic Oncology
Department of Obstetrics and
    Gynecology
University of Michigan Medical Center
Ann Arbor, Michigan

Sally Kope, M.S.W.
Adjunct Professor, Department of
    Human Genetics
University of Michigan Medical Center
Ann Arbor, Michigan

Richard E. Leach, M.D.
Assistant Professor
Division of Reproductive Endocrinology
Department of Obstetrics and
    Gynecology
Wayne State University School of
    Medicine/Hutzel Hospital
Detroit, Michigan

Joseph B. Landwehr, Jr., M.D.
Clinical Instructor
Division of Maternal-Fetal Medicine
Wayne State University School of
    Medicine/Hutzel Hospital
Detroit, Michigan

Michael Leonardi, M.D.
Clinical Instructor
Division of Maternal-Fetal Medicine
Wayne State University School of
    Medicine/Hutzel Hospital
Detroit, Michigan

Frank W. Ling, M.D.
Professor and Chairman
Department of Obstetrics and
    Gynecology
University of Tennessee Medical Group
Memphis, Tennessee

Gary H. Lipscomb, M.D.
Associate Professor and Director
Division of Gynecology
Department of Obstetrics and
    Gynecology
University of Tennessee Medical Group
Memphis, Tennessee

Lisa J. McIntosh, M.D.
Senior Staff
Department of Gynecology
Henry Ford Health System
Detroit, Michigan

S. Gene McNeeley, Jr., M.D., F.A.C.O.G.
Associate Professor
Director, Division of Gynecologic Surgery
Wayne State University School of
    Medicine/Hutzel Hospital
Chief, Department of Gynecology,
    Detroit Receiving Hospital
Detroit, Michigan

Shawn A. Menafee, M.D.
Clinical Instructor
Division of Urogynecology and Pelvic
    Reconstructive Surgery
Department of Obstetrics and Gynecology
Louisiana State University Medical Center
New Orleans, Louisiana

Kamran S. Moghissi, M.D.
Professor of Obstetrics and Gynecology
Division of Reproductive Endocrinology
    and Infertility
Wayne State University School of
    Medicine/Hutzel Hospital
Detroit, Michigan

Dorcas C. Morgan, M.D.
Clinical Instructor
Division of Reproductive Endocrinology
    and Infertility
Department of Obstetrics and Gynecology
Wayne State University School of Medicine
Detroit, Michigan

David Muram, M.D.
Professor and Chief
Pediatric and Adolescent Gynecology
Department of Obstetrics and Gynecology
University of Tennessee
Memphis, Tennessee

**Scott B. Ransom, D.O., F.A.C.O.G.,
    F.A.C.S., C.H.E.**
Assistant Professor
Department of Obstetrics and Gynecology
Division of Gynecology
Wayne State University School of
    Medicine/Hutzel Hospital
Chief, Section of Gynecology
Veterans Administration Medical Center
Detroit, Michigan

R. Kevin Reynolds, M.D.
Assistant Professor
Division of Gynecologic Oncology
Department of Obstetrics and Gynecology
University of Michigan Medical Center
Ann Arbor, Michigan

Acknowledgments

We appreciate the consideration and support received from our families during the many hours that it took us to prepare this manuscript. These include Elizabeth, Susan, Kyle, Kelly, Sarah, and Christopher. We would especially like to note our appreciation to Doris Tolford for the many hours she spent in the preparation, modification, and review of this manuscript. We would like to thank all of the chapter authors for their participation in this work.

Preface

This book is devoted to the primary care provider's understanding, evaluation, diagnosis, and treatment of common gynecologic disorders. As managed care expands and health-care reform progresses, the primary care provider must become knowledgeable of the common disorders of the female patient. With careful study and continued practice, the provider should find this book to be an excellent foundation for the treatment of their common gynecologic disorders. While referral to an appropriate specialist may be necessary, the primary care practitioner should be adequately trained and comfortable treating the majority of these disorders.

Scott B. Ransom, D.O.
S. Gene McNeeley, Jr., M.D.

Contents

CHAPTER 1

Anatomy of the Female Pelvis for the Primary Care Provider

John O. L. DeLancey

SUBCUTANEOUS TISSUES OF THE VULVA

The structures of the vulva lie on the pubic bones and extend caudally under its arch (Fig. 1–1). They consist of the mons, labia, clitoris, and vestibule and associated erectile structures and their muscles. The mons is comprised of hair-bearing skin over a cushion of adipose tissue that lies on the pubic bones. Extending posteriorly from the mons, the labia majora are composed of similar hair-bearing skin and adipose tissue, which contain the termination of the round ligaments of the uterus and the obliterated processus vaginalis (canal of Nuck). The round ligament may give rise to leiomyomas in this region, and the obliterated processus vaginalis can be a dilated embryonic remnant in the adult.

Between the two labia majora, the labia minora, vestibule, and glans clitoris can be seen. The labia minora are hairless skinfolds, each of which splits anteriorly to run over, and under, the glans of the clitoris. The more anterior folds unite to form the hood-shaped prepuce of the clitoris, and the posterior folds insert into the underside of the glans as the frenulum.

In the posterior lateral aspect of the vestibule, the duct of the major vestibular gland can be seen 3 to 4 mm outside of the hymenal ring. The minor vestibular gland openings are found along a line extending anteriorly from this point, parallel to the hymenal ring and extending toward the urethral orifice. The urethra protrudes slightly through the vestibular skin anterior to the vagina and posterior to the clitoris. Its orifice is flanked on either side by two small labia. Skene's ducts open into the inner aspect of these labia and can be cystically dilated in some women.

Within the skin of the vulva are specialized glands that can become enlarged and thereby require surgical removal. The holocrine sebaceous glands in the labia majora are associated with hair shafts, and in the labia minora they are freestanding. They lie close to the surface, and this explains their easy recognition with minimal enlargement. In addition, lateral to the introitus and anus, there are high densities of apocrine sweat glands in addition to the normal eccrine sweat glands. These former structures undergo cyclic change with the menstrual cycle, having increased secretory activity in the premenstrual period. They can become chronically infected as in hidradenitis suppurativa or neoplastically en-

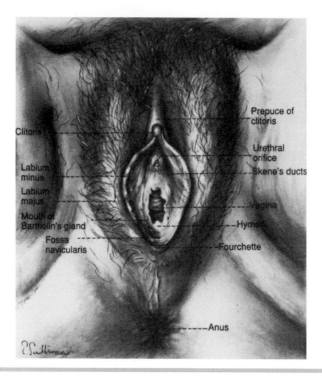

Labels on figure: Clitoris, Labium minus, Labium majus, Mouth of Bartholin's gland, Fossa navicularis, Prepuce of clitoris, Urethral orifice, Skene's ducts, Vagina, Hymen, Fourchette, Anus

Figure 1-1. External genitalia. (From Rock JA, Thompson JD, eds: Te-Linde's Operative Gynecology, 7th ed. Philadelphia, JB Lippincott, 1992.)

larged as in hidradenomas. The eccrine sweat glands in the vulvar skin rarely present abnormalities, but can, on occasion, form palpable masses as syringomas.

Deeper within the vulvar tissues lies the clitoris as well as crura, vestibular bulbs, and the ischiocavernosus and bulbocavernosus muscles (Fig. 1-2). The deep compartment is that region just above the perineal membranes. The erectile bodies and their associated muscles within the superficial compartment are applied to the caudad surface of the perineal membrane. The clitoris is composed of a midline shaft (body) capped with the glans. This shaft is suspended from the pubic bones by a subcutaneous suspensory ligament. The paired aura of the clitoris bend downward from the shaft and are firmly attached to the pubic bones continuing dorsally to lie on the inferior aspects of the pubic rami. The ischiocavernosus muscles originate at the ischial tuberosities and the free surfaces of the crura, to insert on the upper crura and body of the clitoris. A few muscle fibers originate in common with the ischiocavernosus muscle from the ischial tuberosity and run medially to the perineal body. These are called the superficial transverse perineal muscles.

The paired vestibular bulbs lie immediately under the vestibular skin and are composed of erectile tissue. They are covered by the bulbocavernosus muscles, which originate in the perineal body and lie over their lateral surfaces. These muscles, along with the ischiocavernosus muscles, insert into the body of the clitoris and act to pull it downward.

Bartholin's greater vestibular gland is found at the tail end of the bulb of the vestibule and is connected to the vestibular mucosa by a duct lined with squamous epithelium. The gland lies on the perineal membrane and beneath the bulbocavernosus muscle. The intimate relationship between the enormously vascular erectile tissue of the vestibular bulb and Bartholin's gland is responsible for the hemorrhage associated with removal of this latter structure.

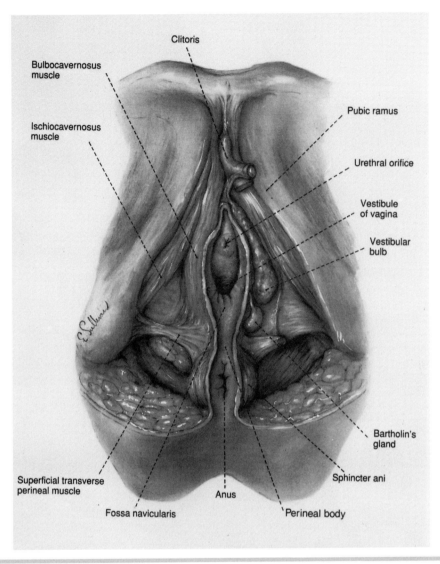

Figure 1–2. Superficial structures of the perineum. (From Rock JA, Thompson JD, eds: TeLinde's Operative Gynecology, 7th ed. Philadelphia, JB Lippincott, 1992.)

PUDENDAL NERVE AND VESSELS

The pudendal nerve is the sensory and motor nerve of the perineum. Its course and distribution in the perineum parallel the pudendal artery and veins, which connect with the internal iliac vessels (Fig. 1–3). The nerve arises from the sacral plexus (S2–4), and the vessels originate from the anterior division of the internal iliac artery.

There are three branches of the pudendal nerve and vessels: the clitoral, perineal, and inferior hemorrhoidal. They supply the clitoris, subcutaneous tissues of the vulva, bulbocavernosus, ischiocavernosus, and transverse perineal muscles. It also supplies the skin of the inner portions of the labia majora, the labia minora, and the vestibule. The inferior hemorrhoidal branch goes to the external anal sphincter and perianal skin. Pudendal nerve block proves useful not only to decrease pain during vaginal birth, but also for local anesthesia during procedures involving the perineal skin.

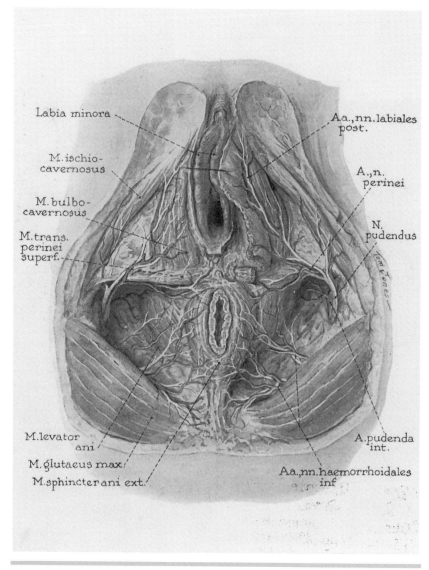

Figure 1–3. Pudendal nerves and vessels. (From Anson BH: Atlas of Human Anatomy. Philadelphia, WB Saunders, 1950.)

LYMPHATIC DRAINAGE

The vulvar lymphatic vessels drain into the superficial inguinal group of lymph nodes. The inguinal lymph nodes are divided into two groups, the superficial and the deep nodes. The superficial nodes are 12 to 20 in number and lie in a T-shaped distribution parallel to and 1 cm below the inguinal ligament, with the stem extending down along the saphenous vein. Lymphatics from the superficial nodes enter the fossa ovalis and drain into the one to three deep inguinal nodes that lie in the femoral canal of the femoral triangle. The superficial nodes are frequently divided into four quadrants with the center of the division at the saphenous opening. The vulvar drainage goes primarily to the medial nodes of the upper quadrant. These nodes lie deep in the adipose layer of the subcutaneous tissues, in the membranous layer, just superficial to the fascia lata. These nodes are frequently enlarged in herpesvirus infections and other inflammatory problems involving the vulvar tissues.

PERINEAL BODY

Within the area bounded by the lower vagina, the perineal skin, and the anus is a mass of connective tissue called the perineal body (see Fig. 1–2). The term *central tendon of the perineum* has also been applied to this structure and is quite descriptive, suggesting its role as a central point into which a number of muscles insert.[1]

The perineal body is attached to the inferior pubic rami and ischial tuberosities through the perineal membrane and superficial transverse perineal muscles. Anterolaterally, it receives the insertion of the bulbocavernosus muscles. On its lateral margins, the upper portions of the perineal body are connected with some of the fibers of the pelvic diaphragm. Posteriorly the perineal body is attached to the coccyx by the external anal sphincter, which is embedded in the perineal body anteriorly and is attached at its other end to the coccyx. All of these connections anchor the perineal body and its surrounding structures to the bony pelvis and help to keep it in place.

ANAL SPHINCTERS

The external sphincter lies in the posterior triangle of the perineum (see Fig. 1–3). It is a single mass of muscle, which has traditionally been divided into superficial and deep portions.[2] The superficial part attaches to the coccyx posteriorly and sends a few fibers into the perineal body anteriorly. The fibers of the deep part generally encircle the rectum and blend indistinguishably with the puborectalis (see later), which forms a loop under the dorsal surface of the anorectum and which is attached anteriorly to the pubic bone.

The internal anal sphincter is a thickening in the circular muscle of the anal wall. It lies just inside the external anal sphincter and is separated from it by a visible intersphincteric groove. It can be identified just beneath the anal submucosa in repair of a chronic fourth-degree laceration of the perineum. The longitudinal layer of the bowel, along with some fibers of the levator ani, separates the external and internal sphincters.

PELVIC MUSCLES

The obturator internus arises from the inner surface of the obturator foramen and membrane and leaves the pelvis through the lesser sciatic foramen to insert into the medial surface of the greater trochanter. The piriformis takes its origin from the anterior aspect of the sacrum and passes through the greater sciatic foramen to insert into the upper border of the greater trochanter. These latter muscles are important to the gynecologist as a cause of deep-seated pain from obturator muscle strains in the piriformis syndrome. Palpating the tender muscle anterolaterally in the case of the obturator internus and posterior and superior to the ischial spine and sacrospinous ligament in the case of the piriformis muscle assists in making this diagnosis. Both of these pelvic wall muscles are lateral rotators and abductors of the thigh.

The opening between the bones and muscles of the pelvic wall is spanned by the muscles of the pelvic diaphragm:[3,4] the pubococcygeus, iliococcygeus, puborectalis, and coccygeus muscles. The most medial of these muscles is the puborectalis/pubococcygeus complex. The pubococcygeus portion of these muscles has an insertion into the anococcygeal raphe and the superior surface of the coccyx, and the puborectalis represents those inferior fibers that pass behind and also insert into the rectum.

The muscle fibers of the pelvic diaphragm form a broad U-shaped layer of muscle with the open end of the U directed anteriorly. The open area within the U through which the urethra, vagina, and rectum pass is called the urogenital hiatus. The normal tone of the muscles of the pelvic diaphragm keep the base of the U pressed against the backs of the pubic bones, keeping the vagina and rectum closed. The region of the levator ani between the anus and coccyx formed by the anococcygeal raphe (see previously) is clinically called the levator plate. It forms a supportive shelf on which the rectum, upper vagina, and uterus can rest. The relatively horizontal position of this shelf is determined by the anterior traction on the fibrous levator plane of the pubococcygeus and puborectalis muscles and is important to vaginal and uterine support.[5] Exercise of the pelvic floor muscles can increase urinary continence and may lessen the symptoms of pelvic organ prolapse. Proper contraction of the levator ani muscles can be insured by checking to see if the anus is pulled upward and inward when the patient attempts to hold gas in the rectum.

PELVIC ORGANS

Vagina

The vagina is a pliable hollow viscus whose shape is determined by the structures that surround it and by its attachments to the pelvic wall. These attachments are to the lateral margins of the vagina, so that its lumen is a transverse slit, with the anterior and posterior walls in contact with one another. The lower portion of the vagina is constricted as it passes through the urogenital hiatus in the levator ani. The upper part is much more capacious. The cervix lies within the anterior vaginal wall, making it shorter than the posterior wall by approximately 3 cm, with the former being approximately 7 to 9 cm in length, although there is great variability in this dimension. The bladder and urethra lie in contact with the anterior vaginal wall, making them accessible to palpation during pelvic examination, and the rectum lies posteriorly and can also be felt through the vaginal wall.

Uterus: Corpus and Cervix

The uterus is a fibromuscular organ whose shape, weight, and dimensions vary considerably depending on both estrogenic stimulation and previous parturition. It has two portions, an upper muscular corpus and lower fibrous cervix (Fig. 1–4). In the reproductive-age woman, the corpus is considerably larger than the cervix, but before menarche and after the menopause, they are relatively similar in size. Within the corpus, there is a triangular-shaped endometrial cavity surrounded by a thick muscular wall. That portion of the corpus which extends

above the top of the endometrial cavity (i.e., above the insertions of the fallopian tubes) is called the fundus.

The uterus is lined by a unique mucosa, the endometrium. It has both a columnar epithelium, which forms glands, and a specialized stroma. The superficial portion of this layer undergoes cyclic change with the menstrual cycle. Spasm of hormonally sensitive spiral arterioles that lie within the endometrium causes shedding of this layer at the end of each cycle, but a deeper basal layer of the endometrium remains to regenerate a new lining. Separate arteries supply the basal endometrium, explaining its preservation at the time of menses.

The cervix is divided into two portions: the portio vaginalis, which is that part protruding into the vagina, and the portio supravaginalis, which lies above the vagina and below the corpus. The substance of the cervical wall is made up of dense fibrous connective tissue with only a small (approximately 10%) amount of smooth muscle. What smooth muscle there is lies on the periphery of the cervix, connecting the myometrium with the muscle of the vaginal wall.[6] The upper border of the cervical canal is marked by the internal os, where the narrow cervical canal widens out into the endometrial cavity. The cervix contains numerous gland clefts. When the orifice of one of these clefts becomes occluded, cystic dilation occurs, resulting in the common nabothian cyst.

Adnexal Structures and Broad Ligament

The fallopian tubes are paired tubular structures, 7 to 12 cm in length. Each has four recognizable portions. At the uterus, the tube passes through the cornu as an interstitial portion. On emerging from the corpus, a narrow isthmic portion begins with a narrow lumen and thick muscular wall. Proceeding toward the abdominal end, next is the ampulla, which has an expanding lumen and more convoluted mucosa. The fimbriated end of the tube has a great number of frondlike projections to provide a wide surface for ovum pickup. The distal

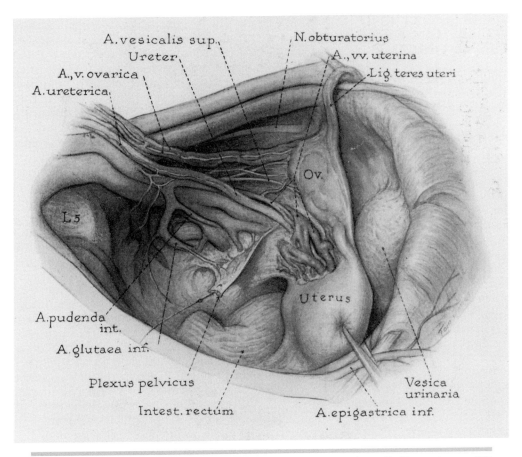

Figure 1–4. Pelvic organs and structures of the pelvic side wall. (From Anson BJ: Atlas of Anatomy. Philadelphia, WB Saunders, 1950.)

end of the fallopian tube is attached to the ovary by the fimbria ovarica, which is a smooth muscle band responsible for bringing the fimbria and ovary close to one another at the time of ovulation. The outer layer of the tube's muscularis is composed of longitudinal fibers; the inner layer has a circular orientation.

The lateral pole of the ovary is attached to the pelvic wall by the infundibulopelvic ligament, and the ovarian artery and vein are contained therein. Medially, it is connected to the uterus through the utero-ovarian ligament. During reproductive life, it measures approximately 2.5 to 5 cm long, 1.5 to 3 cm in thickness, and 0.7 to 1.5 cm in width, varying with its state of activity or suppression, as with oral contraceptive medications. Its surface is mostly free but has an attachment to the broad ligament through the mesovarium, as is discussed subsequently.

The ovary has a cuboidal to columnar covering and consists of a cortex and medulla. The medullary portion is primarily fibromuscular with many blood vessels and connective tissue. The cortex is composed of a more specialized stroma, punctuated with follicles, corpora lutea, and corpora albicantia.

The round ligaments are extensions of the uterine musculature and represent the homologue of the gubernaculum testis. They begin as broad bands that arise on each lateral aspect of the anterior corpus. They assume a more rounded shape before they enter the retroperitoneal tissue where they pass lateral to the deep inferior epigastric vessels and enter each internal inguinal ring. After traversing the inguinal canal, they exit the external ring to enter the subcutaneous tissue of the labia majora. They have little to do with uterine support.

BLOOD SUPPLY AND LYMPHATICS OF THE GENITAL TRACT

The blood supply to the genital organs comes from the ovarian arteries and uterine and vaginal branches of the internal iliac. A continuous arterial arcade connects these vessels on the lateral border of the adnexa, uterus, and vagina (see Fig. 1–4). The blood supply of the upper adnexal structures comes from the ovarian arteries, which arise from the anterior surface of the aorta just below the level of the renal arteries. The accompanying plexus of veins drains into the vena cava on the right and the renal vein on the left. The arteries and veins follow a long mesenteric surface of the ovary to connect with the upper end of the marginal artery of the uterus. As the ovarian artery runs along the hilum of the ovary in addition to supplying the gonad, it sends a number of small vessels through the mesosalpinx to supply the fallopian tube, including a prominent fimbrial branch at the lateral end of the tube.

The uterine artery originates from the internal iliac artery. It usually arises independently from this source but may have a common origin with either the internal pudendal or vaginal artery. It joins the uterus at approximately the junction of the corpus and cervix, but this position varies considerably both with the individual and with the amount of upward or downward traction placed on the uterus. Accompanying each uterine artery are several large uterine veins that drain the corpus and cervix.

On arriving at the lateral border of the uterus (after passing over the ureter and giving off a small branch to this structure), the uterine artery flows into the side of the marginal artery, which runs along the side of the uterus. Through this connection, it sends blood both upward toward the corpus and downward toward the cervix. As the marginal artery continues along the lateral aspect of the cervix, it eventually crosses over the cervicovaginal junction and lies on the side of the vagina.

The vagina receives its blood supply from a downward extension of the uterine artery along the lateral sulci of the vagina and from a vaginal branch of the internal iliac artery. These form an anastomotic arcade along the lateral aspect of the vagina at 3 and 9 o'clock. There are also branches from these vessels that merge along the anterior and posterior vaginal walls. The distal vagina also receives supply from the pudendal vessels, and the posterior wall has a contribution from the middle and inferior hemorrhoidal vessels.

The uterus receives its nerve supply from the uterovaginal plexus (Frankenhäuser's ganglion), which lies in the connective tissue of the cardinal ligament, and through nerves accompanying the ovarian blood vessels. The uterovaginal plexus connects to the central nervous system through the hypogastric nerves and hypogastric plexus. Injection of local anesthetic agents through the lateral vaginal fornix can block conduction of pain through this region and greatly reduces the discomfort of cervical dilation. It does not, however, blunt perception of pain from the uterine corpus.

REFERENCES

1. Oh C, Kark AE: Anatomy of the perineal body. Dis Col Rect 1973; 16:444.
2. Dalley AF: The riddle of the sphincters. Am Surg 1987; 53:298.
3. Lawson JO: Pelvic anatomy: I. Pelvic floor muscles. Ann R Coll Surg Engl 1974; 54:244–252.
4. Lawson JO: Pelvic anatomy: II. Anal canal and associated sphincters. Ann R Coll Surg Engl 1974; 54:288–300.
5. Berglas B, Rubin IC: Study of the supportive structures of the uterus by levator myography. Surg Gynecol Obstet 1953; 97:677–692.
6. Hughesdon PE: The fibromuscular structure of the cervix and its changes during pregnancy and labour. J Obstet Gynaecol Br Commonw 1952; 59:763–776.

CHAPTER 2

History and Physical Examination of the Gynecologic Patient

Scott B. Ransom

S. Gene McNeeley, Jr.

The fundamental purpose of a history and physical examination is to assist the clinician with determining the appropriate diagnosis that may lead to an appropriate therapy. This chapter outlines the essentials of a standard gynecologic evaluation.

GENERAL OFFICE SETTING

The gynecologic history and physical examination should be the initial step in the development of an excellent physician-patient relationship that leads to a satisfactory experience for the patient as well as the development of an accurate diagnosis and therapeutic approach. Although practitioners can complete the general history and physical examination in a number of ways, it is appropriate in the gynecologic evaluation to consider the history and physical examination portions of the evaluation as independent from one another. That is, it may be worthwhile for the practitioner to conduct the history portion of the evaluation in an office-type setting to improve the potential of obtaining an accurate and complete history. On completion of the history from the patient, the patient may be transferred to the examination room

for the remainder of the evaluation. It is important for the physician to develop a methodologic and complete sequence in the evaluation to assess each patient accurately.

GYNECOLOGIC HISTORY

The gynecologic history should allow a general appreciation of the woman's health as well as specific concerns for the office visit. General assessment of health should be obtained through an assessment of previous medical problems, previous surgeries, current medications being used, and drug allergies. A social and family history should be recorded as well. This general health evaluation can prove invaluable to the assessment of specific gynecologic complaints.

Chief Complaint

The patient should be asked to describe the specific reason that brought her to the clinician's office. The circumstances surrounding the onset, duration, severity, and historical significance of the problem should be assessed.

Table 2–1. Obstetrical History Checklist

Date of delivery
Location of delivery
Duration of previous pregnancies
Type of delivery
Duration of labor
Maternal complications
Newborn complications

Menstrual and Reproductive History

An accurate obstetric history should be obtained from the patient, including gravidity, parity, miscarriages, abortions, and living children. While determining the specific events, it is appropriate to discuss each individual pregnancy for problems and outcomes (Table 2–1). The patient's menstrual history should be determined including the age of her first menses (menarche). The last menstrual period should be assessed with specific questions focused on the frequency, duration, and amount of menstrual flow. In addition, it is important to understand whether any change in the menstrual cycle has occurred and subsequently determine what type of change. Following the general menstrual history, problems associated with the reproductive cycle should be specifically addressed, including amenorrhea, dysmenorrhea, menorrhagia, metrorrhagia, mittelschmerz, pelvic pain, and premenstrual syndrome (PMS) symptoms (Table 2–2).

Contraceptive History

If the patient is of reproductive age, contraceptive history is essential to consider in the overall evaluation of the patient. Contraceptive choices should be discussed as well as any contraceptive fail-

Table 2–2. Menstrual Disorders

Amenorrhea	Absent menstruation
Dysmenorrhea	Painful menstruation
Menorrhagia	Profuse menstruation
Metrorrhagia	Intramenstrual bleeding
Mittelschmerz	Midcycle pain associated with ovulation

ures the patient has experienced. In discussing the contraceptive choices the patient has used, the physician should consider aspects of the patient's history in conjunction with the contraceptive choice, including contraceptive efficacy, lifestyle, sexual history, history of sexually transmitted diseases, and long-term family planning considerations (see Chapter 7).

Sexual History

It is important for the patient to understand that during the gynecologic evaluation, an open, discreet, and confidential discussion can be continued regarding sensitive areas such as sexual history. A general assessment of the nature of the patient's sexual health should be considered. Specifically, sexual orientation, marital status, libido, failure to achieve orgasm, dyspareunia, or any other problems of interest to the patient should be discussed. The clinician should invite the patient to bring up for discussion any areas regarding her sexual history. Sexual history should be considered an important aspect of the patient's overall health (see Chapter 17).

Review of Systems

Many problems may be uncovered through a careful and specific review of systems for the patient's condition. An assessment of gastrointestinal symptoms can indicate many problems and should include the presence of pain, nausea, vomiting, food intolerance, hematochezia, diarrhea, and constipation and the relationship to the menstrual cycles. Urinary difficulties should be assessed and discussed, including dysuria, frequency, hematuria, and incontinence should be assessed and discussed. Other gynecologic complaints such as pelvic pain, vaginal discharge, vaginal discomfort or itching, pelvic pressure, and abnormal vaginal bleeding should be discussed. Upon completion of the history the clinician may formulate a differential diagnosis that may enhance the physical examination component of the evaluation. Table 2–3 lists differential di-

Table 2-3. Differential Diagnoses

Symptom	Differential Diagnosis				
Amenorrhea	Pregnancy	Menopause	Polycystic ovarian disease	Hormonal abnormality	Turner's syndrome	Ovarian tumors
Dysmenorrhea	Endometriosis	Pelvic infection	Pelvic neoplasm	Retroverted uterus	Adenomyosis	Fibroid uterus
Menorrhagia	Endometrial polyp	Adenomyosis	Hormonal abnormality	Coagulation defect	Pelvic inflammatory disease	Fibroid uterus
Metrorrhagia	Pregnancy related	Hormonal abnormality	Pelvic inflammatory disease	Pelvic neoplasm	Endometriosis	Hematologic abnormality
Dyspareunia	Pelvic mass	Endometriosis	Pelvic inflammatory disease	Vaginitis	Vestibulitis	Pelvic adhesions

agnoses for many common gynecologic complaints.

PHYSICAL EXAMINATION

Before the physical examination, the patient should empty her bladder. The patient should then be escorted to the examination room and asked to remove all street clothes and dress in an appropriate examination gown. The examination must be completed in the most professional circumstances possible with an assistant present during all aspects of the examination. Although many providers may choose to avoid the cost of a chaperone during the examination, significant medicolegal ramifications can exist for both male and female providers if patient accusations are brought forward.

General Examination

The initial examination should include the patient's height, weight, blood pressure, and other vital signs. A general assessment of physical findings should precede the gynecologic examination, including an evaluation of the head, neck, chest, heart, and lungs. Following the general examination, the gynecologic evaluation may proceed.

Breast Examination

This examination is ideally carried out with the patient in both the sitting and the supine positions. When the patient is sitting, the breast size is noted together with any asymmetry, protuberance, indentation, skin dimpling or edema, abnormal coloration, or other visual abnormalities. After the general inspection, a systematic palpation should be completed on all aspects of the breast bilaterally. Palpation should comprise compression of tissue between thumb and forefinger and pressing the breast against the chest wall with the flat of the hand to determine any significant masses. The examination should be completed in the following positions: sitting with arms down, sitting with arms raised, and sitting with hands pressing hips. The examination may detect breast abnormality in only one of these positions, which emphasizes the importance of the various positions in an effective breast examination. The palpation examination should permit the identification of masses, cysts, nodules, discharge, or any other palpable abnormality. Suspicious lymph nodes should be assessed in both the supraclavicular and the axillary areas. Following the examination in the sitting position, the patient should be placed in a supine position and the same techniques employed (see Chapter 4).

Abdominal Examination

The abdominal examination is critical to the gynecologic evaluation. The abdominal evaluation should assess contour, hair distribution, surgical scars, and obesity. Abdominal tenderness must be determined with concern for rebound, guarding, and rigidity. An abdominal mass should be identified and described for size, location, cystic or solid, smooth or nodular, and fixed or mobile. Further assessment for ascites, abdominal distention, tympany, and dullness should be completed. Bowel sounds must be assessed for presence and pitch. Finally, costovertebral angle tenderness can suggest pyelonephritis, and psoas muscle spasm may indicate pelvic infection.

Pelvic Examination

Inspection and Palpation of the External Genitalia

After the patient is properly positioned and draped on the examining table, the examiner encourages the patient to relax as much as possible for a careful, accurate, and meaningful examination. The vulva should be examined carefully through both inspection and gentle palpation. The examination should evaluate the anal and perianal areas, Bartholin's and Skene's glands, labia majora, labia minora, vestibule, clitoris, and urethra. In addition, the skin should be inspected to identify any abnormalities, including edema, discharge, tumors, leukoplakia, inflammation, atrophy, desquamation, and reddening. After completion of an accurate and careful vulvar examination, the vagina should be inspected by using a speculum. The vagina and cervix should be carefully examined. The speculum should be gently inserted with the blades entering the introitus transversely, then directed posteriorly along the vagina with pressure exerted against the perineum to avoid the sensitive urethra. A general assessment of discharge, lesions, discolorations, and bleeding should be completed. Appropriate evaluations through wet mount, pH testing, cultures, and Papanicolaou (Pap) smear should be completed at this time. On removing the speculum, the blades should be rotated 90 degrees to visualize the anterior and posterior walls of the vagina for abnormalities and lesions. Finally, a general assessment of pelvic support disorders, including cystocele, rectocele, uterine prolapse, and vaginal prolapse, should be completed.

Bimanual Examination

On completion of the speculum examination, a bimanual examination should be completed. The apex of the vagina and the cervix should subsequently be palpated with the size, mobility, consistency, and tenderness noted. Subsequently the internal hand can push the uterus toward the abdominal wall, and the abdominal hand can be used to palpate the fundus of the uterus. On examination of the uterus, the size, consistency, regularity, and significant discomforts should be assessed and noted. Following the palpation of the uterus, a general examination of the ovaries should be completed. The adnexal area should be assessed for masses and tenderness. The pouch of Douglas should be assessed for nodularity and tenderness that may indicate endometriosis, pelvic inflammatory disease, or metastatic carcinoma. Finally a recto-vaginal examination should be undertaken to confirm and expand the findings of the pelvic examination. Subsequently the rectum should be assessed. This examination may improve the evaluation of the cul-de-sac and adnexa if carefully completed. Lubrication should be used liberally and the patient asked to bear down to relax the rectal sphincter. Rectal examination should be used to assess possible rectocele or enterocele as well as rectal masses, polyps, or hemorrhoids. Simultaneously the rectal examination can be used to obtain a stool sample for occult blood loss and guaiac assessment.

CONCLUSION

On completion of the history and physical examination of the patient, the evaluation must be integrated to develop an accurate differential diagnosis. The provider should allow the patient to redress and subsequently complete a review of significant findings for the patient. The provider should outline any abnormalities or concerns noted. At this time, an important dialogue should proceed between the provider and patient. History and physical findings and patient concerns should be discussed in detail to proceed with further diagnostic evaluation or treatment. The patient should be encouraged to ask questions, and the provider should ensure that the patient has a reasonable understanding of all the material presented. In addition, this is an appropriate time to proceed with appropriate patient education including verbal discussion, written material, and audio/visual tapes. It is important to emphasize that the history and physical examination of the female patient are of absolute necessity to develop an accurate diagnosis and appropriate treatment. While the advent of high image radiologic evaluations may be helpful for certain disorders, these tests should not supplant a quality physical examination.

CHAPTER 3

Preventive Gynecologic Care

Joseph B. Landwehr, Jr.

Michael R. Leonardi

Preventive gynecologic care is an important responsibility of the primary care provider. This includes examination and screening for abnormalities and malignancies pertaining to the female reproductive tract, including the breast, as well as counseling and interventions aimed at promoting long-term health and prevention of morbidity.

From a gynecologic standpoint, preventive care is one of the most important roles of the primary care provider, and adequate screening protocols have been developed for abnormalities of the breast and cervix. Unfortunately, ovarian malignancy continues to elude early diagnosis in all screening programs evaluated thus far. Presentation, therefore, tends to be at a much later stage of disease. Evaluation of the cost-effectiveness of screening programs continues, but new modalities for early diagnosis have not emerged over the last decade. Once believed to hold promise for screening and early detection, CA-125 with or without ultrasonography has not proved to be cost-effective and it does not appear to improve patient survival rates.

The newest area of active investigation incorporates genetic testing for markers of malignancy to identify those at high risk. The discovery of the BRCA-1 gene has heightened levels of screening and protocols for early intervention in those identified at high risk, linking genes to some inheritable forms of breast cancer. Familial forms of breast and ovarian cancer do exist, although they contribute a minority of cases. The discovery of the involved gene may lead to earlier detection and treatment of these forms of cancer.

Preventive gynecologic care also presents clinicians with an opportunity to counsel and educate their patients on important health issues, such as preconceptual counseling and smoking cessation. For many women, the annual gynecologic examination is their only encounter with the health care system and may be the only opportunity for the clinician to have a positive impact on long-term health care.

PATIENT EVALUATION

Much of the initial screening of the patient can be done by questionnaire or ancillary personnel while the patient is waiting for her appointment. This allows identification of any high-risk factors that may be present and permits the clinician to focus on specific areas of concern the patient may have. Although some insight into the patient's behavior and risk factors is provided by questionnaires, they do not replace personal interaction by the clinician. Many messages can be conveyed through body language, and what may seem an unimportant response on the questionnaire may provide a gateway to deeper underlying concerns of the patient, such as substance, physical, and sexual abuse. This is especially important because many somatic complaints are linked to an underlying psychosocial problem. Failure to identify that component can result in a needless expensive diagnostic evaluation and fail to address the true cause of the patient's complaint. Such women may be more likely to be lost to follow-up if they interpret the lack of questioning as a lack of caring.

Screening Questionnaires

Development of individualized questionnaires to fit the clinician's patient population is essential. Many good screening questionnaires are available to screen for substance abuse, especially alcoholism. Alcoholism remains one of the most underdiagnosed debilitating conditions because denial is a strong component of the disease process. T-ACE questionnaires[1] and the brief Michigan Alcohol Screening Test (MAST)[2] are simple and effective screening tools (Table 3–1). If a patient is identified at risk, appropriate counseling and referral are required.

Physical trauma and sexual abuse are also areas of great concern, especially in younger reproductive-age women. Although more common in the younger age group, sexual abuse is not unheard of in the elderly population, especially in the institutionalized patient population. The level of questioning has to be individualized and may have to be explored in the patient interview process. Sometimes the patient is looking for permission to discuss these issues, and the questionnaire may provide the patient reassurance that the clinician is genuinely concerned with her total well-being.

High-Risk Factors

Detailed history taking identifies the patient's underlying risk factors. A system-

Table 3–1. T-ACE Screening Test for Possible Alcohol Abuse

T	Tolerance	How many drinks does it take to make you feel high?
A	Annoyed	Have people annoyed you by criticizing your drinking?
C	Cut down	Have you ever felt you should cut down on your drinking?
E	Eye opener	Have you ever had a drink first thing in the morning to steady your nerves or get rid of a hangover?

Scoring:
(+) tolerance is considered 2 drinks or more and scores 2 points

Each of the other categories scores 1 point for a positive response

A score of 2 or more is considered positive for a drinking problem and needs further evaluation

Adapted from Sokol RJ, Martier SS, Ager JW: The T-ACE questions: Practical prenatal detection of risk drinking. Am J Obstet Gynecol 1989; 160:185.

atic approach to this part of the patient interview ensures that no major areas are missed. When searching for high-risk factors, a questionnaire is useful for screening a large list of areas of concern. The questions should be modified to fit the individual patient population and be appropriate for the age, ethnicity, and social mores of the patient.

Ethnicity may suggest investigation of specific disorders that are much more common than in the general population. Patients who are African-American or of Mediterranean descent should have a screening complete blood count and, if a microcytic anemia is noted, a hemoglobin electrophoresis, if not previously performed and documented. The Sickledex screening test is no longer considered an adequate screening examination because many of the hemoglobinopathies are not detected in this manner.[3] In patients who have a history of heavy menstrual flow, a complete blood count and possibly coagulation studies should be performed because many of the childhood coagulopathies are discovered around the time of menarche. Von Willebrand disease, a disease of abnormal platelet function, may be more common than previously thought; therefore, screening a bleeding time may be appropriate along with routine coagulation studies in patients with abnormally heavy menses at the time of menarche.

Any patient who presents for a gynecologic examination should be questioned about her sexuality, including gender preference, practices, and contraception used. In sexually active women, screening for sexually transmitted diseases (STDs) should be performed and human immunodeficiency virus (HIV) testing offered and encouraged. This opportunity should be used to explore and answer questions the patient may have about sexual issues. Barrier contraception should be advised to the appropriate patients as a form of prevention from most STDs in addition to any other form of contraception the patient may use. Patients, especially adolescents, who present for evaluation of pregnancy and have a negative test provide an excellent opportunity for intervention.

The family history and questionnaire should elicit any history of coronary artery disease, hyperlipidemia, or chronic hypertension. If the patient has a positive family history or has diabetes mellitus or smokes, lipid screening should be offered and recommended.

A family history of thyroid disease or an autoimmune disorder should prompt a screening thyroid test. The new thyroid-stimulating hormone (TSH) tests are an adequate screening examination and cost-effective. A clinical suspicion of lupus or other autoimmune diseases or a false-positive rapid plasma reagin (RPR) test warrants a workup for an underlying autoimmune disorder. A screening antinuclear antibody (ANA) and possibly a lupus anticoagulant test should be performed as an initial part of the workup.

If a patient has a family history of familial polyposis coli, colorectal cancer, cancer family syndrome, or a personal history of inflammatory bowel disease, a screening colonoscopy may be necessary at regular intervals. The current recommendations are for the initial screening colonoscopy to be performed at age 40 and then followed as clinically indicated.[4]

AGE-SPECIFIC SCREENING GUIDELINES

Specific screening guidelines have been proposed by many organizations, including the American Heart Association, American Cancer Society, American College of Physicians, National Cancer Institute, and American College of Obstetricians and Gynecologists (ACOG). For the purposes of preventive gynecologic care, ACOG has assigned a task force for primary and preventive health care. Their publication, *The Obstetrician and Gynecologist and Primary-Preventive Health Care*, provides a complete summary for the age-specific screening guidelines for women.[5] Their recommendations are summarized in Table 3–2.

Breast, cervical, uterine, and ovarian screenings are the most important areas of concern to the practicing gynecologist. Many discrepancies exist among the recommendations of these groups. This chapter summarizes these areas and develops a consensus among the current recommendations.

Cervical Screening

Initial screening cytology should be performed at age 18 years or when the patient becomes sexually active. After the initial screening Papanicolaou (Pap) test and pelvic examination, the patient should continue to have annual Pap tests until she has three successive negative Pap tests. At this point, the patient can have less frequent screening at the discretion of the physician.[6,7] Many gynecologists, however, recommend yearly examinations to provide the best screening, allowing for closer follow-up with patients.

Many risk factors are believed to exist for cervical dysplasia and cervical carcinoma. These include factors relating to sexual activity, including early age of onset of sexual activity, multiple sexual partners, nonbarrier contraception, STDs, and possibly HIV. Any history of genital human papillomavirus infection, especially subtypes 16, 18, 31, and 33, or herpes simplex virus type 2 infection increases the relative risk. Also included at higher risk is a previous history of cervi-

Table 3–2. Periodic Screening Tests and Examinations Based on Patient's Age

	Ages 13–18	Ages 19–39	Ages 40–64	Ages 65 and older
Frequency of examination	Yearly*	Yearly*	Yearly*	Yearly*
Pap smear	When sexually active or age 18, then yearly*	Yearly*	Yearly*	Yearly*
Height, weight, blood pressure	Every visit	Every visit	Every visit	Every visit
Pelvic examination	When sexually active or age 18, then yearly*	Yearly*	Yearly*	Yearly*
Immunizations	Initially check all childhood immunizations then DT every 10 y, MMR*, HepB vacc*	DT every 10 y	DT every 10 y, influenza vacc at 55 and yearly, pneumococcal vacc once	DT every 10 y, influenza yearly*, pneumococcal vacc yearly*
Family planning	Yearly	Yearly	Yearly*	N/A
Assess risk factors	Yearly	Yearly	Yearly	Yearly
Mammograms	N/A	Age 35–40 screening exam if (−) family history, then every 2 y, age 35 and yearly if (+) first-degree relative	40–50 every 2 y, in (−) family history, >50 yearly	Yearly
Cholesterol	N/A	Every 5 y	Every 5 y	Every 3–5 y
Fecal occult blood test	N/A*	N/A*	Yearly	Yearly
Sigmoidoscopy	N/A	N/A	Every 3–5 y after age 50*	Every 3–5 y*
Thyroid stimulating test	N/A*	N/A*	N/A*	Every 3–5 y
Urinalysis dipstick	*	*	*	Yearly
Breast self-examination	BSE taught at age 18 then monthly	BSE monthly	BSE monthly	BSE monthly
Clinical breast examination yearly	CBE yearly	CBE yearly	CBE yearly	CBE yearly

*As clinically indicated.
DT = diphtheria-tetanus toxoid; MMR = measles, mumps, rubella; HepB = hepatitis B; vacc = vaccine; N/A = not applicable; BSE = breast self-examination; CBE = clinical breast examination.
Data adapted from American College of Obstetricians and Gynecologists: The Obstetrician-Gynecologist and Primary-Preventive Care. Washington, DC, ACOG, 1993.

cal dysplasia or cervical, vulvar, or vaginal cancer. Smoking and the failure to obtain regular Pap smears have been associated with an increased risk of cervical dysplasia. There is an unclear association between lower socioeconomic status and an increased risk for abnormal cervical cytology. This may be secondary to clustering of other well-known risk factors within this group of individuals.[8]

Previously, any patient who had HIV was thought to be at increased risk for cervical dysplasia and more rapid progression to cervical cancer. Although immunosuppression has been associated with a higher rate of abnormal cytology, the previous assumption that HIV has a more rapid progression to cervical cancer has not been established with further investigation. Colposcopy was initially recommended to screen all patients with HIV. The current recommendation for HIV-positive patients is for at least yearly Pap smears and colposcopy for any abnormalities noted during screening. Once an abnormal Pap smear is identified, colposcopy is the recommended follow-up rather than a repeat Pap smear.

Breast Screening

One in 8 to 1 in 10 women develops breast cancer sometime in her lifetime. Screening mammography remains the only test to screen patients for subclinical or occult breast disease. The current debate is not over the value of mammography, but over what is the most cost-effective screening interval. The level of ionizing radiation used in modern machines is considered negligible and should not be a factor in the consideration of the screening frequency.

Current recommendations are presented by the American Cancer Society and National Cancer Institute. In patients with a first-degree relative who have breast cancer, the initial screening examination should be performed at age 35 and thereafter yearly. In patients with a negative family history, the initial screening mammogram should be performed between the ages of 35 and 40 years. If the initial screening examination is negative, mammography should be repeated at age 40 and then performed every 1 to 2 years for patients between 40 and 49 years of age and then yearly for patients age 50 years and older.[9,10]

The screening mammogram does not replace the need for breast self-examination (BSE) and the yearly clinical breast examination (CBE). Patients should be taught BSE at age 18 so that they become familiar with their own breast and the technique. The most effective method has been developed by the California division of the American Cancer Society. Emphasis must be placed on the importance of the BSE and CSE because the Breast Cancer Detection Demonstration Project demonstrated that approximately 10% of palpable breast cancers are not detected by mammography.[7,9,11]

The incidence of breast cancer increases with increasing age. Other risk factors include a previous history of breast cancer, nulliparity, delayed childbearing (after 30 years of age), early menarche (before age 12), late menopause (after age 53), family history of breast cancer (first-degree relative), and biopsy-proven ductal or lobar hyperplasia, especially in the presence of atypia, obesity, and higher socioeconomic status. The increased incidence of breast cancer appears to be secondary to longer exposure to estrogen. The greatest risk factors remain, however, a previous history of breast cancer and a strong family history. With the discovery and characterization of the BRCA-1 gene in familial breast cancer, new detection modalities may be available to determine the actual risk of patients with a familial inheritance pattern. Patients should be discouraged from having a false sense of security if they do not have risk factors because less than 30% of women with breast cancer have any appreciable risk factors.

Once a mass is suspected, follow-through to resolution is imperative. The management of abnormal breast testing is discussed later.

Uterine Screening

The most common gynecologic malignancy is endometrial carcinoma. Fortunately the presenting sign is usually post-menopausal bleeding; therefore, early diagnosis and therapy are usually possible.

The long-term survival for stage I endometrial cancer exceeds 90%. Currently, no universal screening guidelines exist for endometrial cancer. The most cost-effective management involves screening high-risk patients and patients who have clinical signs and symptoms suggestive of endometrial carcinoma. The availability of endometrial sampling devices (e.g., Pipelle), facilitates safe, efficient office biopsy with minimal patient discomfort. If this does not provide adequate sampling for diagnosis, a more definitive procedure, such as a dilation and curettage and hysteroscopy, must be performed.

Unopposed estrogen remains the most significant risk factor for patients who develop endometrial cancer. Obesity, chronic anovulation, early onset of menarche, late onset of menopause, estrogen-secreting tumors, unopposed estrogen therapy, diabetes, hypertension, infertility, and Lynch II inherited malignancy syndrome all put the patient at increased risk for endometrial cancer. Multiparity, the use of oral contraceptives, and exogenous estrogens seem to have a protective effect on the endometrium.[12–14]

Leiomyomas are a common tumor of the uterine corpus. Rarely are these tumors malignant, necessitating treatment only when they become symptomatic. The best current estimate is that roughly one third of all women over age 30 have these tumors, and leiomyoma is one of the leading causes of morbidity. Once thought to be the site of origin of leiomyosarcomas, the current predominant thought is that sarcomas develop independent from leiomyomas. High-resolution pelvic ultrasound is accurate in the diagnosis of leiomyomas; however, it is unable to differentiate between a leiomyoma and leiomyosarcoma. The history of a rapidly growing fibroid remains the only clinical tool to make the diagnosis of leiomyosarcoma. Unfortunately the survival rate after the diagnosis of a leiomyosarcoma or a rhabdomyosarcoma remains poor.[15]

Ovarian Screening

No currently available techniques are suitable for the routine screening of ovarian cancer. Much debate has been made over the usefulness of CA-125 and routine ultrasound screening; however, these have never been proven accurate or cost-effective. The false-positive rate of these screening protocols may, in fact, put more women at risk than women with ovarian cancer. One in 70 women develops ovarian cancer in her lifetime. Ovarian cancer remains the leading cause of death from a gynecologic malignancy, surpassing both cervical and endometrial cancers combined. This is due largely to the advanced stage of the disease at the time of diagnosis, most commonly found at stage III and above. Only 30% of patients have disease limited to the ovary at the time of diagnosis.[16]

Early diagnosis is hindered by the nonspecific nature of the symptoms associated with early-stage ovarian carcinoma, such as bloating and vague abdominal discomfort. The pelvis of the obese patient is particularly difficult to evaluate. Although not suitable for routine screening, ultrasound may play a role in these patients when the pelvic anatomy cannot be evaluated. Individualization of the use of ultrasound is necessary, and no prospective studies have been performed to assess its accuracy in this setting. Patients should be aware of the limitations of ultrasound, and serial examinations may be necessary. The management of a pelvic mass diagnosed on physical examination or by ultrasound is discussed later.

MANAGEMENT OF ABNORMAL FINDINGS

Abnormal Pap Smears

One of the most frequently encountered abnormal tests the primary care provider encounters when dealing with preventive gynecologic care is the abnormal Pap smear. Difficulty arises in the management of these patients because treatment guidelines are vague and do not set concrete boundaries for treatment. Further difficulty has arisen with newer treatment modalities, such as the laser and loop electrode excision procedure (LEEP). As in other disciplines, treatment should be individualized and performed by a practitioner well versed in the associated pathophysiology and interpretation of findings.

The initial step in determining the treatment options for the patient is assessment of risk factors and patient reliability. Any patient with a history of human papillomavirus or HIV infection is at increased risk for invasive cervical neoplasia as well as those patients who smoke cigarettes. A patient who is not deemed reliable for interval follow-up evaluation may need more definitive therapy earlier in the disease process. Assessment of the individual laboratory is essential because each laboratory has its own subjective means in assessing the Pap smear.

The current reporting scheme for Pap smears is based on the Bethesda System for Reporting Cervical/Vaginal Cytologic Diagnoses.[17] This new system eliminates the old CIN numerical system and includes assessment of the adequacy of the submitted specimen. The abnormal Pap smear is assigned to one of several broad categories: (1) atypical squamous cells of undetermined significance (ASCUS), (2) low-grade squamous intraepithelial lesion (LGSIL), (3) high-grade squamous intraepithelial lesions (HGSIL), and (4) squamous cell carcinoma. Less often, abnormal glandular cells are depicted and evaluated on the Pap smear. The evaluation and treatment of abnormal glandular cells are beyond the scope of this chapter and are better left to a specialist.

ASCUS provides the clinician with a clinical dilemma regarding appropriate follow-up. Because many of these changes are believed to be secondary to reparative changes, treatment usually includes a repeat Pap smear in 4 months. Although the Bethesda System does separate inflammation from ASCUS, the significance of ASCUS on the Pap smear is undetermined at this time. Until more definitive answers become available to define the natural progression of this lesion, a follow-up Pap smear in 4 months is warranted. Treatment of any underlying inflammation should be performed before the repeat Pap smear. If ASCUS persists on the repeat Pap smear, colposcopy is warranted. This treatment plan presumes the patient is deemed reliable for follow-up.

LGSIL incorporate cellular changes associated with human papillomavirus (koilocytosis) as well as the old CIN I designation. The patient must understand that close surveillance is essential because a portion of these lesions progresses to a more high-grade lesion. The patient should be encouraged that most of these lesions spontaneously revert to normal without therapy. If the patient's first abnormal Pap smear is LGSIL, and she has no increased risk factors and is reliable for follow-up, the Pap smear can be repeated in 4 to 6 months. If the lesion persists or progresses on the repeat examination, colposcopy should be performed.

If the colposcopy is adequate and confirms the diagnosis of LGSIL, several treatment options exist. If the entire lesion was identified and the patient is low risk, she can opt for no treatment with close follow-up, understanding that up to 60% of lesions revert spontaneously. She must also be aware that 15% of these progress to HGSIL, making ablation or excision a viable option. Cryotherapy is appropriate in patients with a negative endocervical curettage and potential for future childbearing. Cryotherapy may make future colposcopy more difficult because of the migration of the transition zone up the endocervical canal; however, some have suggested that these may decrease recurrences. A cone biopsy or LEEP provides an excisional biopsy specimen for pathologic examination. No matter what form of therapy is undertaken, the patient needs close follow-up at appropriate intervals. Even if the patient decides on no therapy, definitive therapy is highly recommended if the lesion persists for 1 year.

Women with HGSIL need a colposcopy with directed biopsies and an endocervical curettage (ECC) performed. Ablative therapy can be used selectively in these patients; however, the lesion should be localized and the entire lesion visualized with a negative ECC. Otherwise the most appropriate therapy is conization of the cervix by traditional means or LEEP excision. Close follow-up at 4 months postexcision or postablation is crucial in these patients. Hysterectomy is reserved for patients with HGSIL that cannot be treated with local therapy. Other candidates are those patients who have had previous local therapy and have recurrent or persistent disease. Obviously, this therapy is reserved for those patients who have completed their childbearing.[18]

Breast Lump or Mass

Although mammography has been credited in decreasing the rate of mortality from breast cancer by up to 30%, the false-negative rate of mammography is 10% to 15%. Therefore, any palpable mass found on examination must be evaluated. Fine-needle aspiration remains the cornerstone of evaluation of a palpable breast mass. If a cyst is aspirated, the fluid is clear, and the cyst resolves and does not recur, no further treatment is necessary. If the mass does not completely disappear, the fluid is bloody, or the cyst recurs, an open biopsy should be performed.

If a solid mass is freely mobile and the fine-needle aspiration cytology is benign, the mass can be followed closely. If the mass does not resolve over a reasonable amount of time, an open biopsy should be performed. Open biopsy should also be performed for any of the following findings: (1) bloody nipple discharge, (2) nipple excoriation, or (3) skin edema and erythema suspicious of inflammatory breast carcinoma. The open biopsy should be performed only by specially trained personnel, and estrogen/progesterone receptor status should be assessed and possibly flow cytometry performed where indicated.

Abnormal Mammogram

An abnormal mammogram should be followed by a clinical breast examination performed by a specially trained physician, usually a surgeon. If the patient has a nonpalpable lesion (i.e., an occult lesion), the decision needs to be made whether to perform a needle localized biopsy or to follow the lesion with serial mammograms. If microcalcifications are present, the general consensus is to biopsy the lesion. Ductal dysplasia can be followed by serial mammography if the patient has no risk factors. If the patient

has a history of endometrial or ovarian cancer, she is at high risk and should have a biopsy performed.[10,19,20]

Pelvic Mass on Examination

A pelvic mass or an enlarged uterus on pelvic examination necessitates diagnostic workup. Many gynecologists recommend evaluation by ultrasonography, although this is not universal. In some circumstances, following the patient clinically before obtaining an ultrasound examination is appropriate.

In a young, thin patient who is having normal menses, if an enlarged ovary is palpated that is freely mobile and less than 5 cm in approximate size, the most likely diagnosis is a functional cyst. Follow-up pelvic examination should be scheduled after two to three menstrual cycles. If the cyst has resolved, no further treatment or examination is necessary until the next annual examination. If the cyst persists after several menstrual cycles, it should be evaluated by ultrasound. If the patient is having irregular cycles or shows any signs of hirsutism or virilization, the patient should have an ultrasound to characterize the mass because this may be the presenting findings of an androgen-secreting tumor.

An enlarged uterus that is globular, mobile, and not rapidly enlarging may be followed with serial pelvic examinations. Many gynecologists, however, obtain a baseline ultrasound examination of the uterus to ensure that the palpated mass is the uterus and not an ovary or other pelvic mass adherent to the uterus. Once a leiomyoma is identified, following the patient with serial pelvic examinations is reasonable. If the uterus rapidly enlarges over a 6-month period, the suspicion for a sarcoma is increased, and definitive diagnosis should be made as appropriate for the patient. Any menorrhagia or metrorrhagia that persists in these patients should prompt endometrial sampling before initiating hormone therapy.

Other less common causes of a pelvic mass should be explored in the history with the patient, such as a history of pelvic inflammatory disease or other STDs in the past. These patients are at increased risk for the development of tubo-ovarian complexes/abscesses pyosalpingitis, hydrosalpinx, and pelvic adhesive disease. Another common cause of pelvic masses in patients with cyclic pelvic pain is endometriomas. Consultation with a gynecologist is necessary because many of these patients require surgical evaluation for definitive evaluation and therapy.

COUNSELING

Sexually Transmitted Diseases

During the patient encounter, evaluation and counseling concerning the patient's risks should take place. Patients at increased risk are those with a history of multiple sexual partners or a sexual partner with multiple contacts, sexual contact with a person known to have an STD, and a patient with a recurrent history of STDs.[24] If any high-risk factors are identified, the patient should have the appropriate screening during the physical examination. Serologic testing for hepatitis B and syphilis should be performed when indicated, and the patient should be offered and encouraged to have HIV testing.

The most important part in eliminating STDs is prevention. Perhaps the most important part in counseling the patient is education about the prevention of spread of STDs. Use of the male condom is the most effective form of contraception in the prevention of STDs. Modification of sexual behavior can also be a crucial element in the prevention of STDs. Anal intercourse and orogenital sex are known behavioral factors that increase the risk of spread.

Treating the partners of the patient with STDs is essential to eliminate transfer back to the patient. Difficulty arises in the approach to the treatment of the sexual partner. Providing a partner with a prescription without examining him does carry certain medicolegal risk for the clinician. Even though an adverse reaction to the commonly prescribed antibiotics is rare, reactions do occur and may present as a severe anaphylactoid reaction. More commonly, the partner is referred to his physician of choice for evaluation and treatment. The recommendation to the patient for the partner to be treated should be clearly documented in the chart. Centers for Disease Control in the *1993 Sexually Transmitted Disease Guidelines* requires providers to assist the partners with referral for adequate assessment and treatment.[25]

Contraception

Reproductive-age women should be counseled about family planning. Special attention should be given to the adolescent age group because the rate of unintended pregnancies is high in this group. Across all age groups, approximately 50% of all pregnancies are unintended.[26] All women should receive counseling and be offered appropriate contraceptive options. If a patient wishes contraception, the initial physical examination should include assessment of weight and blood pressure, examination of breasts and pelvic organs, and performance of indicated laboratory tests, which may include random glucose and lipid testing. If a patient smokes, she should be warned of the potential increased risks associated with hormonal contraception, especially after the age of 35.

Domestic Violence

Domestic violence is defined by ACOG as "any act occurring between two individuals who live or have lived together that is intended or perceived to be intended to cause physical or psychological harm."[27] Other definitions and forms of domestic violence are present. The *battered wife syndrome* is defined as violence at any time in which a woman has received deliberate, severe, and repeated (more than three times) physical abuse from her partner, with the presence of at least bruising.

Domestic violence is not limited to physical abuse. Areas also included in domestic violence are psychological abuse, sexual abuse or assault, progressive social isolation, deprivation of essential needs of daily living (e.g., food, shelter), and intimidation alone. Domestic violence is considered a crime in all states, but reporting laws vary by state.

The clinician should ensure the safety of the patient and have available in the office a list of shelters and "safe places" the patient can go to prevent any further harm during or after a dispute. An exit plan can be offered and discussed with the patient, giving her advice on the crucial things she will need to leave expediently and with all the necessary documentation and records she will need (e.g., birth certificates, social security cards), so she will not have to return to an abusive environment.

The incidence of domestic violence is poorly defined. The actual number of reported cases is around 2 million women, but the actual incidence is thought to be twice this figure. Approximately one quarter of all women in the United States are abused by a partner at some time during their lives. A concerning fact is a woman in the United States is more likely to be killed, injured, or raped by a current or former partner than all other forms of assault combined. Rape is a significant form of domestic violence and abuse that is frequently overlooked. Up to 54% of violent marriages have some component of rape present. Battered women may account for one third of all women seeking care in an emergency department.[28] When evaluating a woman, the clinician should be aware and look for evidence and signs of domestic violence. Even more concerning, battered women may account for 25% of suicide attempts in women and 25% of all psychiatric admissions.[28]

Many battered women convey a sense of helplessness and hopelessness when interviewed. The clinician plays a critical role for these women, being able to point out alternatives and options that are available to the patient. The clinician should acknowledge the problem and affirm that this behavior is not acceptable. Any injuries that are noted on the physical examination should be carefully documented in the medical record. These records may be necessary if the case should go to court. If evidence of sexual assault exists, an informed consent should be obtained and evidence collected as for any other case of sexual assault.

The cycle of battering usually occurs in three phases. The first phase consists of the tension-building phase. In this phase, verbal abuse occurs, and mild physical abuse begins. The woman tries to calm her partner down to avoid further aggravating him. As the woman continues to back down from her partner, the partner becomes more aggressive. The second phase begins when minimal stimulus can initiate a hostile or violent act. In this phase, verbal and physical abuse is common, often leading to injuring the women. At this point, the woman believes she has no alternatives but to defend herself, commonly leading to the striking back or even killing the abuser. The third phase is entered when the batterer begins to apologize to the woman, and the woman has a sense of hope that everything can be resolved between the couple. The victim believes the battering has passed, but then phase one begins and the vicious cycle continues. As the cycles become more repetitious, the first phase lasts longer and the second and third stages are shortened.

Sexual Assault

Sexual assault is defined as "any sexual act performed by one person on another without that person's consent."[29] Sexual assault accounts for about 6% of all violent crimes, and the U.S. Department of Justice reports the annual incidence as 73/100,000.[30] Similar to domestic violence, the actual incidence is believed to be much higher than reported because of the reluctance of women to report the crime. As many as 44% of females have been victims of sexual assault, with as many as 50% of these patients having been assaulted on more than one occasion. All age groups and social classes can be victims of sexual assault. The patient should be reassured that the belief she did something to provoke the attack is a myth. Of concern, many attacks are performed by someone the victim knows. *Date rape* is a variant of sexual assault, in which the victim initially is consenting, but the male forces coitus on the victim without her consent. Statutory rape is sexual intercourse with a minor, the definition of which varies by state. It is not dependent on the victim's consent because, by law, she is unable to give consent. Such statutes are infrequently and inconsistently enforced.

A woman may feel violated and out of control of her life. She may experience *rape trauma,* a form of posttraumatic stress disorder. The patient may become emotionally scarred for life. The initial encounter with the health care provider after the assault is critical to her emotional well-being. An empathetic, caring clinician is critical, and many facilities and clinics use a team in the care of the rape victim. The woman experiences the acute phase characterized by denial and numbness of her response mechanism. This phase may last for hours or days, depending on the coping mechanisms of the individual patient. The delayed phase is characterized by flashbacks, nightmares, phobias, and other major life adjustments and may occur months or years after the assault. This may cause the patient a lifelong disability and leave her unable to function in society. Long-term counseling and therapy are necessary for these patients, and they should be referred to a specialist for longitudinal care.

The clinician evaluating the victim of sexual assault has medical and legal responsibilities that vary by state. Several general requirements are universal for the most part, including the collection of evidence. A chaperone should be present during the history and physical examination both to reassure the patient and to verify the information in case the assault goes to trial. An accurate gynecologic history and physical examination are essential, and specific questioning about prior coitus and relations before the assault is necessary evidence. Injuries should be recorded and treated, including prophylaxis for STDs and unintended pregnancy. Centers for Disease Control recommends ceftriaxone 250 mg intramuscularly as a single dose, metronidazole 2 g orally as a single dose, and doxycycline 100 mg orally twice a day for 7 days. The patient should use condoms with her partner until completion of the STD prophylaxis, and morning-after contraception can be offered. HIV testing in these patients as well as an RPR is appropriate; however, the HIV test may be delayed until the follow-up examination when the patient is able to better understand the counseling and give a more informed consent.[30] At the follow-up visit, the patient should have the STD tests repeated and have serology tests for HIV, hepatitis B, and syphilis. The HIV test should be repeated in 3 to 6 months.

The prior pregnancy status should be assessed. The risk of pregnancy in these patients if they are not currently using some form of contraception is 2% to 4%. The two most common morning-after regimens are two combination oral contraceptives at the time of the examination and two tablets 12 hours later.[31] Oral contraceptives containing 50 mcg of ethinyl estradiol are an appropriate choice. If 50 mcg tablets are not available, 4 tablets of an oral contraceptive containing 30 mcg of ethinyl estradiol taken twice 12 hours apart is an acceptable alternative. An alternative to this regimen is a 5-day course of high-dose estrogen such as 5 mg of ethinyl estradiol per day or 20 to 30 mg of conjugated equine estrogen per day. A pregnancy test should be performed at the time of the return visit and, if positive, the patient counseled as to her various options.

Because cases of sexual assault or rape may present as a legal case, appropriate documentation is crucial. Sexual assault and rape are legal, not medical, terms; therefore, their use should be avoided in the medical record. A nonjudgmental description of history and physical findings is crucial, and the proper chain of evidence must be observed or the information is inadmissible in court. The emotional well-being of the patient should also be assessed and recorded. If the patient is a minor, many states have mandatory reporting of sexual assault. The approximate time of the attack should be ascertained from the patient, and the patient should be examined before bathing. The clothing, if it was soiled, should be submitted as possible evidence. A caring and empathetic provider is essential to initiate the process of recovery in these fragile and violated patients. Support groups and counseling should be offered to the patient, and close follow-up is crucial.

Substance Abuse

As previously mentioned, the primary care clinician plays a key role in the identification and treatment of the substance-abusing patient. A questionnaire and patient interview play vital roles in screening the patient population for this frequently ignored area of patient health. The data from the National Household survey on drug abuse indicates that 29% of Americans smoke cigarettes, up to 6.7% abuse alcohol, 2% use psychotherapeutic drugs, and 7% use illicit drugs.[32] Many substance abusers use more than one drug. The use of substances usually coexists with poor health habits, leading to increased health care visits and increased costs to the health care system.

The clinician should educate patients at every opportunity, especially adolescents. Encouraging a healthy lifestyle and behavior modification are essential components of counseling. Emphasis on the detrimental effects of substance abuse may be useful as well as presenting the economic costs an addiction burden places on the patient. Pregnancy presents an ideal opportunity to encourage the patient to discontinue substance use and seek treatment by presenting the adverse effects use may have on the developing fetus. Denial remains a strong component in substance abuse coping mechanisms, making a confession of a problem the first step in treatment.

Screening patients for substance use can be performed only with the patient's consent except in extenuating circumstances. To test a patient without her consent could be a violation of her civil rights. Once the patient is identified as a substance abuser, referrals to help groups are appropriate. Smoking cessation should be attempted by all clinicians; however, the patient should be aware that this involves behavior modification and long-term commitment. Support groups may prove useful for many of these patients.

The final step in treating the substance-abusing patient is the identification of *enablers.* Enablers are defined as people who help the substance abuser work through her problems and smooth things over for her.[32] Physicians should be careful not to become enablers themselves by giving out prescription drugs, writing work and school excuses for days missed because of substance abuse, or ignoring the problem. The patient may interpret the avoidance of the issue by the clinician as a silent approval for her actions. The clinician should take a clear stance that substance abuse is not acceptable and provide empathetic support to help the patient quit her addiction.

Osteoporosis

The old saying "prevention is the best medicine" certainly holds true for osteoporosis. Early education in the adolescent age group is essential and remains key to the prevention of this disease. Adults need 400 IU of vitamin D per day, and this requirement is increased to 800 IU in elderly patients. In adolescents and adults to age 25, the recommended intake of calcium is 1200 mg per day and is decreased to 800 mg per day after age 25. Pregnancy and lactation also increase the necessary intake to 1200 mg per day regardless of age.[34] Calcium carbonate or calcium citrate can be used in patients who are unable to ingest enough calcium-containing foods. Estrogen replacement in the postmenopausal patient remains the most effective therapy in this population in decreasing the rate of osteoporosis. A daily dose of at least 0.625 of conjugated equine estrogen a day or 1 mg of micronized estradiol is recommended. Transdermal estrogen is also acceptable; however, because of the variable absorption of vaginal estrogen, this is not suggested for the prevention of osteoporosis.[35] Health needs of perimenopausal and menopausal women are discussed in depth in Chapter 14.

EVALUATION OF SCREENING PROCEDURES

An essential part of any practice now includes evaluation and assessment of screening evaluations. This allows the clinician to determine the adequacy of the screening procedures and the reliability of the laboratory. Specific guidelines have been established by ACOG. The process of Continuous Quality Improvement is a paradigm directed toward improvement of patient care. The overall approach to Continuous Quality Improvement is beyond the scope of this book, and the reader is referred to other excellent sources.[36]

The first step is for the clinician to identify the indicators of care for quality assessment. These are objective and measurable variables related to the structure, process, or outcome of care. Process indicators are used to monitor and evaluate the standard of care provided. They are intended to answer the questions of access and planning of care the providers give as well as the treatments and procedures provided. Outcome indicators are used to evaluate the quality of care provided and include measurable results that are attributable to the care received from the provider. These can include both the positive and the adverse outcomes that occur.

In the primary care office, an example of this process in action is the evaluation and follow-through of abnormal Pap smears. A log of abnormal Pap smears should be kept in the office along with the date reported. A follow-up and final disposition should be kept on each abnormal Pap smear, and if the patient was not compliant with care, this should also be carefully documented, including the receipt and copies of any certified letters sent. Commercially available software has been developed to facilitate logging and tracking of abnormal Pap smears. Colposcopy results should be correlated with the abnormal Pap smears to evaluate the accuracy of the reporting laboratory. This allows identification of underreporting or overreporting of the laboratory based on the correlation of the Pap smear to biopsy results. Another indicator of the adequacy of screening of the Pap smears is the incidence of invasive squamous cell carcinoma in the patient population. To assess this adequately, correction for patient compliance, date of last Pap smear, and risk factors has to be performed, but invasive squamous cell carcinoma should not appear in a patient with previously normal Pap smears. This raises great suspicion as to the reporting practices of a particular laboratory.

Another indicator that is frequently used in determining the quality of care of a provider is the emergence of endometrial carcinoma in a patient receiving hormone replacement. The clinician should be aware of any change in bleeding patterns in patients who are on hormone replacement. A patient who is on continuous hormone replacement who has been amenorrheic for years requires evaluation if bleeding develops. The clinician should not attribute this bleeding to the hormones alone without performing an adequate sampling of the endometrium.

Breast screening remains one of the most difficult areas to assess. The ultimate care-sensitive indicator is the development of breast carcinoma in a patient with previously negative mammograms and CBEs. These cases should be scrutinized for any breakdown in care, and the radiologist should be contacted so that the previous mammograms can be reviewed. If a problem is detected, a plan of correction should be documented, and further assessment should be followed longitudinally.

REFERENCES

1. Sokol RJ, Martier SS, Ager JW: The T-ACE questions: Practical prenatal detection of risk drinking. Am J Obstet Gynecol 1989; 160:865.
2. Pokorny AD, Miller BA, Kaplan HB: The brief MAST: A shortened version of the Michigan Alcoholism Screening Test. Am J Psychiatry 1972; 129:342–345.
3. American College of Obstetricians and Gynecologists: Hemoglobinopathies in pregnancy. ACOG Technical Bulletin 138. Washington, DC, ACOG, 1996.
4. Hayward RS, Steinberg EP, Ford DE, et al: Preventive care guidelines: 1991. Ann Intern Med 1991; 114:758–783.
5. American College of Obstetricians and Gynecologists: The Obstetrician and Gynecologist and Primary-Preventive Health Care. Washington, DC, ACOG, 1993.
6. American College of Obstetricians and Gynecologists: Standards for Obstetric-Gynecologic Services, 7th ed. Washington, DC, ACOG, 1996.
7. American College of Obstetricians and Gynecologists: Report of the task force on routine cancer screening. ACOG Committee Opinion 68. Washington, DC, ACOG, 1989.
8. American College of Obstetricians and Gynecologists: Guidelines for Women's Health Care. Washington, DC, ACOG, 1996, pp 150–156.
9. American College of Obstetricians and Gynecologists: The role of the gynecologist in the diagnosis of breast disease. ACOG Committee Opinion 67. Washington, DC, ACOG, 1989.
10. Feig SA: Decreased breast cancer mortality through mammographic screen-

ing: Results of clinical trials. Radiology 1988; 167:659–665.

11. American College of Obstetricians and Gynecologists: Guidelines for Women's Health Care. Washington, DC, ACOG, 1996, pp 143–150.

12. American College of Obstetricians and Gynecologists: Carcinoma of the endometrium. ACOG Technical Bulletin 162. Washington, DC, ACOG, 1991.

13. Gallup DG, Stock RJ: Adenocarcinoma of the endometrium in women 40 years of age or younger. Obstet Gynecol 1984; 64:417–420.

14. Davies JL, Rosenshein NB, Antunes CMF, Stolley PD: A review of the risk factors for endometrial carcinoma. Obstet Gynecol Surv 1981; 36:107–116.

15. American College of Obstetricians and Gynecologists: Uterine leiomyomata. ACOG Technical Bulletin 192. Washington, DC, ACOG, 1994.

16. American College of Obstetricians and Gynecologists: Cancer of the ovary. ACOG Technical Bulletin 141. Washington, DC, ACOG, 1990.

17. National Cancer Institute Workshop. The 1988 Bethesda system for reporting cervical/vaginal cytologic diagnoses. JAMA 1989; 262:931–934.

18. American College of Obstetricians and Gynecologists: Cervical cytology: Evaluation and management of abnormalities. ACOG Technical Bulletin 183. Washington, DC, ACOG, 1993.

19. American College of Obstetricians and Gynecologists: Carcinoma of the breast. ACOG Technical Bulletin 158. Washington, DC, ACOG, 1991.

20. Homer MJ, Smith TJ, Marchant DJ: Outpatient needle localization and biopsy for non palpable breast lesions. JAMA 1984; 252:2452–2454.

21. American College of Obstetricians and Gynecologists: Dysfunctional uterine bleeding. ACOG Technical Bulletin 134. Washington, DC, ACOG, 1989.

22. Matsumoto S, Igarashi M, Nagaka Y: Environmental anovulatory cycles. Int J Fertil 1968; 13:15–23.

23. Fries H, Nillus SJ, Petterson F: Epidemiology of secondary amenorrhea: II. A retrospective evaluation of the etiology with special regard to psychogenic factors and weight loss. Am J Obstet Gynecol 1974; 118:473–479.

24. American College of Obstetricians and Gynecologists: Primary and preventive care: A primer for obstetricians and gynecologists. Washington, DC, ACOG, 1994, p 4.

25. Centers for Disease Control and Prevention: 1993 sexually transmitted diseases treatment guidelines. MMWR 1993; 42(RR-14):1–102.

26. American College of Obstetricians and Gynecologists: Guidelines for Women's Health Care. Washington, DC, ACOG, 1996, p 92.

27. American College of Obstetricians and Gynecologists: Domestic violence. ACOG Technical Bulletin 209. Washington, DC, ACOG, 1995.

28. American Medical Association: Diagnostic and Treatment Guidelines on Domestic Violence. Chicago, AMA, 1992.

29. American College of Obstetricians and Gynecologists: Sexual assault. ACOG Technical Bulletin 172. Washington, DC, ACOG, 1992.

30. U.S. Department of Justice: Uniform crime reports for the United States: 1987. Publication No. 14. Washington, DC, U.S. Governmental Printing Office, 1987.

31. Yuzpe AA, Smith RP, Rademaker AW: A multicenter clinical investigation employing ethinyl estradiol combined with dl-norgestrol as postcoital contraceptive agent. Fertil Steril 1982; 37:508–513.

32. National Institute on Drug Abuse: National household survey on drug abuse: Highlights, 1988. DHHS publication 90-1681. Rockville, MD, U.S. Department of Health and Human Services, 1990.

33. Kaplan FS: Osteoporosis: Pathophysiology and prevention. Clin Symp 1987; 39:1–32.

34. National Research Council, Commission on Life Sciences, Food and Nutrition Board, Subcommittee on the 10th Ed. Washington, DC, National Academy Press, 1989.

35. Hammond CB, Jelovsek FR, Lee KL, et al: Effects of long-term estrogen replacement therapy: I. Metabolic effects. Am J Obstet Gynecol 1979; 133:525–536.

36. American College of Obstetricians and Gynecologists: Quality Assessment and Improvement in Obstetrics and Gynecology. Washington, DC, ACOG, 1994.

CHAPTER 4

Breast Disorders

Carolyn Johnston

This chapter reviews a practical approach to the breast examination and evaluation of a palpable mass as well as several common breast disorders, many of which are encountered by the primary care physician. Readers are referred elsewhere for a discussion of breast carcinoma.

BREAST EXAMINATION

A thorough breast examination should be performed as part of the annual gynecologic examination regardless of whether or not a woman has any complaints. This can also provide an opportunity to review the techniques of breast self-examination, which women aged 20 years and older should be encouraged to perform on a regular, monthly basis. If premenstrual, the breast self-examination is best accomplished in the week following the menses, when the breasts are the least nodular and tender. Approximately 50% of all breast cancers are discovered by the patient. In women who are eligible for mammograms, the breast examination is complementary, and neither should be used as a substitute for the other because approximately 16% of breast cancers are detected only on ex-

amination and 45% only by mammogram.[1] The techniques of the breast examination include the following.

Inspection

Look for symmetry. Normal breasts may vary by as much as 10% in size, but larger discrepancies should be assessed.

Assess for nipple number, retraction, inversion, erosions or lesions, and discharge. Accessory nipples (polythelia) occur in approximately 1% to 2% of the population along the midclavicular line (milk line) from the clavicle to the groin.[2] Their appearance may be confused with that of nevi. Nipple inversion increases with age; may be unilateral or bilateral; and can be a normal finding, particularly if of long-standing duration. Nonbloody nipple discharge can be elicited in most women by gently squeezing the nipple; however, both spontaneous and elicited discharge is abnormal if it is bloody or serous and thus requires additional evaluation to rule out carcinoma.[3-5] Greenish discharge, associated with fibrocystic changes, can often be elicited from multiple ducts.

Areas of skin retraction, erythema, thickening, or actual lesions should be noted and considered abnormal until proven otherwise. Retraction may be due to an underlying malignancy or to a previous biopsy scar. Skin retraction that is not immediately apparent may be elicited by the maneuvers of pectoral contraction, raising the hands and arms above the head and gentle, manual molding of the breast tissue around the tumor.[6]

Palpation

Numerous examination techniques have been described with the essential denominator being the establishment of a systematic pattern that evaluates the nodal areas as well as the entire breast and minimizes the number of times the patient has to change position from sitting to supine.

Examination includes the nodes in the supraclavicular, anterior cervical chain, and axillary areas. Having the patient shrug her shoulders slightly facilitates palpation of the supraclavicular area as does support of the patient's arm by the examiner during the axillary portion of the examination. This latter maneuver allows for relaxation of the muscles and thus increases the ease of palpation. Small, rubbery, mobile lymph nodes can often be palpated and are generally considered normal if they are less than or equal to 1 cm in diameter. Nodes that are fixed, matted, firm, or larger than 1 cm are considered pathologic until proven otherwise.

Feel for dominant masses discrete from the surrounding breast tissue. Note any areas of tenderness, and attempt to correlate them with examination findings. Include the axillary tail in the examination. In addition, some women have prominent, and sometimes separate or accessory, breast tissue in the axilla that requires examination as well. The breast of an elderly woman should have scant glandular tissue unless she is on hormone replacement therapy; therefore, asymmetry requires further evaluation and possibly biopsy. Breast augmentation pushes the breast tissue forward and compresses it. Small masses and thickening are best appreciated in the sitting position with bimanual examination. Irregularities may signify rupture of

the implant, which can then be confirmed by mammogram, ultrasound, or magnetic resonance imaging.

Conclusion

Explain the findings to the patient and allow her to ask questions.

PALPABLE MASS

A palpable breast mass must be interpreted in light of the patient's personal and family medical history, breast examination, and age. The risk of a breast cancer within a palpable mass in a woman less than 25 years old is very low, whereas it approaches 75% in a woman over 70 years.[7,8] Physical examination alone is often not sufficient, as noted previously, and should be complemented by radiologic or cytologic evaluation, especially in women older than 25 years.

Establish whether or not the mass is solid or cystic. This is most easily done by fine-needle aspiration (FNA). For a cystic mass, note if the fluid is bloody and if it resolves after aspiration. Nonbloody fluid can be discarded.[9] Residual palpable masses, recurrent cysts (after two to three aspirations), and bloody fluid require histologic evaluation because of a heightened chance of malignancy. Fewer than 20% of simple cysts refill, and only 9% do so after two or three aspirations.[5] Simple cysts with no associated mass or mammographic abnormalities can therefore be managed with repeat aspiration and a follow-up visit at 6 to 8 weeks postaspiration to confirm resolution. Ultrasound can also be used to determine if a mass is cystic or solid if the patient refuses aspiration. If a mammogram is to be performed, it is best to do so before the aspiration so as not to confuse an aspiration-induced hematoma with a true mammographic abnormality.

Solid masses are managed according to size, age, cytologic results, and associated mammographic findings. For example, a confirmed fibroadenoma in a woman younger than 35 years can be safely followed and removed only for patient distress or increase in size or symptoms, whereas those in older women or those associated with mammographic abnormalities should be excised to rule out malignancy. Abnormal or nondiagnostic cytology should lead to biopsy as well. Similarly, if a solid mass has increased with time, biopsy is mandatory. FNA has a specificity of 98% to 100% and a sensitivity of 65% to 99%.[10] False-negative rates are 1% to 35%, and false-positive results are 0 to 18%.[11] Helvie and colleagues[12] also reported a similar sensitivity and specificity for FNA in the diagnosis of mammographically detected, nonpalpable breast lesions: 97% and 94%. This versatile technique is easy to learn and is reviewed well by Wilkinson and colleagues.[13] Diagnostic accuracy is enhanced by using information from three sources: clinical examination, mammogram, and FNA.[11,14] If all three are negative for malignancy, the incidence of a cancer is 0 to 0.7%.[11,14] If, however, all three are positive, the incidence is 97% to 99%.[11,14]

Persistent masses that cannot be clinically characterized as benign with certainty require biopsy, especially in women older than 35 years. Masses that are being followed conservatively should be reevaluated by examination every 3 to 6 months for assessment of stability. Any change, with the exception of shrinkage, should lead to surgical intervention. See Figure 4–1 for a suggested algorithm.

Palpable masses in pregnant or lactating women should undergo similar evaluation. The same range of histologic abnormalities can be found. There does not appear to be an increased incidence of a malignant diagnosis.[15]

INFECTIOUS OR INFLAMMATORY CONDITIONS

Infectious conditions, both puerperal and nonpuerperal, of the breast are most often due to bacterial infections with *Staphylococcus aureus* and streptococci following disruption of the epithelium at the nipple-areola complex. The infection may manifest as a variety of conditions ranging from painful cellulitis to unifocal or multifocal abscesses. If untreated, cellulitis generally progresses to an abscess, especially in the puerperal state. Streptococcal infections are more likely to persist as a diffuse cellulitis, whereas staphylococcal infections present early with suppuration and abscess formation.[16]

The reported incidence of sporadic puerperal mastitis ranges from 1.4% to 8.9% with abscess formation in 4.8% to 11%.[17,18] It is presumed to be due to the presence of nipple fissures and milk stasis, which encourages retrograde bacterial infection.[16,19,20] Although it has been suggested that the determination of milk leukocyte and bacterial counts is diagnostically important,[21] the treatment of puerperal mastitis is best dictated by clinical presentation and the early institution of antibiotics and breast drainage as stated by Bland.[16] The ultimate choice of antibiotic can be guided by the results of Gram stains, cultures, and sensitivities of the infecting organisms.

Cellulitis should be treated early and aggressively with local wound care and oral antibiotics. The application of local heat may also be appropriate. A penicillinase-resistant penicillin is the drug of choice in non–penicillin-allergic patients. Alternatively a first-generation cephalosporin such as cefazolin can be used. Erythromycin can be used in penicillin-sensitive patients. All of these agents can be safely used in lactating or pregnant women. Lactating women should continue to breast-feed or use a breast pump, because it has been shown to shorten the duration of symptoms and improve the outcome with a reduction in the recurrence of infectious mastitis.[22,23] The combination of antibiotics and breast drainage ensures a good outcome as much as 96% of the time in the treatment of puerperal mastitis, whereas no treatment or breast drainage alone leads to successful outcomes 15% and 50% of the time.[21] Furthermore, the bacteria in the milk do not appear to be pathogenic to the breast-feeding infant.[24] Obviously the choice of antibiotics in a lactating mother is then dictated to some degree by the tolerance of both the mother and the infant.

The presence of an abscess necessitates incision and drainage, often under general anesthesia so that adequate débridement of all infected tissue can be performed. Incisions are generally placed in a circumareolar location or in the direction of Langer's lines farther out on

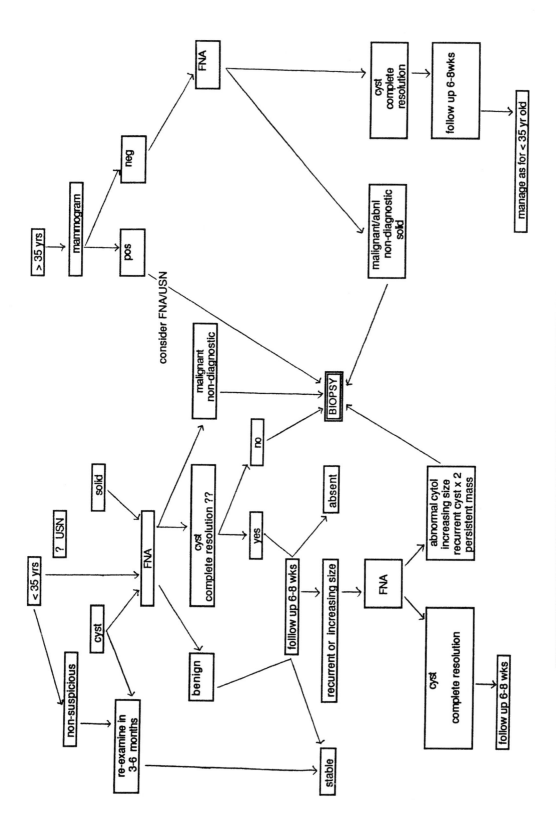

Figure 4-1. Evaluation of a palpable mass. FNA = Fine-needle aspiration. USN = Ultrasound.

the breast. The decision to leave the wound open to heal by secondary intention or to close it primarily with a drain is left to the discretion of the surgeon. Chronic infections generally require healing by secondary intention after surgical débridement.

Women with nonpuerperal mastitis or other inflammatory conditions of the breast should undergo a thorough breast examination and mammogram. Infections not associated with an abscess or underlying mass or mammographic abnormality may initially be treated with antibiotics. Any residual mass, mammographic abnormality, or a failure to respond to antibiotics should lead to a biopsy. Similarly an abscess should be treated with incision and drainage with representative tissue being sent for pathologic analysis. Several authors have documented superior response and decreased recurrence rates with excisional versus incisional techniques.[25–27] The key to successful treatment of periareolar infections is adequate débridement and excision of any sinus tracts from the overlying nipple or areola.[28] Readers are referred to papers by Maier and co-workers[28] and Hartley and colleagues[29] for suggested technical approaches to the treatment of periareolar abscesses. The potential sequelae of this approach include loss of nipple sensation and sloughing as well as recurrent abscesses and deformation; however, potential sequelae should not be a deterrent to surgical management. The biopsy of any inflammatory sites should include a sample of the overlying inflamed skin to assess for dermal infiltration by carcinoma.

The differential diagnosis of nonpuerperal breast inflammation includes malignancy; duct ectasia; chronic or acute periareolar and subareolar infections; inflamed cysts; sarcoidosis; viral, fungal, tubercular, and parasitic infections; thrombophlebitis (see Mondor's disease); and necrosis caused by radiation and anticoagulation.[16] Nonpuerperal breast abscesses tend to be more centrally located than those of the puerperium and are often indolent and chronic in nature.[30] These are often thought to be related to duct ectasia. As with puerperal states, infections are often due to S. aureus and streptococci[16]; however, anaerobic bacteria may also play a role, including Bacteroides species, enterococci, and anaerobic streptococci.[30,31] Persistence of the infection despite surgical débridement and antibiotics should prompt a search for microabscesses, sinus tracts, resistant organisms, and slow-growing organisms such as Mycobacterium species. The presence of foreign bodies in the nipple as a consequence of increasingly popular body piercing has been reported to be associated with a recalcitrant Mycobacterium chelonei infection with sinus tract formation, presumably acquired through contamination of piercing equipment by tap water.[32]

Duct ectasia involves the large and intermediate ductules of the breast.[33] Its main clinical significance is its similarity to invasive carcinoma, from which it must be distinguished by biopsy. It is not associated with an increased risk for carcinoma, and there does not seem to be any relationship to parity or breast-feeding history.[34] Younger patients are more likely to present with breast pain or a mass, whereas older patients more often present with nipple retraction.[34] These presentations correspond to the prominence of periductal inflammation on histologic examination in younger patients and ductal dilatation in older patients.[34] Dixon and colleagues[34] interpreted these findings as evidence that periductal mastitis precedes duct dilatation and is the initial disorder in this condition. Duct ectasia is also in the differential diagnosis of a bloody nipple discharge.

NIPPLE DISCHARGE

Elicited nipple discharge is often a normal finding. It can be elicited by gentle squeezing of the nipple-areolar complex or with a hand-held breast pump. Approximately 48% of all women and 70% of white women produce nipple secretions with manipulation.[35] The amount and presence of nipple discharge depends on race, age, menopausal status, breast disease, and amount of wet ear wax produced.[35–37] It does not appear to vary consistently with the phases of the menstrual cycle, oral contraceptive use, or postmenopausal estrogen use.[35] The color is variable, ranging from green or black to yellow or whitish, and may reflect chemical composition, such as cholesterol content.[38] Cytology of nipple aspiration fluid does not have a role in screening or diagnosis of breast cancer because of the limitations of fluid availability and specimen adequacy.[39]

Spontaneous nipple discharge is rare, constituting only 3% to 5% of breast complaints. Four types of discharge have been found to be associated with breast cancer in increasing frequency: serous, serosanguineous, sanguineous, and watery.[5] These require further evaluation to rule out an underlying malignancy.[4] In a cytologic study of 5305 nipple discharges from 3687 women, bloody discharge was present in 70% of cancer cases.[41] In contrast, two different analyses found cancer to be present in only 4.8% and 5.9% of patients with spontaneous, symptomatic nipple discharge.[40,42] Seltzer and associates[43] evaluated the significance of age and nipple discharges and found that 4.4% of patients under 50 years of age and 32% over the age of 60 years with a bloody nipple discharge had a carcinoma. Cancers present as an isolated abnormal discharge less than 1% of the time.[42] Benign lesions such as duct ectasia, fibrocystic changes, and intraductal papillomas are most often associated with a spontaneous, heme-positive discharge.[40,42] The presence of both an abnormal discharge and a mass should heighten the suspicion for malignancy.[40] Cytology of bloody or serous spontaneous discharge is useful in the absence of an associated mass.[39]

Whether or not the discharge comes from one or multiple ducts, is spontaneous, and is associated with a mass are the three most important parts of the clinical history. Discharge from a single duct is associated with a 4.07 relative risk (Cl 2.7 to 6) of cancer, whereas that from multiple ducts carries the same risk as the general population.[40]

Galactorrhea, or milky discharge, usually from multiple ducts bilaterally, is associated with lactation; elevated serum prolactin; drug intake, especially phenothiazines and oral contraceptives; and, most commonly, idiopathic causes. Thus, a menstrual and drug history should be taken as part of the clinical examination. Other less common systemic disease causes include hypothyroidism, renal failure, and chest trauma, all of which cause an increase in serum prolactin. Cytologic analysis of nipple discharge during pregnancy and lactation can be difficult because blood may be found in the absence of an underlying lesion[44,45] and hence is not indicated. A serum prolactin level should be obtained at a time other than that of the breast examination because breast stimulation can elevate serum levels and lead to a false concern over the presence of a prolactinoma. An estimated 2% of patients with nipple discharge have prolactinomas.[39] Serum prolactin levels greater than 20 ng/mL need further evaluation. Once an abnormality is ruled out, the patient can be reassured.

The treatment of choice for an abnormal nipple discharge is duct excision and removal of any concurrent mass. At times, palpation of a point around the nipple clearly elicits the discharge, and this area should be excised as well. Mammogram should be performed in women over 35 years who are to undergo surgery for a nipple discharge, especially in those without a palpable mass. Galactography has been demonstrated to identify ductal lesions, but because a histologic diagnosis is needed, it is an unnecessary expense.[46]

INTRADUCTAL PAPILLOMAS

Intraductal papillomas are associated with a unilateral, spontaneous serous (48%) or bloody (52%) discharge, which represents the presenting symptom in 76% of patients and the only complaint in 43%.[47] Twenty-four percent of patients present with a palpable, usually subareolar, mass, and 33% present with both a mass and discharge.[47] The mean age of occurrence (47.9 years) is older than that of other benign breast diseases except duct ectasia.[47] There may be an increased risk of carcinomas, especially for the papillomas arising in the periphery of the breast.[48] In addition, multiple papillomas are more likely to be associated with subsequent development of carcinoma, possibly as a result of the co-existent atypical hyperplasia.[49]

The treatment for a solitary intraductal papilloma is surgical duct excision. For a description see Haagensen.[47]

FIBROADENOMAS

Fibroadenoma is the third most common neoplasm of the breast after gross cystic changes and carcinoma, occurring most commonly in premenopausal women at a mean age of 33.9 years.[50] In Haagensen's series,[50] only 2.5% occurred in postmenopausal women. They tend to occur and recur more frequently and at an earlier age in African-American women.[51] Multiple or recurrent fibroadenomas occur in 13% to 16% of women.[50,52] The risk of an associated carcinoma is rare, with approximately 100 cases having been reported by 1985.[53-55] Sixty-five percent to 71% of cancers within a fibroadenoma are lobular carcinoma in situ neoplasms.[53,54] Twenty-nine percent of patients were found to have a contralateral breast carcinoma, which is not surprising given the known associated risk with lobular carcinoma in situ.[53] The prognosis is determined by the type and extent of malignancy and not by the origin within a fibroadenoma.[55]

They usually present as an asymptomatic or slightly tender mass, which if observed grows slowly, taking 6 to 12 months to double in size. Most growth stops after they reach 2 to 3 cm.[50,56] Occasionally, large fibroadenomas develop, particularly in adolescents; hence, their designation as juvenile fibroadenomas.[57] These may grow rapidly but are almost always benign.[58] Similarly, fibroadenomas may increase rapidly in size during pregnancy and be associated with pain and inflammatory changes so as to mimic a carcinoma.[58]

Pathologically, fibroadenomas are characterized by a proliferating connective tissue stroma surrounding multiplication of ducts and acini.[50] Either component may predominate. Grossly, they are well delineated from the surrounding breast tissue and, despite appearances, are not truly encapsulated. On cut section, they have a whitish, whorled appearance, similar to that of uterine leiomyomata. Differing degrees of the adenomatous and fibrous compo-

nents may lead to slightly different appearances.[50] Infarction, although infrequent (1 in 202), may make the differential diagnosis from carcinoma more difficult as well as cause pain for the patient.[59] The pathologic differential diagnosis includes adenomas, phyllodes tumors, and fibromatosis.[60]

Management may be surgical excision or expectant depending on the age of the patient, tumor size, histologic confirmation, mammographic characteristics, and patient desires. Juvenile fibroadenomas are usually excised because of the breast asymmetry they create and to preserve the maximum amount of normal tissue.[57] Although fibroadenomas can be safely followed in women younger than 25 years, only 27% of women chose this option in a longitudinal study of 70 women.[61] If followed conservatively after diagnostic confirmation with FNA, 31% and 52% of fibroadenomas were found to regress after 2 and 5 years.[61,63] Fibroadenomas are more likely to regress in women younger than 20 years and if they are followed conservatively for longer than 1 year.[62] Therefore, age and time course should be discussed when counseling patients about management. Approximately 32% increased in size in both studies; however, no carcinomas occurred.[61,63] FNA was found to be associated with a sensitivity of 84% to 87% and with a specificity of 76% in two longitudinal studies.[61,63] Any associated mammographic finding warrants a biopsy despite the FNA interpretation.[12] Similarly, any suggestion of atypia on cytology necessitates biopsy[64]. Thus, conservative management based on a triple assessment of clinical examination, cytology, and sonogram or mammogram (if indicated) appears to be an appropriate management approach to fibroadenomas in women under 25 years of age.[63] If surgery is indicated, it can usually be performed under local anesthesia as an outpatient. Surgical excision is almost always indicated for women over 35 years to exclude carcinoma.

PHYLLODES TUMOR

Phyllodes tumors, also known as cystosarcoma phyllodes, are uncommon fibroepithelial neoplasms that constitute fewer than 1% of breast tumors in women.[65] They usually present as a palpable mass in premenopausal women. They differ from fibroadenomas by their increased stromal cellularity, occurrence at a later age (median 45 to 50 years), increased tendency toward local recurrence after complete resection, more rapid growth, and higher rate of associated malignancy.[66-68] The most significant difficulty with phyllodes tumors is the inconsistency between histology and clinical behavior.[66,69-72] The treatment of choice is surgical excision. Treatment of any associated cancer is determined by its type and extent. Mammographic findings are not unique and may be confused with those of fibroadenomas.[73]

MASTODYNIA

Mastodynia or mastalgia refers to pain in the breast parenchyma without any specific underlying pathology. The incidence as a presenting breast complaint is 45% to 84%.[74] Typically, it is described as cyclical (40.1%) but may also be noncyclical (26.7%) or due to other causes (33.2%).[76] The association with an underlying breast cancer is reported to be low but may be as high as 24%.[75] Attempts to correlate mastalgia with hormone and gonadotropin levels have been unsuccessful, despite the prominence of cyclicity.[77]

Treatment consists of a history and breast examination and radiologic studies if indicated. An underlying malignancy should be excluded. Any palpable mass should be evaluated and possibly aspirated as indicated by age and consistency. Patients should be reassured as to the normality of the situation.

Most women tolerate the cyclic breast swelling and tenderness associated with menstrual cycles. For those who do not, for whom lifestyle is altered, or for whom the pain becomes constant, no consistently adequate medical therapy currently exists. Symptomatic improvement has been reported with drugs that induce a relative hypoestrogenic state, including danocrine,[78] progestational agents,[79,80] bromocriptine,[81] tamoxifen,[82] and oral contraceptives, but these agents are as-

sociated with side effects that may negate their benefit, such as physiologic stigmata of excessive androgens, altered liver function tests, adverse effects on lipid profiles, symptoms of menopause, nausea, vomiting, orthostasis, and thromboembolic complications. There are also a number of absolute contraindications to their use. Several nonendocrine treatments have also been used with variable results, including vitamin E,[83] evening primrose oil,[84] and abstinence from caffeine.[85] The most consistently beneficial agents in reduction of pain and nodularity are progesterone, danocrine, bromocriptine, tamoxifen, and evening primrose oil. In general, the symptomatic relief from any of these agents is unpredictable and often inadequate or short-lived, leaving the woman and her clinician frustrated. Of interest, most women with severe mastodynia who become menopausal have a rapid improvement in those symptoms.

A report of the successful use of a gonadotropin-releasing hormone analogue, goserelin acetate (Zoladex), for short-term treatment of severe, painful fibrocystic breast disease demonstrated response rates of 81%.[86] Gonadotropin-releasing hormone analogues have been safely used for as long as 6 months with no disruption of serum lipid profiles or induction of irreversible osteoporosis and with the addition of low-dose estrogen may be used for even longer. This may be a viable alternative to the above-mentioned therapies in women with severe refractory cyclic mastalgia.

BENIGN BREAST DISEASE

Lumpiness and diffuse nodular irregularities throughout the breasts have been historically referred to as fibrocystic disease or benign breast disease. Fibrocystic changes is perhaps a better name. The difficulty with the nomenclature results from the lack of a precise clinicopathologic correlation. This problem exists despite the attempt, in 1945, of Foote and Stewart[88] to define components of fibrocystic disease: cysts, sclerosing adenosis, fibrosis, papillomatosis, and apocrine change.[87] Nodular breasts presumably develop because of cyclic proliferative activity with incomplete resolution, caused by either excess hormonal stimulation or an exaggerated proliferative response by hypersensitive breast tissue.[89] These fibrocystic changes are correlated with age and menstrual status and increase in the 10 to 15 years before menopause.[87,90] Patients typically present with complaints of a mass, lumpiness, or pain that may or may not be cyclic.

Some debate has existed over the intrinsic risk of breast cancer in women with fibrocystic changes. Most of the potential for an increased risk comes from the difficulty in examination because of multiple nonspecific nodules. Dupont and Page[91] attempted to clarify the issue by reevaluating specimens from 10,366 breast biopsies done for benign breast disease. They were able to identify 70% of women who were not at high risk for breast cancer and 4% who had atypical proliferating lesions who were.[91] Thus, it appears that for the majority of women with benign breast disease, an increased risk of malignancy is not a valid concern.

Treatment for fibrocystic changes requires a history and breast examination. Mammogram should be performed if the patient is older than 35 and if the palpable changes are new since the last mammogram even if it was performed within the preceding year. The primary goal of the evaluation should be to rule out malignancy. A biopsy may be necessary. Conservative management is discussed under evaluation of the palpable mass. If cyclicity is prominent and oral contraceptives are not contraindicated, they may be useful. If mastalgia predominates, several medical options and non-hormonal remedies exist. See the section on mastalgia. Often, reassurance is the most effective therapy.

HIGH-RISK LESIONS

The high-risk lesions identified by Dupont and Page[91,92] are characterized by degrees of epithelial proliferation and atypia arising within either the ductal or the lobular elements of the breast. For example, mild and moderate hyperplasia have three and five or more nonatypical cell layers above the basement membrane.[92] Atypical hyperplasia is charac-

Table 4–1. Preinvasive Breast Lesions: Associated Risk of Breast Cancer[1]

Lesion	Relative Risk	
	Negative Family History	Positive Family History
No increased risk		
Radial scar		
Sclerosing adenosis		
Intraductal papilloma		
Duct ectasia		
Fibroadenoma		
Fibrocystic changes		
Slight increased risk		
Sclerosing adenosis[2]		
Proliferative disease without atypia	1.5×	2.1×
High risk		
Atypical hyperplasia	3.5–4.0×	8.9×
Atypical hyperplasia with calcifications	6.5×	
Very high risk		
Ductal carcinoma in situ[3]	11×	
Lobular carcinoma in situ[4]	10–12×	

1. Presented with consideration of family history; first degree relative with or without breast cancer. Adapted from Dupont WD, Page DL. NEJM 1985; 312:146–151.
2. Jenson RA, Page DL, et al. Cancer 1989; 64: 1977–83.
3. Regardless of family history. Adapted from Page DL, Dupont WD. Cancer 1982; 49:751–758.
4. Regardless of family history. Adapted from McDivitt RW, Hutter RVP, et al. JAMA 1967; 201:96–100. and Anderson JA. Cancer 1977; 39:2597–2602.

terized by severely abnormal cells within the ductal or lobular unit that do not quite qualify for a diagnosis of carcinoma in situ. Although these lesions are all associated with an increased risk of a subsequent breast cancer, ductal (DCIS) and lobular (LCIS) carcinoma in situ are associated with the highest risk (Table 4–1). Familial and personal risk factors may further modify these risks. Whether it is more likely to occur in the ipsilateral or both breasts depends on the ductal or lobular designation, respectively.

Patients with DCIS have an invasive malignancy discovered 2% to 31% of the time at mastectomy.[93,94] Larger lesions are more likely to be associated with invasive disease.[95–97] DCIS accounts for 5% to 8% of breast cancers and for more than 20% of mammographically detected cancers.[98] It may also present as bloody nipple discharge or a palpable mass.

In contrast, LCIS is usually clinically inapparent and is an incidental finding on biopsy. Unfortunately, it is associated with an 18% to 30% risk of subsequent breast cancer in either breast, in contradistinction to the approximate 10% increased risk of ipsilateral cancer seen with DCIS. It accounts for 3% of invasive cancers.[98]

Radial scars and sclerosing lesions present their largest difficulty in clinical and mammographic similarity to malignancies. Jenson and co-workers,[99] however, found sclerosing adenosis to be an independent risk factor for breast cancer.

Treatment for most of these preinvasive lesions is completed in the process of diagnostic biopsy. Patients should be counseled as to their increased risk of cancer, if any. Estrogen replacement therapy appears to be unassociated with a higher risk of cancer in patients with atypical hyperplasia and LCIS as extrapolated from retrospective studies but has not been studied in a prospective fashion.[100,101] Dupont and colleagues[100] found a lower relative breast cancer risk in patients with atypical ductal hyperplasia who took estrogens versus those who did not: 3.0 versus 4.5. Estrogen should probably be used cautiously in these patients after extensive counseling about the relative personal risks and benefits because of newer information suggesting that estrogen replacement therapy may increase the overall risk of breast cancer for all women regardless of prior pathology.[101–106] For atypical lesions, mammograms and physical examinations are initially conducted on an every-6-month basis. DCIS is treated either with lumpectomy and radiation therapy or simple mastectomy. The latter is associated with a much less than 10% risk of recurrence, whereas the first is associated with a 10% risk of recurrence in the ipsilateral breast. The addition of radiation to surgical excision significantly reduces the recurrence risk of cancer or DCIS by six times.[107] The role of postoperative radiation is less clear for LCIS. LCIS is treated with surgical excision and close observation or ipsilateral mastectomy. Bilateral simple mastectomy may be considered in some instances owing to the bilaterally increased risk of malignancy, such as for patients with strong familial or personal risk factors. This is a decision, however, to be made with input from the patient, medical oncologist, surgeon, and plastic surgeon. Gump and associates[97] surveyed medical oncologists regarding their treatment preferences for LCIS and found 65% in favor of close observation.[98] Patients with LCIS are also candidates for the ongoing National Surgical Adjuvant Breast and Bowel Project (NSABP) prevention trial with tamoxifen versus placebo.

MONDOR'S DISEASE

Mondor's disease, or thrombophlebitis of the superficial veins of the breast, including the lateral thoracic, thoracoepigastric, and, less commonly, the superficial epigastric veins, is an uncommon entity often thought to be associated with antecedent trauma; either surgical or nonsurgical, including biopsies, aesthetic or reconstructive procedures, the use of a body girdle, and intravenous drug use.[108–112] Although not generally associated with a malignancy, a coexistent carcinoma has been reported as much as 12.7% of the time, prompting Catania and associates[109] to recommend a mammogram for any woman with the diagnosis. Furthermore the presence of a mass may necessitate a surgical biopsy to rule out an underlying carcinoma. Four stages of evolution occurring over 2 to 24 weeks have been described consisting of thrombus formation with an associated inflammatory infiltrate (stage 1) followed by the appearance of fibrous cords (stage 2) and multiple sites of recanalization (stage 3) until the entire vein is recanalized with a thick vessel wall and resolution of the perivascular inflammation (stage 4).[113]

The diagnosis of Mondor's disease is easily made by history and examination. Typically, patients present with pain followed by the appearance of a palpable tender cord in the lateral aspect of one breast.[16,114] Physical examination should be performed to rule out an associated mass, which requires biopsy. Treatment consists of nonsteroidal anti-inflammatory drugs and local heat application. Anticoagulants and antibiotics are not generally required.[16] The time course from initial presentation to complete resolution ranges from 2 to 24 weeks.[110,113]

PAGET'S DISEASE

Paget's disease is a skin disorder occurring both on the nipple and in extramammary sites, with the latter being less common. Mammary Paget's disease is thought to arise from gland cells of the lactiferous ducts and thus to represent an ascending carcinoma.[115-118] Histologically, large pale-staining cells are seen above the basement membrane in the epidermis.[119] Various immunohistochemical staining panels have been recommended to differentiate between Paget's disease and other entities, including PAS, CAM 5.2, 21N, S-100, anti-EMA, and anti-c-erbB-2.[120-123]

Paget's disease generally presents as an eczematoid, nonhealing lesion with crusting, scaling, and erythema, sometimes accompanied by a bloody discharge. Highly pigmented lesions have been reported and may be confused with malignant melanoma.[123,124] Other diagnoses in the differential include Bowen's disease, eczema, nipple papillomatosis, and nipple adenoma.[122,123] All nonhealing lesions of the nipple should be biopsied. This is easily performed with a punch biopsy and local infiltration with lidocaine. Scrape cytology has been used in a limited number of patients with excellent diagnostic correlation and may represent a viable alternative to punch biopsy.[125,126] When negative or nondiagnostic, it should be followed by a confirmatory biopsy.

Almost all patients present with an underlying carcinoma or DCIS, although in as many as 40% of patients, this may not be clinically detectable.[122,127] Similarly, 10% of Paget's disease may be diagnosed microscopically in retrospect after removal of a palpable malignancy.[128] Mammography should be performed before biopsy, realizing that as many as 29% may not have a mammographically apparent underlying carcinoma.[129]

Treatment depends on the existence and extent of the underlying carcinoma but usually involves a mastectomy. Excision of the nipple-areolar complex alone is associated with an unacceptably high recurrence rate of 40% to 60% versus a 5% rate with mastectomy.[127,130] More recently, Anelli and colleagues[130] reviewed the role of radiation therapy in conservative management of Paget's disease and found that the addition of 6120 cGy to a central quadrentectomy reduced the recurrence rate from 62% to 11%. Although their numbers were small, this may represent a viable alternative to mastectomy for patients with Paget's disease without invasive disease.

HORMONE USE AND BREAST CANCER

The decision as to whether to use hormone replacement therapy (HRT) in the postmenopausal years is becoming increasingly difficult to make. Often the concern over a possible modest (21%) increased risk of breast cancer outweighs the greater reduction in fatal coronary heart disease (49%) and in deaths from hip fractures (49%).[131] The development of endometrial cancer is avoided by the addition of adequate progesterone. Ultimately the choice to use HRT should include a discussion of these relative risks in light of the patient's family and personal medical history.

Two studies of combined estrogen and progesterone replacement therapy in postmenopausal women failed to find an increased risk of breast cancer and, in fact, found a significantly reduced risk in this cohort.[132,133] Colditz and associates,[105] however, in an update of the Nurses Health Study found an increased risk for users of combination therapy as did Schairer and colleagues.[106] In contrast, three studies, including one meta-analysis, showed an increased relative risk (RR 1.1 to 1.7) of breast cancer in estrogen users.[102-104] Steinberg and colleagues[103] and Bergkvist and co-workers[102] suggested that duration of use was important, greater than 60 and 109 months, respectively. Colditz and associates[104] noted that current users but not past users were at increased risk for breast cancer. Schairer and colleagues[106] confirmed the increased RR and were able to attribute it to an increase in the incidence of in situ cancer.

It also remains unclear as to whether being premenopausal or postmenopausal at the time of exposure to estrogen or the type of exposure, estradiol versus conjugated estrogen, is relevant.[102,103] Although Bergkvist and colleagues[102] reported a 1.8 RR of breast cancer in estradiol users and no increased risk in users of conjugated estrogens, their data were not significant. It is unclear why there should be a difference in RR because both create similar blood concentrations of estrone and estradiol.[134]

The interpretation of the effect of oral contraceptives on the development of breast cancer is difficult especially because of changing formulations. An analysis showed a significant 1.3 RR of breast cancer in oral contraceptive users. This risk was most prominent in the group who developed breast cancer before age 35 and for those who used oral contraceptives for greater than 10 years.[135] Others have not noted an increased risk.[136] Once again the choice to use oral contraceptives needs to include a consideration of this potential risk as well as the multiple well-documented benefits, which seem to outweigh the risks in a young woman without a strong family history of breast cancer.[137]

RADIOLOGIC STUDIES

Mammograms should be used as per the guidelines of the American Cancer Society. Exceptions include additional studies needed in the evaluation of a new palpable mass in women older than 20 years of age and a prior diagnosis of malignancy or a high-risk lesion. Mammography should be used cautiously in pregnancy with appropriate shielding of the fetus and avoidance of the period of organogenesis. Mammography alone has a specificity and a sensitivity of greater than 90%. A hormone or menstrual history should be provided with the mammogram request because of the recognized changes in density patterns secondary to HRT.[138]

Ultrasound is a useful adjunct to mammography. Its roles are as follows: to distinguish a cystic mass from a solid mass, especially in a patient who refuses FNA or in whom it is nonpalpable and seen only on mammogram; to facilitate FNA or core biopsy; and as a diagnostic tool in women younger than 30 years. Ultrasound does not detect small lesions and calcifications well when compared to mammogram.[139,140]

At this time, computed tomography and magnetic resonance imaging have no role in the routine evaluation of the breast.[7]

REFERENCES

1. Moskowitz M: The predictive value of certain mammographic signs in screening for breast cancer. Cancer 1983; 51:1007.
2. Haagensen CD: Anatomy of the mammary glands. *In* Cann C, ed: Diseases of the Breast, 3rd ed. Philadelphia, WB Saunders, 1986, pp 2–7.
3. Haagensen CD: Solitary intraductal papilloma. *In* Cann C, ed: Diseases of the Breast, 3rd ed. Philadelphia, WB Saunders, 1986, pp 141–143.
4. Funderburk WW, Syphax B: Evaluation of nipple discharge in benign and malignant diseases. Cancer 1969; 24:1290–1296.
5. Leis HP Jr: Gross breast cysts: Significance and management. Contemp Surg 1991; 39:13–20.
6. Haagensen CD: Physician's role in the detection and diagnosis of breast disease. *In* Cann C, ed: Diseases of the Breast, 3rd ed. Philadelphia, WB Saunders, 1986, pp 528–543.
7. Donegan WL: Evaluation of a palpable breast mass. N Engl J Med 1992; 327:937–942.
8. Ligon RE, Stevenson DR, Diner W, et al: Breast masses in young women. Am J Surg 1980; 140:779–782.
9. Ciatto S, Cariaggi P, Bulgaresi P: The value of routine cytologic examination of breast cyst fluids. Acta Cytol 1987; 31:301–304.
10. Hammond S, Keyhani-Rofagha S, O'Toole RV: Statistical analysis of fine needle aspiration cytology of the breast. Acta Cytol 1987; 31:276.
11. Layfield LJ, Glasgow BJ, Cramer H: Fine needle aspiration in the management of breast masses. Pathol Annu 1989; 24:23.

12. Helvie MA, Baker DE, Adler DD, et al: Radiographically guided fine needle aspiration of nonpalpable breast lesions. Radiology 1990; 174:657–661.

13. Wilkinson EJ, Franzini DA, Masood S: Cytological needle sampling of the breast: Techniques and end results. *In* Bland KI, Copeland EM, eds: The Breast: Comprehensive Management of Benign and Malignant Diseases. Philadelphia, WB Saunders, 1991, pp 478–480.

14. Butler JA, Vargfas HI, Worthen N, Wilson SE: Accuracy of combined clinical mammographic cytologic diagnosis of dominant breast mass. Arch Surg 1990; 125:893.

15. Byrd BF, Bayer DS, Robertson JC, et al: Treatment of breast tumors associated with pregnancy and lactation. Ann Surg 1962; 155:940.

16. Bland KI: Inflammatory, infectious and metabolic disorders of the mamma. *In* Bland KI, Copeland EM, eds: The Breast: Comprehensive Management of Benign and Malignant Diseases. Philadelphia, WB Saunders, 1991, pp 87–109.

17. Leary WG Jr: Acute puerperal mastitis: A view. Calif Med 1948; 68:147–151.

18. Devereux WP: Acute puerperal mastitis: Evaluation of its management. Am J Obstet Gynecol 1970; 108:78–81.

19. Gibbard GF: Sporadic and epidemic puerperal breast infections. Am J Obstet Gynecol 1953; 65:1038–1041.

20. Newton M, Newton NR: Breast abscess: Result of lactation failure. Surg Gynecol Obstet 1950; 91:651–655.

21. Thompson AC, Espersen T, Maigaard S: Course and treatment of milk stasis, noninfectious inflammation of the breast, and infectious mastitis in nursing women. Am J Obstet Gynecol 1984; 149:492–495.

22. Marshall BT, Hepper JK, Zirbel CC: Sporadic puerperal mastitis: An infection that need not interrupt lactation. JAMA 1976; 233:1377–1379.

23. Niebyl JR, Spence MR, Pharmley TH: Sporadic (non epidemic) puerperal mastitis. J Reprod Med 1978; 20:97–100.

24. Duncan JT, Walker J: *Staphylococcus aureus* in the milk of nursing mothers and the alimentary canal of their infants: Report to the Medical Research Council. J Hyg 1942; 43:474–484.

25. Patey DH, Thackeray AC: Pathology and treatment of mammary-duct fistula. Lancet 1958; 2:871–873.

26. Hadfield J: Excision of the major duct system for benign disease of the breast. Br J Surg 1960; 47:472–477.

27. Urban JA: Excision of the major duct system of the breast. Cancer 1963; 16:516–520.

28. Maier WP, Berger A, Derrick BM: Periareolar abscess in the non lactating breast. Am J Surg 1982; 144:359–361.

29. Hartley MN, Stewart J, Benson EA: Subareolar dissection for duct ectasia and periareolar sepsis. Br J Surg 1991; 78:1187–1188.

30. Benson EA: Management of breast abscesses. World J Surg 1989; 13:753–756.

31. Dixon JM: Periductal mastitis/duct ectasia. World J Surg 1989; 13:715–720.

32. Pearlman MD: *Mycobacterium chelonei* breast abscess associated with nipple piercing. Infect Dis Obstet Gynecol 1995; 3:116–118.

33. Azzopardi JG: Problems in Breast Pathology. Philadelphia, WB Saunders, 1979, pp 59–71.

34. Dixon JM, Anderson TJ, Lumsden AB, et al: Mammary duct ectasia. Br J Surg 1983; 70:601–603.

35. Petrakis NL, Mason L, Lee R, et al: Association of race, age, menopausal status, and cerumen type with breast fluid secretion in nonlactating women, as determined by nipple aspiration. J Natl Cancer Inst 1975; 54:829–834.

36. Wynder EL, Lahti H, Laakso K, et al: Nipple aspirates of breast fluid and the epidemiology of breast disease. Cancer 1985; 56:1473–1478.

37. Sartorius OW, Smith HS, Morris P, et al: Cytologic evaluation of breast fluid in the detection of breast disease. J Natl Cancer Inst 1977; 59:1073–1080.

38. Petrakis NL, Lee RE, Miike R, et al: Coloration of breast fluid related to concentration of cholesterol, cholesterol epoxides, estrogen and lipid peroxides. Am J Clin Pathol 1988; 89:117–120.

39. King EB, Goodson WH: Discharges and secretions of the nipple. *In* Bland KI, Copeland EM, eds: The Breast: Comprehensive Management of Benign and Malignant Diseases. Philadelphia, WB Saunders, 1991; pp 61–62.

40. Murad TM, Contesso G, Mouriesse H: Nipple discharge from the breast. Ann Surg 1982; 195:259–264.

41. Ciatto S, Bravetti P, Cariaggi P: Significance of nipple discharge clinical patterns in the selection of cases for cytologic examination. Acta Cytol 1986; 30:17–20.

42. Chaudary MA, Millis RR, Davies GC, Hayward JL: The diagnostic value of testing for occult blood. Ann Surg 1982; 196:651–655.

43. Seltzer MH, Perloff LJ, Kelley RI, et al: The significance of age in patients with a nipple discharge. Surg Gynecol Obstet 1970; 131:522.

44. Kline TS, Lash SR: Nipple secretion in pregnancy: A cytologic and histologic study. Am J Clin Pathol 1962; 37:626–632.

45. Kline TS, Lash SR: The bleeding nipple of pregnancy and postpartum period: A cytologic and histologic study. Acta Cytol 1964; 8:336.

46. Johanson A, Sager EM: Contrast mammography in spontaneous bloody secretion from the nipple. Tidsskr Nor Laegeforen 1990; 110:3750–3752.

47. Haagensen CD: Solitary intraductal papilloma. In Cann C, ed: Diseases of the Breast, 3rd ed. Philadelphia, WB Saunders, 1986, pp 138–162.

48. Ohuchi N, Abe R, Kasai M: Possible cancerous change of intraductal papillomas of the breast: A 3-D reconstruction study of 25 cases. Cancer 1984; 54:605–611.

49. Carter D: Intraductal papillary tumors of the breast: A study of 78 cases. Cancer 1977; 39:1689–1692.

50. Haagensen CD: Adenofibroma. In Diseases of the Breast, 3rd ed. Philadelphia, WB Saunders, 1986, pp 267–283.

51. Organ CH Jr, Organ BC: Fibroadenoma of the female breast: A critical clinical assessment. J Natl Med Assoc 1983; 75:701–704.

52. Semb C: Pathologico-anatomical and clinical investigations of fibroadenomatosis cystica mammae and its relation to other pathological conditions in the mamma, especially cancer. Acta Chir Scand 1928; 64(suppl 10):1.

53. Fondo EY, Rosen PP, Fracchia AA, Urban JA: The problem of carcinoma developing in a fibroadenoma: Recent experience at Memorial Hospital. Cancer 1979; 43:563–567.

54. Pick PW, Iossifides IA: Occurrence of breast carcinoma within a fibroadenoma: A review. Arch Pathol Lab Med 1984; 108:590–594.

55. Ozzello L, Gump FE: The management of patients with carcinomas in fibroadenomatous tumors of the breast. Surg Gynecol Obstet 1985; 160:99–104.

56. Wilkinson S, Anderson TJ, Rifkind E, et al: Fibroadenoma of the breast: A follow-up of conservative management. Br J Surg 1989; 76:390–391.

57. Pike AM, Oberman HA: Juvenile (cellular) adenofibromas: A clinicopathologic study. Am J Surg Pathol 1985; 9:730–736.

58. Page DL, Simpson JF: Benign, high-risk, and premalignant lesions of the mamma. In Bland KI, Copeland EM, eds: The Breast: Comprehensive Management of Benign and Malignant Diseases. Philadelphia, WB Saunders, 1991; pp 126–128.

59. Majmudar B, Rosales-Quintanta S: Infarction of breast fibroadenomas during pregnancy. JAMA 1975; 231:963–964.

60. Wargotz ES, Norris HJ, Austin RM, Enzinger FM: Fibromatosis of the breast: A clinical and pathological study of 28 cases. Am J Surg Pathol 1987; 11:38–45.

61. Dent DM, Cant PJ: Fibroadenoma. World J Surg 1989; 13:706–710.

62. Cant PJ, Madden MV, Coleman MG, Dent DM: Non-operative management of breast masses diagnosed as fibroadenoma. Br J Surg 1995; 82:792–794.

63. Carty NJ, Carter C, Rubin C, et al: Management of fibroadenoma of the breast. Ann R Coll Surg Engl 1995; 77:127–130.

64. Benoit JL, Kara R, McGregor SE, Duggan MA: Fibroadenoma of the breast: Diagnostic pitfalls of fine needle aspiration. Diagn Cytopathol 1992; 8:643–647.

65. Norris HJ, Taylor HB: Relationship of the histologic appearance to behavior of cystosarcoma phyllodes: Analysis of ninety-four cases. Cancer 1967; 20:2090–2091.

66. Kario K, Maeda S, Mizuno Y, et al: Phyllodes tumor of the breast: A clinicopathologic study of 34 cases. J Surg Oncol 1990; 45:46–51.

67. Bernstein L, Deapen D, Ross RK: The descriptive epidemiology of malignant cystosarcoma phyllodes tumors of the breast. Cancer 1993; 71:3020–3024.

68. Cohn-Cedermark G, Rutqvist LE, Rosendahl I, et al: Prognostic factors in cystosarcoma phyllodes: A clinicopathologic study of 77 patients. Cancer 1991; 68:2017–2022.

69. Al-jurf A, Hawk WA, Crile G: Cystosarcoma phyllodes. Surg Gynecol Obstet 1978; 146:358–364.

70. Hajdu SI, Espinosa MH, Robbins GF: Recurrent cystosarcoma phyllodes: A clinicopathologic study of 32 cases. Cancer 1976; 38:1402–1406.

71. Bennett IC, Khan A, DeFreitas R, et al: Phyllodes tumors: A clinicopathological review of 30 cases. Aust NZ J Surg 1992; 62:628–633.

72. Chua CL, Thomas A: Cystosarcoma phyllodes tumors. Surg Gynecol Obstet 1988; 166:302–306.

73. Cosmacini P, Zurrida S, Veronesi P, et al: Phyllodes tumor of the breast: Mammographic experience in 99 cases. Eur J Radiol 1992; 15:11–14.

74. Souba WW: Evaluation and treatment of benign breast disorders. In Bland KI, Copeland EM, eds: The Breast: Comprehensive Management of Benign and Malignant Diseases. Philadelphia, WB Saunders, 1991, pp 723–724.

75. River L, Silverstein J, Grout J, et al: Carcinoma of the breast: The diagnostic significance of pain. Am J Surg 1951; 82:733–735.

76. Preece PE, Mansel RE, Bolton PM, et al: Clinical syndromes of mastalgia. Lancet 1976; 2:670–673.

77. Wang DY, Fentiman IS: Epidemiology and endocrinology of benign breast disease. Breast Cancer Res Treat 1985; 6:5–36.

78. Tobiassen T, Rasmussen T, Doberl A, Rannevik G: Danazol treatment of severely symptomatic fibrocystic breast disease and long-term follow-up—the Hjorring project. Acta Obstet Gynaecol Scand 1984; 123(suppl):159–176.

79. Dennerstein L, Spencer-Gardner C, Gotts G, et al: Progesterone and the premenstrual syndrome: A double blind crossover trial. Br Med J (Clin Res Ed) 1985; 290:1617–1621.

80. Lafaye C, Aubert B: The effect of local progesterone on benign breast diseases: 500 case studies. J Gynecol Obstet Biol Reprod 1978; 7:1123–1139.

81. Hughes LE, Mansel RE, Webster DJT: Breast pain and nodularity. In Benign Disorders and Diseases of the Breast: Concepts and Clinical Management. London, Balliere Tindall, 1989, pp 75–92.

82. Ricciardi I, Ianniruberto A: Tamoxifen-induced regression of benign breast lesions. Obstet Gynecol 1979; 54:80–84.

83. Ernster VL, Goodson WH 3d, Hunt TK, et al: Vitamin E and benign breast "disease": A double-blind, randomized clinical trial. Surgery 1985; 97:490–494.

84. Pashby NL, Mansel RE, Hughes LE, et al: A clinical trial of evening primrose oil in mastalgia. Br J Surg 1981; 68:801–805.

85. Parazzini F, LaVecchia C, Rlundi R, et al: Methylxanthine, alcohol-free diet and fibrocystic breast disease: A factorial clinical trial. Surgery 1986; 99:576–581.

86. Hamed H, Caleffi M, Chaudary MA, Fentiman IS; LHRH analogue for treatment of recurrent and refractory mastalgia. Ann R Coll Surg Engl 1990; 72:221–224.

87. Page DL, Simpson JF: Benign, high-risk, and premalignant lesions of the mamma. In Bland KI, Copeland EM, eds: The Breast: Comprehensive Management of Benign and Malignant Diseases. Philadelphia, WB Saunders, 1991; pp 113–116.

88. Foote FW, Stewart FW: Comparative studies of cancerous versus noncancerous breasts: I. Basic morphologic characteristics. II. Role of so-called chronic cystic mastitis in mammary carcinogenesis: Influence of certain hormones on human breast structure. Ann Surg 1945; 121:6–53.

89. Hutter RVP: Goodbye to fibrocystic disease (editorial). N Engl J Med 1985; 312:179–181.

90. Frantz VK, Pickren JW, Melcher GW, Auchincloss H Jr: Incidence of chronic cystic disease in so-called "normal breasts": A study based on 225 postmortem examinations. Cancer 1951; 4:762–783.

91. Dupont WD, Page DL: Risk factors for breast cancer in women with proliferative breast disease. N Engl J Med 1985; 312:146–151.

92. Page DL, Simpson JF: Benign, high-risk, and premalignant lesions of the mamma. In Bland KI, Copeland EM, eds: The Breast: Comprehensive Management of Benign and Malignant Diseases. Philadelphia, WB Saunders, 1991; 117–124.

93. Swain SM: Ductal carcinoma in situ. Cancer Invest 1992; 10:443–454.

94. Swain SM: Ductal carcinoma in situ—incidence, presentation and guidelines to treatment. Oncology 1989; 3:25–42.

95. Lagios MD, Margolin FR, Westdahl PR, et al: Mammographically detected duct carcinoma in situ: Frequency of local

recurrence following tylectomy and prognostic effect of nuclear grade on local recurrence. Cancer 1989; 63:618–624.

96. Lagios M: Duct carcinoma in situ: Pathology and treatment. Surg Clin North Am 1990; 70:853–871.

97. Gump FE, Jicha DL, Ozella L: Ductal carcinoma in situ (DCIS): A revised concept. Surgery 1987; 102:790–795.

98. Moore MP, Kinne DW: Diagnosis and treatment of in situ breast cancer. Contemp Oncol 1992; 46–51.

99. Jensen RA, Page DL, Dupont WD, Rogers LW: Invasive breast cancer (IBC) risk in women with sclerosing adenosis (SA). Cancer 1989; 64:1977–1983.

100. Dupont WD, Page DL, Rogers LW, Parl FF: Influence of exogenous estrogens, proliferative breast disease, and other variables on breast cancer risk. Cancer 1989; 63:948–957.

101. Rosen PP, Senie RT, Farr GH, et al: Epidemiology of breast carcinoma: Age, menstrual status, and exogenous hormone usage in patients with lobular carcinoma in situ. Surgery 1979; 85:219–224.

102. Bergkvist L, Adami HO, Persson I, et al: The risk of breast cancer after estrogen and estrogen-progestin replacement. N Engl J Med 1989; 321:293–297.

103. Steinberg KK, Thacker SB, Smith J, et al: A meta-analysis of the effect of estrogen replacement therapy on the risk of breast cancer. JAMA 1991; 265:1985–1990.

104. Colditz GA, Stampfer MJ, Willett WC, et al: Prospective study of estrogen replacement therapy and risk of breast cancer in postmenopausal women. JAMA 1990; 264:2648–2653.

105. Colditz GA, Hankinson SE, Hunter DJ, et al: The use of estrogens and progestins and the risk of breast cancer in postmenopausal women. N Engl J Med 1995; 332:1589–1593.

106. Schairer C, Byrne C, Keyl PM, et al: Menopausal estrogen and estrogen-progestin replacement therapy and risk of breast cancer (United States). Cancer Causes Control 1994; 5:491–500.

107. Fisher ER, Leeming R, Anderson S, et al: Conservative management of intraductal carcinoma (DCIS) of the breast. J Surg Oncol 1991; 47:139–147.

108. Marin-Bertolin S, Gonzalez-Martinez R, Velasco-Pastor M, et al: Mondor's disease and aesthetic breast surgery: Report of case secondary to mastopexy with augmentation. Aesthetic Plast Surg 1995; 19:251–252.

109. Catania S, Zurrida S, Veronesi P, et al: Mondor's disease and breast cancer. Cancer 1992; 69:2267–2270.

110. Green RA, Dowden RV: Mondor's disease in plastic surgery patients. Ann Plast Surg 1988; 20:231–235.

111. Chiedozi LC: Mondor's disease: Relationship to use of body girdle. Trop Geogr Med 1990; 42:162–165.

112. Cooper RA: Mondor's disease secondary to intravenous drug abuse. Arch Surg 1990; 125:807–808.

113. Johnson WC, Wallrich R, Helurg EB: Superficial thrombophlebitis of the chest wall. JAMA 1962; 180:103–108.

114. Camiel MR: Mondor's disease in the breast. Am J Obstet Gynecol 1985; 152:879–881.

115. Tsuji T: Mammary and extramammary Paget's disease: Expression of Ca 15-3, Ka-93, Ca 19-9, and CD44 in Paget cells and adjacent normal skin. Br J Dermatol 1995; 132:7–13.

116. Wolber RA, Dupuis BA, Wick MR: Expression of c-erbB-2 oncoprotein in mammary and extramammary Paget's disease. Am J Clin Pathol 1991; 96:243–247.

117. Kanitakis J, Thivolet J, Claudy A: p53 protein expression in mammary and extramammary Paget's disease. Anticancer Res 1993; 13:2429–2433.

118. Nadji M, Morales AR, Girtanner RE, et al: Paget's disease of the skin: A unifying concept of histogenesis. Cancer 1982; 50:2203–2206.

119. Shehi LJ, Pierson KK: Benign and malignant epithelial neoplasms and dermatological disorders. In Bland KI, Copeland EM, eds: The Breast: Comprehensive Management of Benign and Malignant Diseases. Philadelphia, WB Saunders, 1991, pp 227–228.

120. Sitakalin C, Ackerman AB: Mammary and extramammary Paget's disease. Am J Dermatopathol 1985; 7:335–340.

121. Hitchcock A, Topham S, Bell J, et al: Routine diagnosis of mammary Paget's disease: A modern approach. Am J Surg Pathol 1992; 16:58–61.

122. Vielh P, Validire P, Kheirallah S, et al: Paget's disease of the nipple without clinically and radiologically detectable breast tumor: Histochemical and immunohistochemical study of 44 cases. Pathol Res Pract 1993; 189:150–155.

123. Reed W, Oppedal BR, Eeg Larsen T:

Immunohistology is valuable in distinguishing between Paget's disease, Bowen's disease and superficial spreading malignant melanoma. Histopathology 1990; 16:583–588.

124. Peison B, Benisch B: Paget's disease of the nipple simulating malignant melanoma in a black woman. Am J Dermatopathol 1985; 7(suppl):165–169.

125. Lucarotti ME, Dunn JM, Webb AJ: Scrape cytology in the diagnosis of Paget's disease of the breast (meeting abstract). Cytopathology 1994; 5:9.

126. Samarasinghe D, Frost F, Sterrett G, et al: Cytological diagnosis of Paget's disease of the nipple by scrape smears: A report of five cases. Diagn Cytopathol 1993; 9:291–295.

127. Dixon AR, Galea MH, Ellis IO, et al: Paget's disease of the nipple. Br J Surg 1991; 78:722–723.

128. Dabski K, Stoll HL: Paget's disease of the breast presenting as a cutaneous horn. J Surg Oncol 1985; 29:237–239.

129. Sawyer RH, Asbury DL: Mammographic appearances in Paget's disease of the breast. Clin Radiol 1994; 49:185–188.

130. Anelli A, Anelli TF, McCormick B, et al: Conservative management of Paget's disease of the nipple (meeting abstract). Proc Annu Meet Am Soc Clin Oncol 1995; 14:A100.

131. Gorsky RD, Koplan JP, Peterson HB, Thacker SB: Relative risks and benefits of long-term estrogen replacement therapy: A decision analysis. Obstet Gynecol 1994; 83:161–166.

132. Gambrell RD, Maier RC, Sanders BI: Decreased incidence of breast cancer in postmenopausal estrogen-progestogen users. Obstet Gynecol 1983; 62:435–443.

133. Stanford JL, Weiss NS, Voigt LF, et al: Combined estrogen and progestin hormone replacement therapy in relation to risk of breast cancer in middle aged women. JAMA 1995; 274:137–142.

134. Whitehead MI, Campbell S: Endometrial histology, uterine bleeding and oestrogen levels in women receiving oestrogen therapy and oestrogen/progesterone therapy. *In* Taylor R, Brush M, King R, eds: Endometrial Cancer. London, Balliere Tindall, 1978; pp 65–80.

135. Brinton LA, Daling JR, Liff JM, et al: Oral contraceptives and breast cancer risk among younger women. J Natl Cancer Inst 1995; 87:827–835.

136. Sattin RW, Rubin GL, Wingo PA, et al: Oral contraceptive use and the risk of breast cancer: The cancer and steroid hormone study of the Centers for Disease Control and the National Institute of Child Health and Human Development. N Engl J Med 1986; 315:405–411.

137. American College of Obstetricians and Gynecologists: Hormonal contraception. ACOG technical bulletin. No. 198, October 1994 (replaces No. 106, July 1987). Int J Gynecol Obstet 1995; 48:115–126.

138. Stomper PC, Bradley J, Voorhis V, et al: Mammographic changes associated with postmenopausal hormone replacement therapy: A longitudinal study. Radiology 1990; 174:487–490.

139. Sickles EA, Filly RA, Callen RW: Breast cancer detection with sonography and mammography: Comparison using state of the art equipment. Am J Roentgenol 1983; 140:843–845.

140. Sickles EA: Sonographic detectability of breast calcifications. SPIE 1983; 419:51–52.

141. Page DL, Dupont WD, Rogers LW, et al: Intraductal carcinoma of the breast. Cancer 1982; 49:751–758.

142. McDivitt RW, Hutter RVP, Foote FW, et al: In situ lobular carcinoma: A prospective follow-up study indicating cumulative patient risks. JAMA 1967; 201:96–100.

143. Andersen JA: Lobular carcinoma in situ of the breast: An approach to rational treatment. Cancer 1977; 39:2597–2602.

CHAPTER 5

Lower Genital Tract Infections

S. Gene McNeeley, Jr.

Scott B. Ransom

Genital tract infections are among the most common gynecologic conditions treated by the primary care provider. Owing to the vast array of infections, this chapter serves as a concise review of risk factors, physical findings, office laboratory evaluation, and common treatments of the most common genital tract infections.

VULVOVAGINAL INFECTIONS

Common vulvovaginal infections are listed in Table 5–1. Although many patients and health care providers alike think yeast infections are the most common genital tract infection occurring in women, definitive studies have found that bacterial vaginosis is the most common microbiologically confirmed infection. Fungal infections, most caused by *Candida albicans*, are a distant second, and *Trichomonas vaginalis* accounts for approximately 10% of vulvovaginal infections.[1]

BACTERIAL VAGINOSIS

The vagina is normally colonized by the low-virulence bacteria *Lactobacillus* and *Corynebacterium* species. The lactobacilli are most important in maintaining a pH of 3.8 to 4.2 and preventing overgrowth of bacteria and yeast. Patients with bacterial vaginosis (BV) are less likely to be colonized with lactobacilli, and the vagina is more likely to be colonized with anaerobic pathogens such as *Bacteroides, Peptostreptococcus, Mobiluncus,* and *Gardnerella vaginalis.* There is a 10-fold to 100-fold increase in the concentration of these pathogens. The BV-associated pathogens produce organic acids (primarily succinic acid), which are converted to amines thus producing the malodorous discharge often described as *fishy.* Bacterial byproducts also alter white blood cell migration into the vaginal secretions resulting in the clinical picture of infection without inflammation. The presence of white blood cells precludes the diagnosis of BV.[2]

Risk factors for developing BV include the presence of sexually transmitted diseases (STDs), greater number of sexual partners, long history of sexual activity, and the presence of an intrauterine contraceptive device (IUD).[3] Although BV is seen more frequently in heterosexual women, it can occur in virgins and lesbians.

The standard tests for diagnosing the

Table 5–1. Common Genital Tract Infections

Vulvovaginitis
   Bacterial vaginosis
   Yeast vaginitis
   Trichomonas vaginitis
Ulcerative diseases
   Genital herpes
   Syphilis
   Chancroid
   Lymphogranuloma venereum
Cervical infections
   Chlamydia
   Gonorrhea
Pelvic inflammatory disease

most common vulvovaginal infections are the saline and potassium hydroxide (KOH) wet mount, pH testing of vaginal fluids, and the whiff test for detecting amines in the vaginal secretions. These findings are summarized in Table 5–2. In BV a homogeneous gray or slate-colored discharge is noted on physical examination. The pH exceeds 4.5, and the whiff test is positive. A saline wet mount should be examined for the presence of clue cells. The presence of three of four criteria confirms the diagnosis of BV. The presence of white blood cells suggests other infections such as chlamydia or

gonorrhea as the likely cause of the infection. The predictive value of various tests and test combinations for bacterial vaginosis is noted in Table 5–3.[4] Genital cultures for *G. vaginalis* are not recommended because approximately 50% of women culture positive for *G. vaginalis* are asymptomatic.

Treatment consists of oral or topical antibiotics. Oral metronidazole (250 mg three times daily or 500 mg twice daily) for 5 to 7 days is a standard therapy. Metronidazole gel 0.75% (one applicator twice daily for 5 days) and clindamycin cream 2% (one applicator daily for 7 days) demonstrate comparable efficacy and avoid systemic side effects of oral metronidazole. Recurrence is common and is a difficult management problem. Treatment with a 14-day course of metronidazole gel 0.75% followed by weekly applications has been modestly effective (J. Sobel, personal communication). There is no evidence that treating sexual partners reduces recurrences.

Although many health care providers consider BV a trivial infection, there is a growing body of evidence that BV is associated with pelvic inflammatory disease (PID), abnormal Papanicolaou (Pap) smear and is readily recognized as an important risk factor for postoperative gynecologic infections. Preoperative treat-

Table 5–2. Vaginal Infections

	Patient Concern	Discharge	Vaginal pH	Amine odor	Microscopic
Normal	None	White flocculent	3.8–4.2	Absent	Lactobacilli
Candida vulvovaginitis	Itching Burning Discharge	White cottage cheese–like May be increased	<4.5	Absent	Mycelia Budding yeast Pseudohyphae with KOH preparation
Bacterial vaginosis	Discharge Bad odor, may be worse after intercourse	Thin, homogeneous White-gray Adherent Often increased	>4.5	Present Fishy	Clue cells Coccoid bacteria No WBCs
Trichomonas vaginitis	Itching Frothy discharge Bad odor Dysuria	Yellow, green, frothy Adherent Increased	<4.5	Present Fishy (not always)	Trichomonads WBCs >10/hpf

KOH = Potassium hydroxide; WBCs = white blood cells.

Table 5–3. Bacterial Vaginosis

Excellent Predictors	Predictive Value (%) +	Predictive Value (%) −	Poor Predictors	Predictive Value (%) +	Predictive Value (%) −
Odor on alkalinization	94	93	Homogeneous discharge	42	88
Clue cells on saline suspension	90	99	pH >4.5	52	94
Mobiluncus species on saline suspension	99	57	Background bacteria	61	97
Clue cells and odor	99	92			

Adapted from Thomason JL: Statistical evaluation of diagnostic criteria for bacterial vaginosis. Am J Obstet Gynecol 1990; 162:155–160.

ment of BV has been shown to decrease the incidence of postabortion endometritis. BV is also associated with preterm labor, preterm premature rupture of membranes, and postpartum endometritis. Treatment during pregnancy has not consistently improved pregnancy outcome.[5–13]

FUNGAL INFECTIONS

Fungal or *yeast* infections account for approximately 35% of vulvovaginal infections. The vast majority of infections are caused by *C. albicans*. Over the past two decades, there has appeared to be a trend toward a greater prevalence of non-*albicans* species causing vulvovaginal infections (*Candida tropicalis, Candida glabrata*).[14] *Saccharomyces cerevisiae* (bakers' yeast) accounts for 1% of vulvovaginal infections. Postmenopausal women who are not taking hormone replacement are not colonized with yeast, and symptomatic infections are uncommon. Infections are common in women on hormone replacement and in women receiving tamoxifen for breast cancer. *C. glabrata* is a common pathogen in the latter group of women. The clinical significance of recovering non-*Albicans* species is not clear. Some species tend to be less susceptible to over-the-counter medications (miconazole, clotrimazole), and prescription antifungal medications may be required.

Approximately 15% to 20% of women are colonized with yeast. Carriage rates range from 20% to 40% in pregnancy and are higher following antibiotic therapy and in a STD clinic setting. Contraceptive method plays an important role in vaginal colonization rates, with carriage occurring more frequently in women using IUDs and condoms. The colonization rate is not increased in women on low-dose oral contraceptives.[15] Other important risk factors for vulvovaginal infection include diabetes, recent antibiotic use, chronic corticosteroid use, and immunodeficiency conditions. Tight-fitting underclothes and pantyhose have been associated with increased vaginal colonization and symptomatic infections.[16,17]

Women most often complain of vulvovaginal pruritus and a cottage cheese–like vaginal discharge. Erythema, vaginal discharge, and edema of the vulva and vagina are readily apparent. Excoriation is frequently present. Results of the wet mount examination and pH are noted in Table 5–2. Cultures are not routinely recommended. For women with recurrent symptoms, however, culture confirms recurrent infection and may identify pathogens that tend to be more resistant to over-the-counter medications. A negative culture identifies women who need to be investigated more thoroughly for other causes of vulvovaginal burning and pruritus, including a hypersensitivity to topical antifungals.

Once the diagnosis is confirmed, topical or systemic therapy is highly effective in treating most infections (Table 5–4). Recurrent infections are a challenge to the provider. Self-diagnosis and self-therapy are not acceptable. Underlying medical conditions need to be controlled, soaps need to be changed because they

Table 5–4. Treatment of Vulvovaginal Candidiasis

Therapy of Acute Infection

Butoconazole	2% cream	5 g at bedtime × 3 d
Clotrimazole	1% cream	5 g at bedtime × 7–14 d
Miconazole	10%	5 g at bedtime × 7 d
	100 mg vaginal supp	1 suppository at bedtime × 7 d
	200 mg vaginal supp	1 suppository at bedtime × 3 d
	1200 mg vaginal supp	1 suppository single dose
Econazole	150 mg vaginal tablet	1 tablet at bedtime × 3 d
Fenticonazole	2% cream	5 g at bedtime × 7 d
Tioconazole	2% cream	5 g at bedtime × 3 d
	6.5% cream	5 g at bedtime single dose
Terconazole	2%	5 g at bedtime × 3 d
Fluconazole	Oral tablet	150 mg single dose
Ketoconazole	200 mg tablet	400 mg daily × 5 d

Therapy of Recurrent Infection

Ketoconazole	100 mg	1 tablet orally, daily × 6 mo
Fluconazole	150 mg	1 tablet orally daily, days 1–4– 8, then 100 mg orally, weekly × 6 mo if asymtomatic and culture negative on day 15

Data from refs. 17, 18, and 19.

may be an irritant, and loose-fitting undergarments should be worn. Once a recurrent infection is proven, it is best managed with oral long-term suppression with systemic antifungals as noted in Table 5–4. Although ketoconazole has been shown to be safe and effective in reducing recurrences, long-term suppression with fluconazole minimizes the risk of hepatotoxicity[18, 18a] (J. Sobel, personal communication).

TRICHOMONAS VAGINITIS

T. vaginalis causes approximately 10% of cases of vulvovaginitis. *T. vaginalis* does not invade the vaginal tissues but incites an intense inflammatory response in the vaginal lumen. This flagellated protozoan swims freely in this vaginal discharge and also can attach to the vaginal epithelium.

Because trichomonas vaginitis is a sexually transmitted infection, risk factors for acquiring the infection include multiple partners, the presence of other sexually transmitted diseases, and use of a nonbarrier contraceptive.

Approximately 50% of women with trichomonas vaginitis are asymptomatic. Common symptoms include vaginal discharge, dysuria, and dyspareunia.[19]

Physical examination reveals erythema of the vulva and vagina. A profuse frothy, yellow-to-green vaginal discharge is typical. The pH is commonly greater than 4.5. Examination of the wet mount reveals the flagellated protozoan, and white blood cells are also frequently noted. Culture for *T. vaginalis* is not necessary unless one is trying to document metronidazole resistance. As with other sexually transmitted infections, treatment of the patient and her partner is necessary. Recommended treatment consists of a single dose of 2 g metronidazole or 500 mg given twice daily for 7 days or 250 mg orally three times a day for 7 days. The side effects, particularly nausea and a metallic taste, preclude long-term therapy, and, hence, the single-dose regimen significantly increases patient compliance. For women with documented metronidazole treatment failures, the following regimen is recommended: 1 g orally twice daily for 7 to 14 days plus a 500-mg vaginal suppository twice daily for 7 to 14 days.[20] Treatment of asymptomatic women is recommended as a means of STD control. Because trichomonas can produce inflammatory atypia on Pap smears, treatment may cause an abnormal smear report and the unnecessary expenses incurred in the evaluation of an abnormal Pap smear. As with BV, an association has been noted between trichomoniasis and poor obstetric outcome and other gynecologic infections.

GENITAL HERPES INFECTIONS

Herpes simplex virus (HSV) infections account for up to 60% of genital ulcerations in women and must be differentiated from syphilis and chancroid. The prevalence of genital herpes infections depends on the clinical characteristics of the patients studied. In the general private practice population, HSV can be isolated from the genital tract of less than 1% to 5% of women. The prevalence is doubled or tripled in the STD clinic setting. Most genital HSV infections are due to HSV II. In general, anti–HSV II antibodies do not appear until sexual activity has begun. The prevalence of HSV II antibodies parallels those findings of HSV isolation in the population studied. In obstetric populations, 30% of women have detectable antibodies to HSV II. HSV II antibodies can be detected in greater than 50% of women attending STD clinics.[21-26]

Genital HSV infections most often follow intimate contact with a person shedding the virus. Transmission via fomites is an uncommon means of transmitting HSV infections. Following an incubation period of approximately 5 to 7 days, small vesicles appear, which may coalesce with adjacent vesicles forming larger ulcers. During this initial infection, the HSV ascends the peripheral nerves and enters the dorsal route ganglion of the sacral plexus. Recurrent infections represent reactivation of the virus from a latent stage. Although uncommon, reinfection with different HSV strains can occur resulting in new primary episodes.[26-28]

Genital herpes infections are divided into three clinical settings: first episode of genital herpes, primary genital herpes, and recurrent genital herpes. Antibody studies have documented that many HSV II infections are initially asymptomatic. Up to 25% of women who are experiencing the first episode of symptomatic genital herpes have serologic evidence of prior HSV II infection. Symptoms may be mild, especially in patients with prior HSV in-

fection. The first episode of HSV infection is usually associated with systemic symptoms, such as malaise, regional lymphadenopathy, and fever. The systemic symptoms begin approximately with the onset of lesions and resolve 8 to 10 days after onset. The lesions with the initial episode of genital herpes usually heal within 21 days. Viral shedding lasts for approximately 12 to 14 days with the first episode of genital herpes. HSV I accounts for approximately 5% to 10% of first episode genital herpes infections, and most infections are primary infections. Primary genital HSV infections are characterized by more intense systemic and local symptoms. As with first episode infections, systemic symptoms occur on day 2 to 3 of the infection and resolve within 1 week. Genital lesions tend to be more numerous and pain more severe with primary herpes when compared to other first episode genital infections. Infection of the urethra and cervix is common (approximately 70% to 90%). More lesions appear to occur with primary HSV I compared to primary HSV II and other first episode HSV II infections. The duration of viral shedding and duration of lesions is also somewhat longer in primary infections.[21]

Although the first episode and primary herpetic infections usually involve multiple lesions and systemic symptoms, recurrent infections exhibit relatively mild local symptoms and an absence of systemic symptoms. Most recurrent infections are preceded by a prodrome described as a numbness or paresthesia at the site of recurrence. The mean duration of viral shedding is approximately 4 days with recurrent genital herpes infections, and the mean duration of time to healing is approximately 10 days. Of those women with recurrent genital lesions, approximately 12% shed virus from the cervix.[21,26]

Systemic antiviral treatment is effective in managing primary and recurrent HSV infections. For primary infections, acyclovir 200 mg orally five times a day for 7 to 10 days or until clinical resolution decreases the duration of viral shedding and shortens the healing time. Some patients with recurrent HSV infections benefit from administration of a 5-day course of acyclovir 200 mg five times a day, or 400 mg three times a day, or 800 mg twice a day. New antiviral medications indicated for treating recurrent infections include famciclovir 125 mg twice daily for 5 days and valacyclovir 500 mg twice daily for 5 days, both taken orally. All regimens have been shown to reduce the duration of viral shedding and speed lesion healing by approximately 1 day. For patients with multiple frequent occurrences, long-term suppression reduces the number of recurrences. Safety and efficacy data have been obtained from persons taking acyclovir up to 5 years. Recommended suppression consists of acyclovir 400 mg orally twice a day. It is recommended that acyclovir be discontinued after 1 year of continuous suppressive therapy to assess the patient's rate of recurrent infections.[29] Treatment of the primary infection with acyclovir has not been shown to reduce the incidence or frequency of recurrences. Approximately 70% of women with HSV infections experience a recurrence within 1 year.

SYPHILIS

Syphilis is a chronic infectious disease caused by *Treponema pallidum* and clinically is divided into primary, secondary, early latent, late latent, and tertiary syphilis. Except for congenital syphilis, transmission is by intimate sexual contact. The spirochete enters the body through breaks in the skin, and the primary chancre appears at the site of entry into the body. Untreated the chancre resolves in 4 to 6 weeks. Secondary syphilis is a result of hematogenous spread of *T. pallidum* that lasts 2 to 6 weeks. Clinical manifestations include generalized lymphadenopathy and rash. The patient then enters the latent phase in which she is asymptomatic. Early latent syphilis is defined as an infection of less than 1 year's duration. Approximately one third of untreated patients develop tertiary syphilis, occurring anywhere from 1 to 20 years or more after the secondary stage. Tertiary manifestations consist of gumma formation; cardiovascular changes, including aneurysm of the aorta or other great vessels, aortic insufficiency, and

Table 5–5. Treatment of Syphilis

Primary, Secondary, and Early Latent Syphilis	
Benzathine penicillin G	2.4 million units IM in a single dose
Late Latent Syphilis or Latent Syphilis of Unknown Duration	
Benzathine penicillin G	7.2 million units total, administered as 3 doses of 2.4 million units IM each, at 1-wk intervals

heart failure; and a variety of neurologic manifestations.

The primary chancre appears as a nontender, indurated ulcer. Most chancres go unnoticed in women and resolve in 2 to 4 weeks. Maculopapular mucocutaneous lesions are the most common clinical manifestation of secondary syphilis. Lesions on the palms of hands and soles of feet are seen in about one half of patients. Inguinal adenopathy may be present in up to 85% of patients.[30]

Dark field examination is the most accurate means of diagnosing primary and secondary syphilis. Most women, however, are diagnosed by antibody testing. Confirmatory tests following a positive Venereal Disease Research Laboratory (VDRL) or rapid plasma reagin (RPR) include fluorescent treponemal antibody absorption (FTA-ABS) or microhemagglutination–*Treponema pallidum* (MHA-TP). Treatment recommendations for syphilis are given in Table 5–5. Therapy should be monitored with serial VDRL titers with a fourfold decline in titer over a 3-month period. Treatment failures should be retreated. Sexual partners must be treated.[31]

CHANCROID

Chancroid is the third most common ulcerative STD and is caused by *Haemophilus ducreyi*, a small, nonmotile, gram-negative rod. Chancroid is much more common in developing nations and in tropical climates. Infections occur more often in men than in women and are transmitted by intimate sexual contact. Fomites are not a means of transmission of chancroid. In the United States, most outbreaks are endemic, and the reservoir tends to be prostitutes. Coinfection with other sexually transmitted pathogens is common including HIV.[32]

Approximately 4 to 7 days after inoculation, a genital ulcer appears. Inguinal tenderness or adenopathy may be present. The ulcer is painful and surrounded by erythema, is covered with necrotic exudate, and is not indurated. In contrast, the syphilitic ulcer is nontender and indurated. Inguinal adenitis is a characteristic feature of chancroid occurring in up to 50% of patients and is most often unilateral. The bubos may become fluctuant and rupture through the skin. Gram-negative rods that form chains are seen on Gram stain. The diagnosis can be confirmed with culture for *H. ducreyi* or biopsy. It is imperative that one exclude the presence of other infectious organisms causing genital ulcers. The treatment of choice is azithromycin 1 g orally single dose or ceftriaxone 250 mg intramuscularly. Multidose regimens include erythromycin, trimethoprim/sulfamethoxazole, and amoxicillin/clavulanate.[33]

LYMPHOGRANULOMA VENEREUM

Lymphogranuloma venereum is one of the sexually transmitted infections caused by *Chlamydia trachomatis*. This infection is caused by the L_1, L_2, and L_3 strains. These are antigenically distinct from the other chlamydial serotypes causing STDs. Clinical manifestations include genital ulceration, lymphadenopathy, and proctitis. Late manifestations include genital elephantitis, genital fistulas, rectal strictures, and anal fistulas.[34]

Following an incubation period of 3 days to 3 weeks, a primary lesion appears. In women, this is most often in the posterior fourchette. This lesion appears as a vesicle or papule that may ulcerate. This primary lesion is often not recognized. One to 4 weeks after the primary lesion appears, systemic symptoms such as fever, malaise, and headache occur. The lymphadenopathy is unilateral (66%), and the lymph nodes are firm to palpa-

tion. The nodes become matted together, and the inflammatory response involves the overlying soft tissues. The bubo enlarges with pain and fever. Rupture through the skin usually heralds resolution of the infection. Significant scarring may subsequently occur. Disappearance of the bubo usually indicates the end of the disease. Approximately 20% of untreated patients have recurrences. The inguinal syndrome is most commonly seen in men and noted in only 20% to 30% of women with lymphogranuloma venereum. More often, women complain of proctitis and low abdominal pain. Colorectal symptoms are more common in women because of the lymphatic drainage of the posterior fourchette to the pelvic and perirectal nodes. The diagnosis of lymphogranuloma venereum is confirmed with culture or monoclonal antibody testing of the nodal aspirate.[34] Treatment includes a 21-day course of doxycycline 100 mg twice daily. Alternative medications include erythromycin 500 mg four times a day for 21 days or sulfisoxazole 500 mg four times a day for 21 days.[35] Surgical intervention is not indicated except for management of late sequelae such as fistulas or strictures.

CONDYLOMA ACUMINATA

Genital warts are epidermal tumors caused by the human papillomavirus (HPV) and are the most common viral STD. Clinical and subclinical infections with HPV may be associated with the development of preinvasive and invasive cancer. Approximately 1% of Pap smears may contain evidence of human papillomavirus infection. Genital warts have been reported to occur in 6% or more of women ages 20 to 34.[36] HPV 6 and 11 are most frequently associated with genital condyloma, whereas types 16, 18, 31, and 33 have been associated with dysplasia of the cervix and invasive genital cancers. Most warts occur in young adults. Many patients with genital warts have other sexually transmitted infections, including gonorrhea, chlamydia, and trichomoniasis. Multiple sex partners have been associated with increased risk of HPV infection. Immunosuppressed women are at increased risk of condyloma acuminatum and cervical intra-epithelial neoplasia.[37–39]

Exophytic warts usually appear in the fourchette and adjacent labia. Condyloma may appear on other areas of the perineum in approximately 20% of women. Subclinical infection may be evident with colposcopy after the application of acetic acid. Although the diagnosis of genital warts is rather straightforward, one must rule out vulvar intraepithelial neoplasia in atypical appearing warts or in those warts that fail conventional medical therapy. These lesions must also be distinguished from condyloma lata of secondary syphilis.

Treatment of genital warts is determined by site and extent of wart growth and patient preference. Podofilox 0.5% is applied by the patient daily for 3 days followed by 4 days of no therapy. This can be repeated for a total of four cycles. Podophyllin is easily applied in the office setting. The area should be washed 4 hours after application. Weekly treatments may be necessary. Trichloroacetic acid (80% to 90%) can also be applied to warts in the office setting also and should be performed weekly. For warts persisting after four to six applications, other therapeutic modalities should be used. Treatment efficacy for topical therapy varies from 30% to 80%, and recurrences occur in up to 65% of patients. Podophyllin and podofilox are contraindicated in pregnancy.[40–43]

Warts may be removed in the outpatient setting with cryotherapy therapy, electrodesiccation, and electrocautery. Local anesthesia is required for these methods. Extensive warts should be treated with ablative rather than topical therapy. Multifocal disease is common; vaginal and cervical warts are treated in similar fashion. A Pap smear should be obtained to rule out cervical neoplasia and dysplasia. Persistent or recurrent warts should be biopsied and treated with other methods.

Subclinical genital tract infection is more common than exophytic warts. Infection is often diagnosed on the cervix by Pap smear, colposcopy, or biopsy. Tests for detecting HPV DNA type are available; however, the clinical utility has not been determined. Screening for subclinical genital HPV using DNA tests and acetic acid/colposcopy is not recommended. HPV infection may persist throughout the patient's lifetime in a dormant state and may become infectious or clinically apparent on a sporadic basis.

CERVICITIS

Cervicitis is a common clinical infection. It is the most common clinical manifestation of infection with *C. trachomatis*. Infection with either *C. trachomatis* or *N. gonorrhoeae* is the most important risk factor for developing upper tract infections, including PID, which is called endometritis, salpingitis, and peritonitis by some authors. The cervix appears erythematous and friable, as evidenced by bleeding induced when placing the vaginal speculum or touching the cervix with a swab or spatula. Mucopurulent discharge appears yellow to green on an endocervical swab and contains greater than 10 polymorphonuclear cells per oil emersion field on a Gram stain specimen. Approximately 50% of women are asymptomatic with a grossly normal appearing cervix.[44,45]

CHLAMYDIA TRACHOMATIS

C. trachomatis is the most common sexually transmitted pathogen in the United States causing more than 4 million new infections annually, and cervicitis is the most common clinical manifestation. There are 15 serotypes of *C. trachomatis*. Strains L_1, L_2, and L_3 cause lymphogranuloma venereum and were discussed previously. Eight serotypes (D, E, F, G, H, I, J, K) cause a spectrum of infections in women, including Bartholin's gland infections, cervicitis, and PID including Fitz-Hugh-Curtis syndrome (perihepatitis associated with PID). *C. trachomatis* also causes conjunctivitis and oropharyngeal infections in women. Vertical transmission to the infant can produce similar syndromes. *C. trachomatis* has a cell wall similar to gram-negative bacteria and is an obligate intracellular pathogen. The chlamydia attach to columnar and cuboidal epithelium and are phagocytized by the host cell. Intracellular replication occurs with subsequent lysis of the host cell in approximately 48 hours.[33,44]

Overall, approximately 5% of nonpregnant women are infected with *C. trachomatis.* Infection occurs more frequently in women seen in STD clinics. Younger age, nonwhite race, socioeconomic status, multiple sexual partners, and new sex partner are important risk factors for chlamydial infections. Thirty percent to 70% of women whose partner has nongonococcal urethritis test positive for *C. trachomatis.*[46] Coinfection with *N. gonorrhoeae* is common. Approximately 50% of women with gonococcal infection of the cervix test positive for chlamydia. Other important risk factors for chlamydial infection include use of oral contraceptives or nonbarrier contraceptives and the presence of urethral syndrome (frequency, dysuria with sterile pyuria).[47–50]

Before the 1980s, the ability to diagnose chlamydial infections was limited to a small number of laboratories that had appropriate facilities and personnel for tissue culture. Although tissue culture has been the gold standard, most laboratories use an antigen detection test. Highly sensitive and specific nucleic acid probes are readily available for the clinician. The complement fixation test is most useful in diagnosing lymphogranuloma venereum. Serologic tests otherwise have limited utility in the outpatient management of chlamydial infections. The poor sensitivity and specificity of the Pap smear limits the utility of a Pap smear for diagnosing chlamydial infections.

Treatment of uncomplicated cervical infections includes doxycycline 100 mg orally twice daily for 7 days. A single dose of azithromycin 1 g orally or ofloxacin 300 mg orally twice daily for 7 days is equally effective. Repeat testing after completion of therapy is not indicated.[35]

GONORRHEA

There are approximately 2 million gonococcal infections in the United States annually. Genital tract infections in women caused by *N. gonorrhoeae* include Bartholin's gland infections, cervicitis, and PID. Systemic infections include sepsis, migratory polyarthritis, and endocarditis.[51] Risk factors for infection are similar to those with other sexually transmitted infections, including the number of sex partners, younger age, use of a nonbarrier method of contraception, lower socioeconomic status, nonwhite race, and unmarried status. As with *C. trachomatis,* male-to-female transmission occurs more frequently than female-to-male transmission.[61] Although men are usually symptomatic with gonococcal urethritis, the same cannot be said for women, in whom the vast majority of cervical infections are asymptomatic. Symptoms of lower genital tract infection include dysuria, vaginal discharge, and abnormal bleeding. Approximately 15% of women with uncomplicated gonococcal cervicitis develop PID (endometritis, salpingitis, peritonitis).[51–54] Physical findings suggestive of gonococcal infection include urethral or endocervical discharge. The cervix may appear normal or may show evidence of hypertrophy and a mucopurulent cervicitis. Other sites of lower genital tract infection include the Bartholin's glands and urethra. Anal infection also occurs. The diagnosis of cervical infection can be made with Gram stain of the cervical specimen showing intracellular gram-negative diplococci. As with chlamydial infections, DNA probe technology has supplanted culture in many institutions for the diagnosis of *N. gonorrhoeae.*

Treatment of uncomplicated gonococcal infections consists of ceftriaxone 125 mg intramuscularly, cefixime 400 mg orally, ciprofloxacin 500 mg orally, or ofloxacin 400 mg orally. All patients with gonococcal infections should receive empiric treatment of *C. trachomatis* with doxycycline 100 mg orally, twice daily for 7 days or an alternative regimen listed previously. [55]

PELVIC INFLAMMATORY DISEASE

There are approximately 1 million cases of PID in the United States on an annual basis. As with other sexually transmitted infections, risk factors include the presence of a sexually transmitted infection, instrumentation of the uterus (endometrial biopsy or dilatation and curettage), multiple partners, age less than 24 years, use of nonbarrier contraceptive, and the presence of BV. Approximately one quarter of all women diagnosed with PID require inpatient treatment. The organisms associated with PID include *N. gonorrhoeae* (approximately 40% to 50%), *C. trachomatis* (approximately 20%), and nongonococcal/nonchlamydial infections (approximately 40%). The nongonococcal/nonchlamydial infections are usually caused by a variety of pathogens consisting of aerobic and anaerobic gram-positive and gram-negative bacteria normally found in the vagina. The role mycoplasmas and ureaplasmas play in PID is not clearly defined. *Mycobacterium tuberculosis* is an uncommon cause of PID in the United States. Endometritis, often asymptomatic, is a common manifestation of chlamydia infection in women. Approximately 50% of women with chlamydial cervicitis also harbor *C. trachomatis* in the endometrial cavity.[56–60] Chlamydial endometritis persists in women treated with beta-lactam antibiotics alone for PID, emphasizing the importance of properly selecting antibiotics when treating PID.[61]

PID is classically described as an ascending infection beginning at the cervix and progressing to the upper genital tract. In some way, the functional barrier that prevents ascending infection is breached. The infection spreads from the endometrium into the tubes and adjacent structures. The infection can ascend intra-abdominally to produce perihepatitis (Fitz-Hugh-Curtis syndrome).

PID can present with few symptoms or as a life-threatening infection. Vaginal discharge, abnormal bleeding, fever, and lower abdominal pain are the most common symptoms. The development of symptoms often coincides with onset of menses, and symptoms are more common with gonococcal PID.[62] Physical findings include abdominal tenderness with or without rebound, mucopurulent cervical discharge, cervical motion tenderness, unilateral or bilateral adnexal tenderness, and uterine tenderness. A mass may or may not be palpable on examination. Frequently a satisfactory examination is not possible because of severe pain.

The patient with chlamydial PID may be asymptomatic or complain of mild or atypical lower abdominal pain and abnormal uterine bleeding. The pelvic examination may be entirely normal or reveal minimal uterine tenderness or pain with cervical motion.[58,59,63] Right upper quadrant abdominal tenderness may be indicative of Fitz-Hugh-Curtis syndrome. Patients with diffuse rebound tenderness require a more in-depth evaluation to exclude other causes of an acute abdomen.

Tests to aid in the clinical diagnosis include cultures or probe tests of the cervix for *N. gonorrhoeae* and *C. trachomatis*, culdocentesis with culture for aerobic and anaerobic bacteria, and endometrial biopsy. Other required tests include complete blood count with differential and sensitive pregnancy test. The erythrocyte sedimentation rate and C-reactive protein have been shown to be elevated in women with acute salpingitis; however, they may also be elevated in other conditions and are not diagnostic for PID. Ultrasound is helpful particularly in women in whom a satisfactory pelvic examination is not possible and should be performed on all patients with a suspected mass or abscess.

Clinical criteria for the diagnosis of acute PID is noted on Table 5–6. All three major criteria must be present for the diagnosis of PID and one of the minor criteria should be present.[64] The major criteria for PID are nonspecific. In prospective studies in which laparoscopy confirmed the diagnosis of PID, the diagnosis was incorrect in approximately 35% of women with the clinical diagnosis of PID.[65] Thus, patients who do not respond promptly following treatment of PID require further

Table 5–6. Clinical Criteria for Diagnosis of Pelvic Inflammatory Disease

Major Criteria (All 3 must be present)
Lower abdominal tenderness
Adnexal tenderness
Cervical motion tenderness

Minor Criteria (At least 1 must be present)
Oral temperature >38.3°
Abnormal cervical or vaginal discharge
Elevated erythrocyte sedimentation rate
Elevated C-reactive protein
Laboratory documentation of cervical infection with *N. gonorrhoeae* or *C. trachomatis*

Table 5–7. Treatment of Pelvic Inflammatory Disease

Inpatient Treatment Options

Regimen A
1. Cefoxitin	2 g IV every 6 hours
or	
Cefotetan	2 g IV every 12 hours
2. Doxycycline	100 mg orally or IV every 12 hours

Regimen B
1. Clindamycin	900 mg IV every 8 hours
2. Gentamicin	Loading dose IV or IM - (2 mg/kg body weight) followed by maintenance dose of 1.5 mg/kg every 8 hours

Outpatient Treatment Options

Regimen A
1. Cefoxitin	2 gm IM
2. Probenecid	1 g orally in single dose concurrently
3. Doxycycline	100 mg orally every 12 hours for 14 days

Regimen B
1. Ceftriaxone	250 mg IM
2. Doxycline	100 mg orally every 12 hours for 14 days

Regimen C
1. Ofloxacin	400 mg orally every 12 hours for 14 days
2. Metronidazole	500 mg orally every 12 hours for 14 days

Regimen D
1. Ofloxacin	400 mg orally every 12 hours for 14 days
2. Clindamycin	450 mg orally 4 times daily

evaluation. The differential diagnosis includes acute salpingitis, acute appendicitis, endometriosis, symptomatic ovarian cyst, ectopic pregnancy, ovarian neoplasm, and symptomatic fibroid uterus.

An important decision the clinician must make when managing PID is determining whether the patient will be treated as an outpatient or inpatient. Traditional indications for inpatient management include younger age, nulliparity or low parity, significant leukocytosis, suspected pregnancy, unsatisfactory examination and mass noted on pelvic examination. Each patient must be individualized to determine the best treatment regimen. A patient with an uncertain diagnosis or who fails to show prompt clinical improvement with therapy must proceed to invasive procedures to confirm the diagnosis. Specifically the patient should be referred for consultation in the event that laparoscopy is necessary. Treatment recommendations are given in Table 5–7.[66] Complications of PID are common and account for significant morbidity. Approximately 15% of women with PID develop tubo-ovarian abscess, and approximately 70% of women with tubo-ovarian abscess respond to initial antimicrobial therapy. Of those failing to respond, prolonged hospitalization is necessary for additional antibiotics, and frequently surgical intervention is required.[67] Approximately 15% of women who have had one episode of PID are infertile. The risk for infertility approximately doubles with each episode of PID and is more common with chlamydial PID.[65] There is a six- to tenfold increased risk for ectopic pregnancy following one episode of salpingitis.

REFERENCES

1. Kent HL: Epidemiology of vaginitis. Am J Obstet Gynecol 1991; 165:1168.
2. Eschenbach DA, Hillier SL, Critchlow C, et al: Diagnosis and clinical mani-

festations of bacterial vaginosis. Am J Obstet Gynecol 1988; 158:819.

3. Thomason JL, Gelbart SM, Scaglione NJ: Bacterial vaginosis: Current review with indications for asymptomatic therapy. Am J Obstet Gynecol 1991; 165:1210.

4. Thomason JL: Statistical evaluation of diagnostic criteria for bacterial vaginosis. Am J Obstet Gynecol 1990; 162:155.

5. Paavonen J, Teisala K, Heinonen PK, et al: Microbiological and histopathological findings in acute pelvic inflammatory disease. Br J Obstet Gynaecol 1987; 94:454–460.

6. Larsson PG, Platz-Christensen JJ, Thejis H, et al: Incidence of pelvic inflammatory disease after first trimester legal abortion in women with bacterial vaginosis after treatment with metronidazole: A double-blind, randomized study. Am J Obstet Gynecol 1992; 166:100–103.

7. Larrson PG, Platz-Christensen JJ, Forsum U, Pahlson C: Clue cells in predicting infections after abdominal hysterectomy. Obstet Gynecol 1991; 77:450–453.

8. Soper DE, Bump RC, Hurt WG: Bacterial vaginosis and trichomoniasis vaginitis are risk factors for cuff cellulitis after abdominal hysterectomy. Am J Obstet Gynecol 1990; 163:1016–1023.

9. Hillier SL, Nugent RP, Krohn MA, et al: The association of bacterial vaginosis with adverse pregnancy outcome. Presented at ICAAC, Chicago 1991.

10. McGregor JA, French JI, Richter R, et al: Antenatal microbiologic and maternal risk factors associated with prematurity. Am J Obstet Gynecol 1990; 163:1465–1473.

11. Silver HM, Sperling RS, St. Clair PJ, Gibbs RS: Evidence relating bacterial vaginosis to intra-amniotic infection. Am J Obstet Gynecol 1989; 161:808–812.

12. Watts DH, Krohn MA, Hillier SL, Eschenbach DA: Bacterial vaginosis as a risk factor for post-cesarean endometritis. Obstet Gynecol 1990; 75:52–58.

13. Hillier SL, Nugent RP, Eschenbach DA, et al: Association between bacterial vaginosis and preterm delivery of a low-birth-weight infant. N Engl J Med 1995; 333:1737–1742.

14. Odds FC: Candida and Candidosis, 2nd ed. London, Baillier-Tindall, 1988.

15. Davidson F, Oates JK: The pill does not cause "thrush." Br J Obstet Gynaecol 1985; 92:1265.

16. Sobel JD: Vulvovaginal candidiasis. In Holmes K, ed: Sexually Transmitted Diseases. New York, McGraw-Hill, 1990, p 515.

17. Fleury FJ: Adult vaginitis. Clin Obstet Gynecol 1981; 24:407.

18. Sobel JD: Recurrent vulvovaginal candidiasis: A prospective study of the efficacy of maintenance ketoconazole therapy. N Engl J Med 1986; 315:1455.

18a. Sobel JD: Fluconazole maintenance therapy in recurrent vulvovaginal candidiasis. Int J Gynecol Obset 1997; 37:17–24.

19. Wolner-Hansen P, Kreuger JN, Stevens CE, et al: Clinical manifestations of vaginal trichomoniasis. JAMA 1989; 261:571.

20. Centers for Disease Control: 1993 Sexually transmitted diseases treatment guidelines. MMWR 1993; 42:71.

21. Corey L: Genital herpes. In Holmes K, ed: Sexually Transmitted Diseases. New York, McGraw-Hill, 1990, p 515.

22. Stavraky KM, Rawls WE, Chiavelta J, et al: Sexual and socioeconomic factors affecting the risk of past infections with herpes simplex virus type 2. Am J Epidemiol 1983; 118:109–121.

23. Rauh JL, Brookman RR, Schiff GM: Genital surveillance among sexually active adolescent girls. J Pediatr 1977; 90:844.

24. Sumaya CV, Marx J, Villis K, et al: Genital infections with herpes simplex virus in university student populations. Sex Transm Dis 1980; 7(1):16–20.

25. Sullivan-Bolyai J, Hill HF, Willson C, et al: Neonatal herpes simplex virus infection in King County, Washington: Increasing incidence and epidemiological correlates. J Am Med Asso 1983; 250(22):3059–62.

26. Corey L, Spear PG: Infections with herpes simplex viruses. N Engl J Med 1986; 314:686–749.

27. Barringer JR, Swoveland P: Recovery of herpes simplex virus from human trigeminal ganglions. N Engl J Med 1973; 188:648.

28. Warren KG, Brown SM, Wroblewska Z, et al: Isolation of latent herpes simplex virus from the superior cervical and vagus ganglions of human beings. N Engl J Med 1978; 298:1068.

29. Centers for Disease Control: 1993 Sexually transmitted diseases treatment guidelines. MMWR 1993; 42:22.

30. Chapel TA: The signs and symptoms of

secondary syphilis. Sex Transm Dis 1980; 7:161.

31. Centers for Disease Control: 1993 Sexually transmitted diseases treatment guidelines. MMWR 1993; 42:33.

32. Schmid GP, Sanders LL, Blount JH, et al: Chancroid in the United States, reestablishment of an old disease. J Am Med Associate Professor 1987; 258:3265.

33. Centers for Disease Control: 1993 Sexually transmitted diseases treatment guidelines. MMWR 1993; 42:21.

34. Pearlman MD, McNeeley SG: A review of the microbiology, immunology and clinical implications of *Chlamydia trachomatis* infections. Obstet Gynecol Surv 1992; 47:448–461.

35. Centers for Disease Control: 1993 Sexually transmitted diseases treatment guidelines. MMWR 1993; 42:27.

36. Daling JR, Weiss NS, Sherman KJ: History of genital warts in a selected population. Lancet 1984; 1:157.

37. Daling JR, Weiss NS, Sherman KJ: Risk factors for condyloma acuminatum in women. Sex Transm Dis 1986; 13:16.

38. Koss JG: Carcinogenesis in the uterine cervix and human papillomavirus infection. *In* Syrjanen K, et al, eds: Papillomaviruses and Human Disease. Berlin, Springer-Verlag, 1987, p 235.

39. Schneider V, Kay S, Lee HM: Immunosuppression as a high-risk factor in the development of condyloma acuminatum and squamous neoplasia of the cervix. Acta Cytol 1983; 27:220.

40. Kinghorn GR: Genital papillomavirus infections: Treatment. *In* Oriel JD, et al, eds: Recent Advances in Sexually Transmitted Diseases 3. Edinburgh, Churchill-Livingstone, 1986, p 147.

41. Dretler SP, Klein LA: The eradication of intraurethral condylomata acuminata with 5 percent 5-fluorouracil cream. J Urol 1975; 113:195.

42. Simmons PD, Langlet F, Thin RN: Cryotherapy versus electrocautery in the treatment of genital warts. Br J Vener Dis 1981; 57:273.

43. Centers for Disease Control: 1993 Sexually transmitted diseases treatment guidelines. MMWR 1993; 42:84.

44. Schachter J: Chlamydial infections. N Engl J Med 1978; 298:428.

45. Harrison HR, Costin M, Meder JB, et al: Cervical *Chlamydia trachomatis* infection in university women: Relationship to history, contraception, ectopy and cervicitis. Am J Obstet Gynecol 1985; 153:244.

46. Tait IA, Rees E, Hobson D, et al: Chlamydial infection of the cervix in contacts of men with non-gonococcal urethritis. Br J Vener Dis 1980; 56:37–45.

47. Richmond SJ, Paul ID, Taylor PK: Value and feasibility of screening women attending STD clinics for cervical chlamydial infections. Br J Vener Dis 1980; 56:92.

48. Brunham R, Iwin B, Stamm WE, et al: Epidemiological and clinical correlates of *C. trachomatis* and *N. gonorrhoeae* infection among women attending an STD clinic. Clin Res 1981; 29:47A.

49. Saltz GR, Linneman CC Jr, Brookman RR, et al: Chlamydia trachomatis cervical infections in female adolescents. J Pediatr 1981; 98:981.

50. Bowie WR, Borrle-Hume CJ, Manzon LM, et al: Prevalence of *C. trachomatis* and *M. gonorrhoeae* in two different populations of women. Can Med Associate Professor J 1981; 124:1477.

51. Suleiman SA, Grimes EM, Jones HS: Disseminated gonococcal infections. Obstet Gynecol 1983; 61:48–51.

52. Spence MR: Gonorrhea. Clin Obstet Gynecol 1983; 25:111–124.

53. Hook EW III, Holmes KK: Gonococcal infections. Ann Intern Med 1985; 102:229–243.

54. Sweet RL: Acute salpingitis: Diagnosis and management. J Reprod Med 1977; 19:21–30.

55. Centers for Disease Control: 1993 Sexually transmitted diseases treatment guidelines. MMWR 1993; 42:56.

56. Eschenbach DA: Epidemiology and diagnosis of acute pelvic inflammatory disease. Obstet Gynecol 1980; 55:142.

57. Mardh PA, Moller BR, Ingerselv HJ, et al: Endometritis caused by *Chlamydia trachomatis*. Br J Vener Dis 1981; 57:191.

58. Gump DW, Dickstein S, Gibson M, et al: Endometritis related to *Chlamydia trachomatis* infection. Ann Intern Med 1981; 95:61.

59. Paavonen J, Kiviat N, Brunham RC, et al: Prevalence and manifestations of endometritis among women with cervicitis. Am J Obstet Gynecol 1985; 152:280.

60. Centers for Disease Control: Chlamydia trachomatis infections: Policy guidelines for prevention and control. MMWR 1985; 34:53.

61.   Sweet RL, Schachter J, Robbie MO: Failure of beta-lactam antibiotics to eradicate *Chlamydia trachomatis* in the endometrium despite apparent clinical cure of acute salpingitis. JAMA 1983; 250:2641.

62.   Sweet RL, Blankfort-Doyle M, Robbie MO, et al: The occurrence of chlamydial and gonococcal salpingitis during the menstrual cycle. J Am Med Associate Professor 1986; 255:2062.

63.   Svensson L, Westrom L, Ripa K, et al: Differences in some clinical and laboratory parameters in acute salpingitis related to culture and clinical findings. Am J Obstet Gynecol 1980; 138:1017.

64.   Hager WD, Eschenbach DA, Spence MR, Sweet RL: Criteria for diagnosis and grading of salpingitis. Obstet Gynecol 1983; 61:113–114.

65.   Westrom L: Incidence, prevalence and trends of acute pelvic inflammatory disease and its consequences in industrialized countries. Am J Obstet Gynecol 1980; 138:880.

66.   Centers for Disease Control: 1993 Sexually transmitted diseases treatment guidelines. MMWR 1993; 42:78.

67.   Landers DV, Sweet RL: Tubo-ovarian abscess: Contemporary approach to management. Rev Infect Dis 1983; 5:876–884.

CHAPTER 6

Disorders of the Cervix Including Colposcopy and Management

R. Kevin Reynolds

NORMAL CERVICAL DEVELOPMENT, ANATOMY, AND THE TRANSFORMATION ZONE

During embryogenesis, the vagina is lined by columnar müllerian epithelium, which is later replaced by cuboidal epithelium migrating up from the urogenital sinus. The urogenital epithelium is destined to become squamous epithelium later during gestation. By the end of pregnancy, the squamocolumnar junction dividing the two epithelial types normally resides on the cervix.

Cervical epithelium evolves significantly during a woman's lifetime. In the prepubertal years, the squamocolumnar junction is located on the ectocervix. Once the ovaries begin to produce estrogen, the vaginal and cervical squamous mucosa develop glycogen-rich cells, which favor bacterial colonization of the vagina with *Lactobacillus* species. This, in turn, results in an increase of vaginal acidity and is thought to be the stimulus for development of squamous metaplasia whereby the columnar epithelium is undermined and replaced by squamous epithelium. As a woman ages, the squamocolumnar junction migrates centrally toward the external os, where protection from vaginal acidity by cervical mucus causes the migration to stop. By the time menopause occurs, the squamocolumnar junction is typically located slightly within the cervical canal. The area of the cervix where the process of squamous metaplasia has occurred is referred to as the transformation zone. Most cervical human papillomavirus lesions and squamous cervical cancers occur within the transformation zone. Nabothian cysts are frequently observed within the transformation zone. They represent obstructed cervical gland clefts overgrown by metaplastic squamous epithelium resulting in accumulation of mucinous secretions. They are typically 2 to 5 mm in diameter and are hemispheric in shape. Prominent, arborized blood vessels are seen across the surface of the nabothian cysts. Although nabothian cysts are not pathologic, the differential diagnosis of vascular nodules includes cervical dysplasia and cancer. An experienced colposcopist should have little difficulty in discerning the difference, but biopsy is mandated if any uncertainty exists.

DISORDERS OF THE CERVIX

The clinician who detects a cervical abnormality on examination should have a logical approach to developing a differential diagnosis, confirming the diagnosis, and planning treatment. Cervical disorders can be divided into nonneoplastic and neoplastic disorders. This chapter briefly reviews the former and examines the latter in detail.

CONGENITAL NONNEOPLASTIC ABNORMALITIES

Nonneoplastic disorders can be congenital or acquired. Congenital abnormalities include such diagnoses as duplicated cervix with or without vaginal septum, congenital absence of the cervix, and adenosis extending from the cervix onto the vagina. The duplicated cervix usually indicates the presence of uterine anomalies such as didelphic or complete bicornuate uteri. These anomalies are uncommon, occurring in less than 0.1% to 2% of women. Urinary tract anomalies are present in up to 40% of these women. Accurate diagnosis has important ramifications for future fertility and genetic counseling. In some cases, the septate vagina may form a blind vaginal pouch below the duplicated cervix resulting in obstruction of menstrual outflow. The resultant hematocolpos may cause pain, abdominal distention, and injury to pelvic viscera. Ultrasound is a reasonable test to evaluate the suspected abnormal cervix and uterus, although hysterosalpingography is the definitive test for confirmation and classification of these congenital abnormalities.

The congenitally absent cervix and uterus is also frequently associated with urinary tract abnormalities. Two reported syndromes have been linked to congenital absence, including Rokitansky-Küster-Hauser syndrome with a normal 46,XX karyotype and androgen insensitivity syndrome (testicular feminization). In the latter instance, a 46,XY karyotype is present, the significance of which is the high likelihood of gonadoblastoma development. Gonadoblastoma may, in turn, lead to development of malignant germ cell tumors. These gonadal neoplasms can be prevented by timely removal of the abnormal gonad after pubertal development is complete. Karyotyping of the patient with congenital absence of the uterus is necessary to detect the androgen insensitivity syndrome.

Cervical and vaginal adenosis refers to extension of the glandular epithelium, which normally lines the cervical canal, out onto the cervical portio and vagina. In utero exposure to diethylstilbestrol (DES) inhibits the normal migration of the squamocolumnar junction, resulting in persistence of the glandular epithelium on the cervix and vagina. Recognition of this clinical entity is important because the incidence of vaginal and cervical clear cell carcinoma is significantly increased in the patient with in utero DES exposure, although only 1 DES-exposed woman out of 1000 ever develops this neoplasm. Recommended evaluation should include Papanicolaou (Pap) smears every 6 months with colposcopic examination at least every 2 years. Careful palpation of the adenosis is important because a palpable nodule is often the first indication of a developing clear cell carcinoma. Opinions vary as to whether or not the area of adenosis is at increased risk for developing squamous dysplasia. Additional cervical abnormalities associated with in utero DES exposure include the so-called collared cervix and the cock's comb cervix, in which redundant vaginal epithelium forms visible folds around the cervix.

ACQUIRED NONNEOPLASTIC ABNORMALITIES

Polyps are the most common of acquired growths on the cervix and are most likely to occur in patients in their 30s to 50s. Polyps vary in size from a few millimeters to lesions that can fill the vagina. Vaginal discharge and irregular vaginal bleeding are common symptoms. Cervical polyps are most commonly of the endocervical mucosal type, although fibrous, vascular, inflammatory, and pseudodecidual types are also reported. Biopsy for histologic diagnosis is indicated because the differential diagnosis includes condyloma, leiomyoma, microglandular endocervical hyperplasia, adenocarcinoma, squamous carcinoma, and sarcoma. Treatment of symptomatic polyps is removal. Small polyps are usually removed in the office using cervical biopsy instruments or curettes. Large polyps and cervical leiomyomas are more safely removed in the operating room. Malignant growths are clinically staged and treated accordingly.

Obstetric delivery with or without lacerations, in addition to cervical surgical procedures, often result in distortions of cervical symmetry when healed. In the nullipara, the cervix and the external os are generally circular, whereas after obstetric delivery the os may be linear or stellate. Although these changes can be extensive, they are of little functional significance.

CERVICITIS

Cervicitis can be grouped into infectious and noninfectious categories. Infectious causes include bacterial, viral, fungal, protozoal, and parasitic infections. Sexually transmitted diseases are an important subset of these infectious causes. Genital tract infections and sexually transmitted diseases are discussed in detail elsewhere in this book.

Noninfectious cervicitis refers to inflammatory changes caused by mechanical or chemical irritants. Mechanical causes include tampons, intrauterine devices, diaphragms, cervical caps, or pessaries. Chemical irritants include disinfectant, deodorant, or perfumed feminine hygiene products such as douches as well as lubricants, latex allergy (condoms), and spermicide allergy.

Cervicitis results in clinically apparent swelling, erythema, friability, and mucopurulent discharge. If the mechanical or chemical irritant causes prolonged cervicitis, scar tissue, ulceration, and loss of endocervical secretions can occur. Appropriate evaluation includes careful history to identify likely mechanical or chemical irritants and obtaining cultures to rule out infectious causes.

CERVICAL DYSPLASIA AND CANCER

Incidence

In much of the world, cervical cancer is the most common cancer diagnosis in women. Only in nations with health care systems that provide screening and treatment of preinvasive lesions is the incidence of cervical cancer substantially lower. Worldwide, cervical cancer is the second most common cancer diagnosis in women, whereas in the United States it is the seventh most common cancer diagnosis. Over the last four decades, the incidence of squamous cervical cancer in the United States has fallen by 80%. Although the reasons for this drop in mortality are complex, the trend clearly followed the widespread acceptance of Pap smear screening to identify patients with treatable preinvasive disease. Currently, 15,000 new diagnoses of cervical cancer and 4600 cervical cancer deaths occur in the United States each year.

Epidemiology

The risk of developing cervical cancer has long been known to be associated with sexual behavior, even before the link to a specific sexually transmitted disease was identified. Risk factors, as summarized in Table 6–1, include early first intercourse, multiple sexual partners, high-risk male partners, and genital condyloma. It is hypothesized that the active squamous metaplasia that is present on the cervix of the adolescent may be a developmental *open window* favoring human papillomavirus (HPV) infection and subsequent development of dysplasia and cancer in women with early onset of sexual activity. Multiple partners increase the statistical likelihood of exposure to sexually transmitted diseases and, in particular, HPV. High-risk men may have a history of penile condyloma, dysplasia, or cancer as well as multiple sexual partners or partners with a history of cervical cancer. Women with high-risk partners have increased risk of cervical cancer independent of their own behavioral risk factors.

Table 6–1. Risk Factors for Development of Cervical Cancer

High Risk
Early first intercourse, especially if less than age 16 or within 1 year of menarche
Multiple sexual partners, especially if greater than 3
High-risk male partner
History of genital condyloma
Smoking history, dose dependent
Immunosuppression

Increased Risk
History of genital herpes infection
Low socioeconomic status
African-American, Hispanic or Native American race

Possible Increased Risk (Controversial)
Oral contraceptive use
Diet deficient in vitamin A

Decreased Risk
Nuns
Jewish, Amish, Mormon, or Muslim faith
Barrier contraceptive use

Smoking increases cervical cancer risk in a dose-dependent fashion: Cervical mucus in smokers contains elevated levels of nicotine and tars from cigarette smoke, thereby exposing cervical mucosa to topical chemical carcinogens. Women who require treatment with immunosuppressive drugs, such as patients with transplanted organs or with rheumatologic disorders such as lupus, are three to five times more likely to develop cervical cancer, presumably because of impairment of the immune response to HPV. Similarly, human immunodeficiency virus (HIV)–infected patients are at increased risk to develop cervical neoplasia. Cervical cancer is now one of the Centers for Disease Control criteria for diagnosis of acquired immunodeficiency syndrome (AIDS). Low socioeconomic status is thought to be a risk factor because of poor access to medical care, including screening Pap smears. The higher incidence of cervical cancer in several racial minority groups is also thought to be related to health care access.

Low-risk groups include nuns and members of some religious groups who are significantly less likely to have multiple sexual partners, thereby reducing the likelihood of exposure to sexually transmitted diseases. Use of condoms has been shown in two retrospective studies to reduce HPV transmission by about 80%. Because HPV may reside on skin of the vulva in women and the scrotum in men, barrier contraceptives do not cover all affected surfaces and do not offer complete protection.

Human Papillomavirus

In past decades, many sexually transmitted diseases have been proposed as the causative agent for cervical cancer. In years past, many researchers identified herpes simplex virus as a likely candidate based on several studies demonstrating an association with genital herpes infection and cervical cancer incidence. In 1976, Meisels observed the similarity of cells from genital warts with those from lesions now called dysplasia. HPV was found to be prevalent in low-grade dysplastic lesions but not in high-grade dysplasia or cancer when antibodies to HPV capsid proteins were used in immunoperoxidase reactions. With the advent of Southern blot and polymerase chain reaction (PCR) techniques to identify specific DNA sequences, more than 90% of squamous cervical cancers have been found to contain HPV viral DNA. The discordance with earlier immunoperoxidase study data is explained by noting that in low-grade lesions, the virus remains in its native circular DNA form and produces intact virions that are infective and easily identified with anticapsid antibodies. High-grade dysplasia and cancer cells incorporate the HPV DNA into the host-cell genome. Expression of viral genes can be identified, but assembly of infective virions does not occur.

To date, more than 70 different HPV types have been identified. Although they resemble each other genetically, each type has significant specificity regarding sites of infection and clinical manifestations. For example, HPV types 1, 2, and 4 are associated with verruca vulgaris (common warts) but not with genital infections. HPV types 6 and 11 are most often associated with genital condyloma in both men and women, although DNA from types 6 and 11 is identified in a small proportion of cervical cancers.

Some oncogenic types, including HPV types 16, 18, 31, 45, and 51–53, are much more likely to be found in cervical cancer than in condyloma or dysplastic lesions. The oncogenic HPV types are known to have mutations in several identified gene sequences, including genes E6 and E7, which code for oncoproteins that are linked to development of transformed and immortalized phenotypes in infected squamous cells. Proteins E6 and E7 have been shown to interact with tumor suppressor gene products P53 and Rb (retinoblastoma gene). Binding of the tumor suppressor gene product inactivates the normal regulatory processes in the cell in favor of promoting DNA synthesis. Although this mechanism is not in itself sufficient to explain the development of cervical cancer, it may provide the first hit in a *two-hit* model for carcinogenesis.

Natural History of Dysplasia

The prevalence of HPV in the general population is surprisingly high. Use of the PCR technique to identify HPV DNA in asymptomatic populations in the United States and the Netherlands demonstrated a prevalence of 22% to 33%. The virus is transmitted through sexual contact, primarily genital-genital, although rare cases of oral-genital transmission are reported. Between 60% and 70% of persons with an infected partner develop HPV infection, although only about 5% of women develop HPV-associated lesions. The incubation period varies between 3 weeks and 9 months, but prolonged latent periods in excess of one to two decades are also reported. The HPV types with a proclivity for genital skin are found on the vulva, vagina, and cervix in women as well as the penis and scrotum in men. Many lesions regress spontaneously, and some progress to develop cancer. Cofactors such as smoking and immune function are undoubtedly significant regarding the likelihood of progression. Infection with an innocuous HPV type such as 6 or 11 is less likely to recur after treatment. Infection with an oncogenic strain of HPV is more likely to recur after treatment. Because HPV types 6 and 11 can progress to cancer in some cases, knowledge of the viral type does

not at this time permit selective management of preinvasive lesions. Although viral typing tests are commercially available, the indications for their use are limited to protocols rather than standard of care. All current therapies are directed at removal or ablation of dysplastic epithelium: No current treatment to eradicate the virus exists.

When Pap smears became accepted for screening large numbers of women, Reagan noted that the mean age of women with dysplasia was 34 years, the mean age for those with carcinoma in situ was 42 years, and the mean age for invasive cervical carcinoma was 48 years. This suggested a stepwise progression from low-grade lesions to high-grade dysplasia and then invasive cancer. A number of studies observing the natural history of dysplasia were published, including the work of Barron and Richart, which supported the hypothesis of stepwise progression. They reported that the time required for a dysplastic lesion to progress to carcinoma in situ varied by the severity of the lesion at time of diagnosis. Mild dysplasia averaged 58 months' time to progression, whereas moderate dysplasia averaged 38 months, and severe dysplasia averaged 12 months. The time required to progress from carcinoma in situ to invasive cancer has been reported in the range of less than 1 year to 20 years, although Kottmeier showed a 72% likelihood of progression within 12 years. Nasiell demonstrated that a significant proportion of dysplastic lesions either regress spontaneously or remain stable, depending on the grade at time of diagnosis (Table 6–2). The American College of Obstetricians and Gynecologists (ACOG) based their recommendation for expectant

Table 6–2.   Natural History of Dysplasia

Mild Dysplasia	
Regression	62%
Persistence	22%
Progression	16%
Moderate Dysplasia	
Regression	54%
Persistence	16%
Progression	30%

Adapted from K. Nasiell, 1983, and 1986.

management of mild lesions on these data showing the low likelihood of progression of mild dysplasia. In contrast, the high likelihood of progression of moderate and severe dysplasia has led ACOG to recommend ablation or excision of these lesions.

Screening and Diagnosis for Cervical Dysplasia

Papanicolaou developed the field of exfoliative cytology and popularized the use of the Pap smear as a screening test for cervical cancer. Data from numerous public health screening programs show a correlation between falling cervical cancer rates and regular cytologic screening. The accuracy of Pap smears has been a topic of interest both in the medical world and in the lay press. False-negative rates for Pap smears have been reported in the range of 8% to 50%. Sampling error accounts for the greatest number of missed diagnoses. Modifications of the original Pap smear technique have been incorporated to minimize the likelihood of a false-negative report. These include use of the Ayre spatula and cytobrush for specimen collection, instead of the older techniques of vaginal pool aspiration or use of cotton-tipped applicators for the endocervical specimen. The Ayre spatula collects a much more cellular and representative cytologic sample from the transformation zone than vaginal pool aspiration does. Furthermore, pool aspiration has a reported false-negative rate of 40%. Use of the cytobrush yields 7 to 10 times more endocervical cells than a cotton-tipped applicator and has been demonstrated to be safe for use in pregnancy. Rapid fixation minimizes drying artifact, which, if present, can obscure accurate diagnosis. By incorporating these modifications, the accepted false-negative rate for Pap smears is 10% to 20%.

Pap Smear Technique

Proper technique minimizes the risk of sampling error. A number of investigators in addition to ACOG have published

Table 6–3. Optimal Pap Smear Technique

Instruct patient to refrain from douching or intercourse 24 h before test
Do not perform Pap smear during menses
Collect cells before bimanual examination
Do not use lubricant or acetic acid before collecting cells
Collect cells before obtaining cultures for sexually transmitted infections
Copious vaginal discharge may be carefully removed before collecting cells
Treat vaginitis before obtaining Pap smear if no signs of cancer are present
Visualize the entire portio and identify the squamocolumnar junction
Obtain portio sample with spatula, two full turns with firm pressure
Insert cytobrush gently into os, rotate 90 to 180 degrees, and remove
Apply cells from spatula and brush evenly on one fully labeled slide
Fix cells immediately to prevent air drying using spray fixative or alcohol

lists of recommendations for obtaining an adequate Pap smear. These recommendations are outlined in Table 6–3. When the cervix is scraped with the Ayre spatula (Fig. 6–1), two 360-degree turns with firm pressure on the cervical portio should be made. The squamocolumnar junction, which is generally visible to the naked eye, may be displaced laterally on the cervix in adolescents, pregnant women, and in utero DES-exposed women. It is important that the spatula scrape the squamocolumnar junction and the adjacent transformation zone because this is the site where most squamous cervical dysplasia and cancer develop. The endocervical sample is optimal when a cytobrush (Fig. 6–2) is used. Proper technique is to insert the brush gently, turn 90 to 180 degrees, and remove. More vigorous spinning of the cytobrush is likely to cause bleeding that may obscure cytologic detail, not to mention causing discomfort. Both samples are then spread promptly onto a single slide and fixed immediately. For in utero DES-exposed patients in whom vaginal dysplasia or cancer may be present, a second smear from the walls of the upper two thirds of the vagina is indicated.

mal findings, the Pap test may be performed less frequently in a low-risk woman at the discretion of her physician. ACOG went on to define the high-risk factors that would be more likely to lead to continued annual screening (Table 6–4). Several epidemiologic studies suggest that more women are likely to be in the high-risk category than not. In the ACOG Committee Opinion for recommendations on frequency of Pap test screening, support of the consensus agreement was tempered by the observation that "theoretical models may show this strategy to be cost saving; however, a reduction in the frequency of Pap test screening in England has been accompanied by an increased incidence of cervical cancer cases and deaths from cervical cancer. In contrast, . . . British Columbia has had a continuing reduction in morbidity and mortality from invasive squamous cell

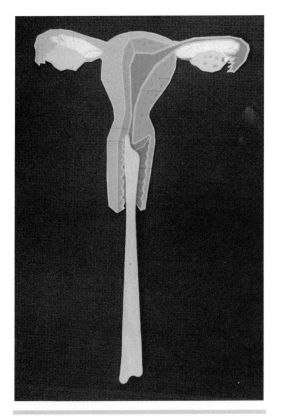

Figure 6–1. Pap smear technique. Use the Ayre spatula to scrape the ectocervix on the transformation zone.

Screening Interval

The appropriate interval for cytologic screening has been scrutinized in recent years. On the one hand, regular cytologic screening has unquestioned benefits regarding decreased cervical cancer incidence and mortality; on the other hand, cost has become a central issue. In 1988, ACOG, the National Cancer Institute, the American Cancer Society, the American Medical Association, the American Academy of Family Physicians, the American Nurses Association, and the American Medical Women's Association developed a consensus recommendation regarding frequency of cervical cancer screening. The consensus recommendation stated that all women who are or who have been sexually active or who have reached age 18 should undergo an annual Pap test and pelvic examination. After a woman has had three or more consecutive, satisfactory annual examinations with nor-

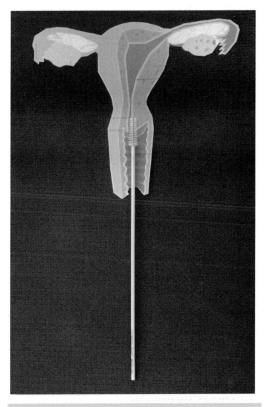

Figure 6–2. Pap smear technique. Use the cytobrush to obtain the endocervical specimen. Insert gently and turn only 90 to 180 degrees to minimize bleeding and discomfort.

Table 6–4. American College of Obstetricians and Gynecologists Recommendations on Frequency of Pap Test Screening

All women who are or who have been sexually active or who have reached age 18 should undergo an annual Pap test and pelvic examination. After a woman has had 3 or more consecutive, satisfactory annual examinations with normal findings, the Pap test may be performed less frequently in a *low-risk* woman at the discretion of her physician

High-Risk Factors

Women who have had multiple sexual partners or whose male partners have had multiple partners

Women who began sexual intercourse at an early age

Women whose sexual partners have had other sexual partners with cervical cancer

Women with current or prior human papillomavirus infection or condyloma or both

Women with current or prior genital herpes simplex virus infections

Women who are infected with the human immunodeficiency virus

Women with a history of other sexually transmitted diseases

Women who are immunosuppressed (e.g., transplant recipients)

Smokers and abusers of other substances, including alcohol

Women who have a history of cervical dysplasia; cervical cancer; or endometrial, vaginal, or vulvar cancer

Author's note: Multiple partners refers to more than one to three partners, and *early age* refers to first intercourse at 16 years of age or less.

cancers of the cervix, which is directly attributable to the province's 30-year history of performing annual Pap tests." Bearman and Shy, working independently, suggest that screening intervals of greater than 24 months lead to increased risk of cervical cancer and that the stage of disease is higher the longer the screening interval is. Therefore, unless a woman is clearly in the low-risk category, it is reasonable to continue annual Pap smear examinations.

Bethesda System

The original nomenclature devised by Papanicolaou for reporting cytology results has changed dramatically. The current reporting system in the United States is referred to as the Bethesda System for Reporting Cervical/Vaginal Cytologic Diagnoses. The Bethesda System (TBS) arose in 1988 from multidisciplinary conferences under the auspices of the National Cancer Institute and was revised in 1991. TBS has replaced the original class system of Papanicolaou and the more recent cervical intraepithelial neoplasia (CIN) system. TBS has not, as yet, been adopted by the World Health Organization (WHO) and is not in widespread use outside of the United States. In contrast to previous reporting systems, TBS cytologic categories are designed to be correlated with histologic diagnosis, and the number of diagnostic categories have been reduced to reflect current understanding of the biologic behavior of HPV and dysplasia. Pap smear reporting systems previously and currently in use are outlined in Table 6–5. Standardization of reporting criteria in TBS (Table 6–6) is intended to reduce confusing cytologic diagnoses because of differences of interpretation. A cytologic report using TBS provides a statement of specimen adequacy, a general categorization that may be used to suggest triage, and a descriptive diagnosis.

Before the advent of TBS, the term *atypia* was overused and vague. Under the new system, the diagnosis of atypical squamous cells of uncertain significance (ASCUS) and atypical glandular cells of uncertain significance (AGCUS) is limited to cases in which the cytopathologist is unable to determine significance. Cellular changes related to reactive changes such as inflammation, atrophy, and radiation are diagnosed as such and are not placed in either the ASCUS or AGCUS categories. Cytopathologists are encouraged to avoid this diagnosis when a more specific diagnosis is possible. A widely recommended management schema for ASCUS includes repeating the Pap smear after a 3-month interval. If the abnormality persists, colposcopic examination is warranted. A number of studies published before the development of TBS reported that when atypical Pap smear results were followed up with colposcopic examination, dysplasia was identified in 20% to 35% of patients. It is not yet clear

Table 6-5. Comparison of Pap Smear Reporting Terminology

Papanicolaou Class System	World Health Organization System	Bethesda System
Class I	Normal	Within normal limits

Class II	Atypia
	    Inflammatory
	    Squamous, glandular
		Benign cellular changes
		    Inflammation
		ASCUS, AGCUS

Class III	Mild dysplasia CIN-1	LSIL (koilocytosis and con- dyloma included)
	Moderate dysplasia CIN-2	HSIL
Class IV	Severe dysplasia CIN-3 Carcinoma in situ	HSIL HSIL
Class V	Squamous cell carcinoma Adenocarcinoma	Squamous cell carcinoma Adenocarcinoma

CIN = Cervical intraepithelial neoplasia; ASCUS = atypical squamous cells of uncertain significance; AGCUS = atypical glandular cells of uncertain significance; LSIL = low-grade squamous intraepithelial lesion; HSIL = high-grade squamous intraepithelial lesion.

Table 6-6. Bethesda System for Reporting Cervical/Vaginal Cytologic Diagnoses

Format of the Report
Statement of specimen adequacy
General categorization, which may be used to assist with clerical triage (optional)
Descriptive diagnosis

Adequacy of Diagnosis
Satisfactory for evaluation
Satisfactory for evaluation, but limited by (state reason)
Unsatisfactory for evaluation (state reason)

General Categorization
Within normal limits
Benign cellular changes
Epithelial cell abnormality

Descriptive Diagnoses
Benign cellular changes: infection
Trichomonas vaginalis
Fungal organisms consistent with *Candida*
Predominance of coccobacilli consistent with shift in vaginal flora
Bacteria consistent with *Actinomyces*
Cellular changes associated with herpes simplex virus
Other
Reactive cellular changes associated with:
Inflammation (includes typical repair)
Atrophy with inflammation (atrophic vaginitis)
Radiation
Intrauterine device
Other

Epithelial cell abnormalities
Squamous cell
Atypical squamous cells of undetermined significance (qualify as to whether a reactive or premalignant/malignant process favored)
Low-grade squamous intraepithelial lesion encompassing HPV (koilocytic atypia), mild dysplasia/CIN-1
High-grade squamous intraepithelial lesion encompassing moderate dysplasia and severe dysplasia, CIN-2, CIN-3, CIS
Squamous cell carcinoma
Glandular cell
Endometrial cells, cytologically benign, postmenopausal woman
Atypical glandular cells of undetermined significance (qualify as to whether a reactive or premalignant/malignant process favored)
Endocervical adenocarcinoma
Endometrial adenocarcinoma
Extrauterine adenocarcinoma
Adenocarcinoma, not otherwise specified
Other malignant neoplasms (specify)
Hormonal evaluation (vaginal smears only)
Hormonal pattern compatible with age and history
Hormonal pattern incompatible with age and history (specify)
Hormonal evaluation not possible due to (specify)

if TBS classification of ASCUS will substantially reduce the likelihood of dysplasia at the time of colposcopic examination. Until that time, it is wise to know more about the probability of dysplasia in the ASCUS group based on the past track record of the local laboratory as well as local prevalence of both HPV and dysplasia.

The lack of significant morphologic differences between koilocytosis and mild dysplasia on the one hand and moderate dysplasia from severe dysplasia and carcinoma in situ on the other has resulted in poor interobserver reproducibility among cytopathologists. In TBS, the two-tier grouping of koilocytosis with mild dysplasia in the low-grade squamous intraepithelial lesion (LSIL) category and moderate dysplasia with severe dysplasia and carcinoma in situ in the high-grade squamous intraepithelial lesion (HSIL) category has been reported to improve interobserver and intraobserver reproducibility. The natural history of the LSIL lesions (koilocytosis, condyloma, mild dysplasia, and CIN-1) are similar in terms of predominance of HPV types 6 and 11 as well as high likelihood of spontaneous regression. Because the probability that an LSIL will progress is only 16%, whereas 60% spontaneously regress, follow-up is an appropriate form of management for this group. ACOG has formalized these recommendations and has recommended that follow-up include Pap smears every 3 months. LSIL in the endocervical canal can be managed expectantly with Pap smear and endocervical curettage (ECC) on the same schedule. Expectant management assumes that the patient is likely to comply with surveillance. If the lesion persists for more than 1 year or if progression to HSIL occurs, treatment is indicated.

HSIL lesions are much more likely to progress to invasive cancer and are more likely to harbor oncogenic HPV types. Colposcopy with directed biopsies is indicated, and if HSIL is confirmed on histology, ACOG recommendations include ablative or excisional therapy aimed at destruction or removal of the entire transformation zone. The entire transformation zone must be destroyed rather than selectively removing the lesion because of the unacceptably high failure rates that occur. Cartier showed that selective removal of lesions was accompanied by a 55% recurrence rate. Wright reported a 25% recurrence rate when lesions were removed in strips rather than as a single specimen. This is in contrast to a 90% success rate when the entire transformation zone is treated. A cervical dysplasia management flow chart is shown in Figure 6–3.

Colposcopy

When a squamous intraepithelial lesion is diagnosed on Pap smear (either LSIL or HSIL) or if a visible lesion is identified on the cervix, the standard of care includes visual and colposcopic inspection of cervix and vagina with directed biopsy, ECC, and bimanual pelvic examination. Colposcopy, when combined with directed biopsy, approaches a diagnostic accuracy of 100% but is not considered a cost-effective screening test for the general population with no history of abnormal cytology because of the time and cost involved. The colposcope (Fig. 6–4) is a binocular operating microscope with magnification in the range of 16×, a high-intensity light source, and a blue or green color filter. There are two premises on which colposcopy is based. The first is that most squamous cervical cancers develop in the transformation zone, which is visible in the majority of colposcopic examinations. For a colposcopic examination to provide a meaningful evaluation of the cervix, the area at risk for development of the cancer (i.e., the transformation zone) must be seen in its entirety. By definition, if the squamocolumnar junction, which defines the medial border of the transformation zone, is seen in its entirety, the colposcopic examination is satisfactory, and if the squamocolumnar junction cannot be seen, the colposcopic examination is unsatisfactory. The colposcopic examination technique and the International Federation of Cervical Pathology and Colposcopy recommendations for colposcopic terminology are summarized in Table 6–7. A colposcopic examination is more likely to be adequate in young women and is often inadequate in postmenopausal women because the squa-

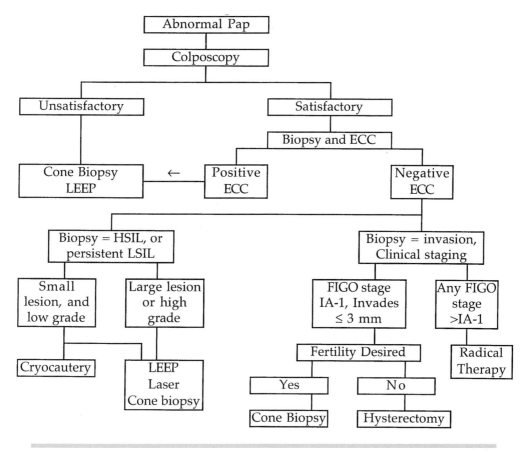

Figure 6–3. Flow chart for management of the abnormal Pap smear. LEEP = Loop electrosurgical excision procedure; ECC = endocervical curettage; HSIL = high-grade squamous intraepithelial lesion; LSIL = low-grade squamous intraepithelial lesion.

mocolumnar junction is often within the endocervical canal following menopause. Use of the largest vaginal speculum that is comfortable for the patient improves the chances of easily identifying the squamocolumnar junction. Maneuvers to aid in visualization of the squamocolumnar junction if it enters the endocervical canal include use of either a small endocervical speculum, such as the Kogan speculum, or a small cotton-tip applicator to evert the cervical os.

The second premise on which colposcopy is based is the observation that dysplastic lesions and cancers have visually distinct morphology that can be recognized by the skilled colposcopist. The expectation that the worst lesion on the cervix can be identified allows a directed biopsy to be performed using specialized

biopsy instruments shown in Figures 6–5 and 6–6.

After obtaining a Pap smear and inspecting the cervix with the colposcope, the cervix is washed with 3% to 5% acetic acid. The acetic acid application is an essential component of the complete colposcopic examination. Rinsing with acetic acid removes mucus and provides a clearer view of the cervical portio and lower endocervical canal. More importantly, the acetic acid dehydrates the epithelial cells, causing areas with abnormal keratinization, parakeratosis, or nuclear crowding to become less transparent and more reflective than normal cells. Abnormal areas therefore appear white on colposcopic examination after staining with acetic acid. White lesions seen after staining with acetic acid are

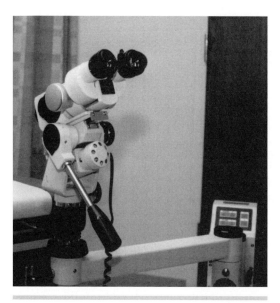

Figure 6–4. Colposcope. A binocular operating microscope for evaluation of the lower genital tract.

referred to as *acetowhite lesions* (Fig. 6–7). The cervix should be remoistened with acetic acid throughout the colposcopic examination because acetowhite change is lost if the cervix dries. Acetowhite change usually represents condyloma or dysplasia, especially if the boundaries are distinct. Faint or wispy borders of acetowhite epithelium generally indicate squamous metaplasia, a normal process within the transformation zone. White lesions seen before application of acetic acid are called *leukoplakia* and usually are found to be condyloma on biopsy, although some invasive lesions also appear as leukoplakia.

The color filter on the colposcope aids in visualizing the subepithelial capillary network. After initially inspecting the cervix with white light, either green or blue filtered light is used to evaluate vessels in the transformation zone. Normal capillaries are fine in caliber and evenly

Table 6–7.   Colposcopy

Optimal Colposcopy Technique	International Federation of Cervical Pathology and Colposcopy Terminology
Insert speculum and position colposcope	Normal colposcopic findings
Repeat Pap smear, if indicated	Original squamous epithelium
Inspect briefly with colposcope on low power. Look for leukoplakia	Columnar epithelium
	Normal transformation zone
Stain cervix with 3%–5% acetic acid. Frequently remoisten mucosa	Abnormal colposcopic findings
	Within the transformation zone
Inspect with colposcope using 15× objective and white light	Acetowhite epithelium
	Punctation
Identify squamocolumnar junction	Mosaic
Use endocervical speculum or evert os with swab if needed to see SCJ within endocervix	Iodine-negative epithelium
	Leukoplakia
Look for acetowhite epithelium and vascular patterns. Assess for ability to visualize entire border of lesion	Atypical blood vessels
	Outside the transformation zone
Using green light, inspect the transformation zone	Colposcopically suspect frank cancer
	Unsatisfactory colposcopy
Perform endocervical curettage under colposcopic guidance. Be careful not to curette lesions on cervical portio. ECC contraindicated if patient is pregnant	SCJ not visible
	Severe inflammation or atrophy
	Cervix not visible
	Miscellaneous
Biopsy abnormal appearing areas under colposcopic guidance	Nonacetowhite micropapillary surface
	Exophytic condyloma
Apply Monsel's solution to control bleeding	Inflammation
Inspect vagina and vulva with colposcope when speculum is withdrawn	Atrophy
	Ulcer
	Other

SCJ = Squamocolumnar junction; ECC = endocervical curettage.

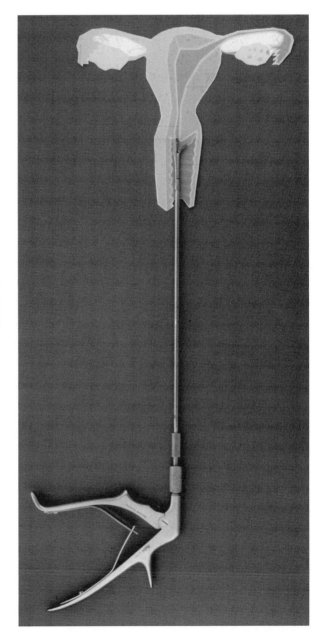

Figure 6–5. Cervical biopsy forceps. The long handle and fine tip are well suited for colposcopically directed biopsy of the cervix. Anesthetic is not required.

spaced. Dysplastic epithelium often exhibits vascular patterns such as punctation or mosaicism. A punctation pattern (Fig. 6–8) resembles red polka dots, typically within an acetowhite lesion. They represent dilated vertical capillaries seen on end. The coarser the vessel caliber and the wider the intercapillary distance, the higher the degree of associated dysplasia. In contrast, a mosaic pattern (Fig. 6–9) resembles a tile floor, in which the borders of each polygonal tile are blood vessels that typically arise in acetowhite lesions. Vessel caliber and intercapillary spacing have the same significance with mosaic patterns as with punctation.

When invasive cancer develops, the colposcopic findings differ from the acetowhite epithelium with or without the punctation or mosaic vascular patterns usually seen with dysplastic lesions. Invasion is suspected based on color change, irregular contour, and presence of atypical vessels. The color change seen in the presence of invasive disease reflects increased vascularity

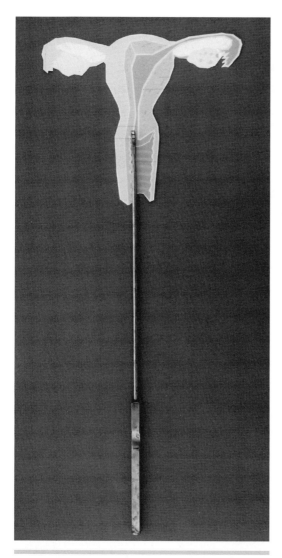

Figure 6–6. Endocervical curette. The small rectangular tip is inserted into the cervical canal, and scrapings are made with care to avoid colposcopically identified ectocervical lesions.

vasion or high-grade dysplasia should always be suspected when atypical vessels are identified. Nabothian cysts are often vascular but should not be mistaken for atypical vascular patterns because of the normal pattern of vessel arborization present and the characteristic hemispheric contour of the cyst.

Staining of the transformation zone with Lugol's iodine solution can be a useful adjunct to the colposcopic examination. The iodine stains mature glycogenated squamous cells but is poorly taken up by dysplastic cells and columnar epithelium. Lugol's solution can be helpful in establishing the lateral border of cervical lesions, which are sometimes difficult to visualize with acetic acid staining alone. The disadvantage of Lugol's solution is its messiness and tendency to stain clothing.

Although an expert colposcopist may become adept at predicting lesion severity based on colposcopic appearance, biopsy is still required for accurate triage and diagnosis. The colposcopist should evaluate all abnormal appearing lesions and perform biopsies of the highest-grade lesions identified. Figure 6–11 is a diagram of the histologic characteristics of dysplasia and cancer as they would appear on biopsy. An ECC provides additional information about the cervical canal and is particularly important in the evaluation of patients with inadequate colposcopic examinations, lesions extending into the canal, and Pap smears showing AGCUS or adenocarcinoma cells. After obtaining the biopsy specimens, topical application of Monsel's solution (ferric subsulfate) or silver nitrate controls spotting from the biopsy sites.

Squamous Epithelial Lesions in Pregnancy

The primary goal of colposcopic evaluation during pregnancy is to exclude the presence of invasive disease. Dysplasia has little likelihood of progression to invasion during gestation. Colposcopic surveillance during pregnancy with delay of definitive treatment until postpartum is safe. Biopsy of the cervical portio does not increase the likelihood of fetal wastage but can cause significant blood loss

and tissue necrosis, resulting in an orange-tan appearance. Invasive lesions may grow in an exophytic manner, resulting in a raised or irregular surface contour. Invasive lesions may also be endophytic, resulting in ulceration. Atypical vessels are distinct from the punctation and mosaic vessel patterns described with dysplasia. The atypical vessels are horizontal surface capillaries that assume unusual patterns, such as hairpin loops, corkscrews, abnormal branching, and commas (Fig. 6–10). In-

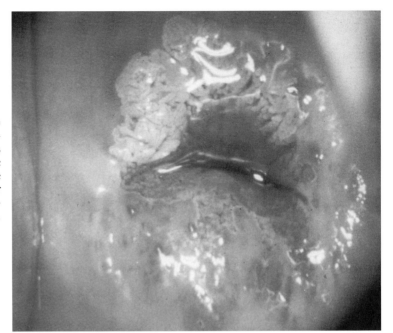

Figure 6–7. Colpophotograph (16×). Cervix has been stained with acetic acid, revealing acetowhite epithelium on the anterior lip of the cervix. Biopsy revealed moderate dysplasia.

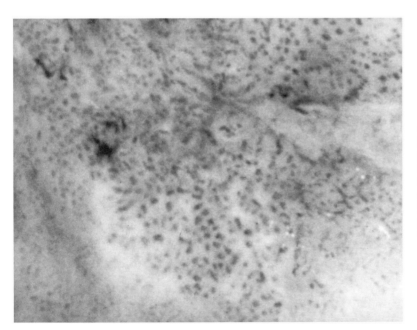

Figure 6–8. Colpophotograph (close-up of 24×). Cervix has been stained with acetic acid, revealing punctated vascular pattern in an acetowhite background. Biopsy revealed severe dysplasia.

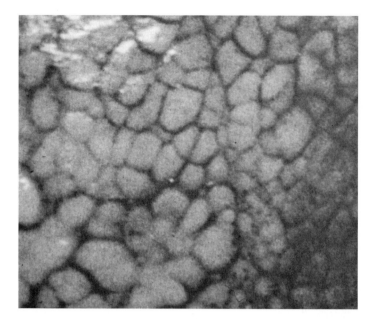

Figure 6–9.   Colpophotograph (close-up of 24×). Cervix has been stained with acetic acid, revealing mosaic vascular pattern in an acetowhite background. Biopsy revealed severe dysplasia.

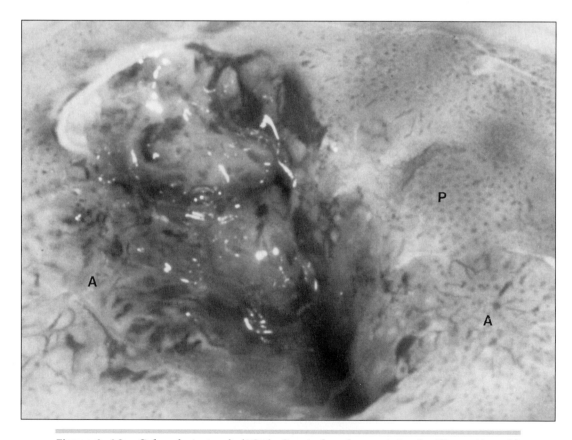

Figure 6–10.   Colpophotograph (16×). Cervix has been stained with acetic acid, revealing punctated vascular pattern in an acetowhite background (P) and atypical vessels (A). Biopsy revealed invasive squamous carcinoma.

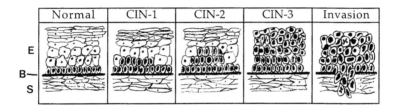

Normal	CIN-1	CIN-2	CIN-3	Invasion

Figure 6–11.   Histologic characteristics of squamous cervical neoplasia. The epithelial layers are represented by *E*, the basement membrane by *B*, and the cervical stroma by *S*. There is a progressive increase in the proportion of neoplastic cells, arising from the epithelial base and extending toward the surface, as the grade of dysplasia increases. Penetration of the basement membrane signifies invasion, and both local inflammation and keratinization of the invasive cells are commonly seen.

because of the vascularity of the gravid cervix. An *expert* colposcopist may be able to avoid the need for biopsy in many circumstances. ECC is contraindicated during pregnancy because of the risk of bleeding and rupture of amniotic membranes.

If an abnormal Pap smear is obtained during pregnancy, colposcopic evaluation is performed, and the Pap smear is repeated. Lesions with the appearance of HSIL or invasive disease should be biopsied. Findings consistent with LSIL, if in agreement with the cytologic diagnosis, can be managed with serial colposcopic inspection without biopsy. Examinations are repeated every 8 weeks, and definitive evaluation, biopsy, and treatment are deferred until 6 to 8 weeks' postpartum.

A cone biopsy during pregnancy is indicated if punch biopsy suggests microinvasion (FIGO stage IA-1). This procedure should be done only by an experienced clinician because of the risks involved. Patients with documented dysplasia or microinvasion may deliver vaginally, if otherwise indicated. Although rare vertical transmission of HPV to the fetus has been reported, there is no apparent benefit of prophylactic cesarean section. Macroscopic invasive lesions are more likely to hemorrhage during labor: Cesarean delivery, sometimes with concurrent radical hysterectomy, is warranted.

Treatment of Cervical Dysplasia

Treatment indications have been discussed earlier and are dependent on ac-curate histologic diagnosis as well as colposcopic evaluation of extent of disease. Treatment modalities can be divided into two groups: ablation and resection. In each case, the entire transformation zone is treated, rather than the focal lesion, to reduce the likelihood of recurrent dysplasia. Regardless of treatment modality, recurrence of dysplasia occurs in about 10% of patients. With the exception of cold knife cone biopsy (CKC) and hysterectomy, the treatments for cervical dysplasia can be carried out in an office setting. Ablation modalities include cryocautery and carbon dioxide (CO_2) laser photoablation. Resection modalities include loop electrosurgical excision procedure (LEEP), cold knife conization, and, in limited instances, simple hysterectomy. Indications for each modality are summarized in Table 6–8. Ablative treatment modalities are never appropriate for treatment of microinvasive or invasive cervical cancer, and resection modality treatments are indicated for carefully selected cases of microinvasive squamous cervical carcinoma.

Cryocautery

Cryocautery is an inexpensive and easily learned procedure. Abnormal cells are frozen using a nitrous oxide refrigerant (−90°C), and the resultant intracellular ice crystals cause cell death. The cryoprobe should be large enough to cover the cervical lesion. Patients with lesions involving more than two quadrants of the cervix, HSIL histology, or irregular cervical contours owing to nabothian

Table 6–8.   Treatment of Cervical Dysplasia

Indications for Ablative Therapy (Cryocautery and CO_2 Laser Photoablation)	Indications for Resection (LEEP and Cone Biopsy or Simple Hysterectomy)
Satisfactory colposcopic examination (entire transformation zone visible)	Unsatisfactory colposcopic examination (entire transformation zone not visible)
Lesion fully visualized with no endocervical extension	Lesion with endocervical extension or not fully visualized
Endocervical curettage negative for dysplasia or microinvasive cancer	Endocervical curettage positive for dysplasia or microinvasion
Cytology and histology concordant	Microinvasion on directed punch biopsy
Contraindications for Ablative Therapy	Cytologic evidence of HSIL or squamous carcinoma in the absence of a consistent biopsy diagnosis
Frank malignancy, either squamous or adenocarcinoma. Proceed to clinical staging and appropriate cancer therapy	Cytologic or biopsy evidence of endocervical adenocarcinoma
	Contraindications for Resection
	Frank malignancy, either squamous or adenocarcinoma. Proceed to clinical staging and appropriate cancer therapy

HSIL = High-grade squamous intraepithelial lesion.

cysts or old obstetric lacerations are poor candidates for cryocautery.

Before starting the procedure, cervical secretions should be removed, after which the cryoprobe is applied to the cervix with a small amount of lubricant to improve thermal transfer. The freeze is carried out until the ice ball extends 5 mm beyond the cryoprobe. The lesion is allowed to thaw completely and is then frozen a second time. The double-freeze technique is associated with a significantly lower risk of treatment failure than single-freeze methods (10% versus 40%). Cryocautery methods based on timing of the freeze, rather than anatomic distribution of the freeze, are inadequate. The 5-mm ice ball correlates with destruction of the underlying gland clefts, which are often reservoirs of dysplastic epithelium. Care must be taken not to freeze adjacent vaginal epithelium because this can be painful.

Patients should be told to expect copious, watery vaginal discharge for several weeks after the procedure. They should refrain from intercourse for several weeks to allow the friable eschar to heal. Cryocautery complications include a 30% incidence of obscured squamocolumnar junction, rendering any future colposcopic examinations unsatisfactory. In addition, cryocautery can cause cervical stenosis and bleeding in about 1% of cases. Cryocautery must not be performed during pregnancy or on any lesion in which invasion is diagnosed or suspected.

Carbon Dioxide Laser Photoablation

The CO_2 laser produces a beam of infrared light that is invisible to the naked eye. The infrared wavelength is absorbed by intracellular water, resulting in vaporization of the target cells. Although there are many different types of lasers in medical use, the CO_2 laser is particularly well suited to ablation of abnormal epithelium because of the excellent cutting properties of the beam with minimal thermal injury or coagulation to adjacent or underlying tissue. This allows the clinician to destroy dysplastic epithelium precisely while sparing normal adjacent epithelium and stroma. Laser photoablation is well suited to treatment of geographically large lesions, including lesions that extend onto the vagina. It is also a good technique for the irregularly shaped cervix distorted by nabothian cysts or old obstetric lacerations. Disadvantages of laser photoablation include the expense of equipment and the high level of expertise required.

Briefly the technique begins with placement of a nonreflective speculum, followed by colposcopic inspection and injection of lidocaine-containing epinephrine at several sites around the perimeter of the transformation zone. The laser is set to a spot size of 2 mm and a power density of 750 to 1000 watts/cm^2. A smoke evacuator must be used during ablation to remove the laser plume. All of the transformation zone is vaporized by moving the beam in a continuous circular fashion using colposcopic guidance. Beginning on the posterior lip and moving anteriorly minimizes loss of visibility as a result of bleeding. To destroy the underlying cervical glands that often harbor dysplastic epithelium, the ablation is carried out to a depth of 7 mm. This depth exceeds the deepest likely extension of 99% of cervical glands in the transformation zone. After completing the procedure, Monsel's solution (ferric subsulfate) is applied to prevent delayed bleeding.

Patients should expect clear vaginal discharge and spotting for up to 2 weeks after the procedure. Tampon use and sexual intercourse should be delayed for 1 month to allow healing. Laser photoablation complications include a 1% incidence of stenosis and delayed bleeding. The squamocolumnar junction is much more likely to remain visible after laser photoablation than with cryocautery. Laser photoablation is contraindicated in pregnancy and on any lesion in which invasion is identified or suspected.

Loop Electrosurgical Excision Procedure

LEEP is the most recently developed of the dysplasia treatment modalities. A radiofrequency current (350 KHz to 3.3 MHz) is used to energize a fine tungsten wire loop (Fig. 6–12), which is shaped to allow excision of the transformation zone in a single pass in most cases. The loops are 7 to 8 mm deep, which facilitates removal of the underlying glands that may harbor dysplasia. LEEP has quickly become popular for several reasons. First, LEEP provides a biopsy specimen for histologic diagnosis, in contrast to ablative cryocautery and laser procedures. In two large series, LEEP specimens detected unrecognized microinvasive squamous carcinoma in 2% to 3% of cases treated by expert colposcopists. A second advantage is that the equipment is relatively inexpensive, and training is much simpler than for laser photoablation procedures. The procedure is well suited to treatment of dysplastic lesions of any grade as long as they are confined to the cervical portio. Because the procedure is relatively new, little long-term follow-up is available in the medical literature. Many clinicians have virtually replaced all CKC procedures with LEEP, even though there is virtually no published information re-

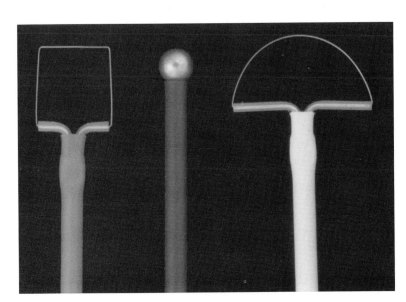

Figure 6–12. Loop electrosurgical excision procedure (LEEP) electrodes. The tungsten loop on the right is 2 cm wide and 8 mm deep, allowing removal of the transformation zone in a single pass for most patients. The square electrode on the left is 1 cm wide and 1 cm deep. It is used for resection of lesions extending into the cervical canal. The ball electrode, in the center of the photograph, is used to cauterize the base of the biopsy to attain hemostasis.

garding use of LEEP for treatment of dysplasia in which the colposcopic examination is inadequate or when the ECC is positive for dysplasia.

LEEP is begun by inserting an insulated speculum with a smoke evacuator attachment. The abnormal epithelium is identified with the colposcope, and an anesthetic containing lidocaine and epinephrine is injected circumferentially around the transformation zone. A loop is selected that allows removal of the transformation zone in a single pass (usually 2 cm wide and 8 mm deep). The tissue is excised using radiofrequency current at a power of 40 watts for a 2-cm loop. The colposcope is used to evaluate the cervix for any evidence of persistent abnormal epithelium after the specimen is removed. A second, smaller segment of the endocervical canal can be removed if extension of the lesion into the canal makes this step necessary, by using a 1-cm by 1-cm square loop at a power setting of 30 watts. An ECC should be performed if the lesion extended into the canal before the procedure. The biopsy site is cauterized using a ball-shaped electrode at 50 watts in the coagulation mode. Monsel's solution should always be applied after removal of the specimen because this reduces the likelihood of postoperative bleeding from 10% to 1%.

Discharge and spotting after a LEEP are common. Postoperative instructions are identical to laser photoablation instructions. Postoperative complications include bleeding and stenosis, each occurring in about 1% of cases. Use of overly large loops (>8 mm from crossbar to deepest point) can result in excessive shortening of the cervix, bleeding, and subsequent problems with cervical incompetence.

Some clinicians have advocated performing the initial colposcopic evaluation of an abnormal Pap smear followed by immediate treatment of abnormal appearing epithelium with LEEP. The advantage of *see and treat care* is timeliness of treatment and associated improvement in patient compliance. Critics point out, however, that many LSIL lesions would be overtreated using this regimen. To minimize overtreatment, LEEP should be delayed until colposcopically directed biopsies confirm an appropriate treat-

ment indication. Ferenczy summarized by saying that LEEP does not mean "let's excise every patient." LEEP is contraindicated in pregnancy and should not be used for biopsy or removal of an obvious malignancy.

Cold Knife Cone Biopsy

CKC has been the gold standard for evaluating lesions in which the colposcopic examination is inadequate or the ECC is positive for dysplasia. The use of CKC for treatment of dysplasia with adequate colposcopy and negative ECC has largely been replaced with cryocautery, laser photoablation, and LEEP. Primary advantages of the CKC include customization of biopsy shape and size to fit the location and size of the lesion and the cervix. The CKC remains the best diagnostic choice when a punch biopsy shows microinvasive squamous carcinoma that must be evaluated to rule out deeper invasion. Similarly, if an endocervical adenocarcinoma or adenocarcinoma in situ is suspected, CKC is the preferred method of evaluation. CKC is a surgical procedure and is performed in the operating room with anesthesia. The higher cost and morbidity of CKC have relegated this procedure to a select group of patients who should not be treated with any of the office-based treatments noted previously. The likelihood of stenosis and cervical incompetence following CKC is 2% to 10% of cases, and the likelihood of postoperative bleeding is 5%.

Hysterectomy

Hysterectomy is the most invasive and costly treatment for cervical dysplasia and is appropriate for only a small subset of patients. Less invasive treatment modalities should be recommended preferentially. Nevertheless, patients with recurrent HSIL, HSIL at the endocervical margin of a cone biopsy when fertility is no longer desired, and previously untreated but colposcopically evaluated HSIL in patients with other valid reasons for hysterectomy are candidates for hysterectomy. Dysplasia can recur in the vagina in 1% to 2% of hysterectomy patients.

Follow-up After Treatment

None of the treatment modalities discussed has a 100% success rate with respect to eradication of dysplasia, and none are likely to eradicate the HPV infection. Laser photoablation, LEEP, and cone biopsy all result in successful treatment outcomes in about 90% of cases. Cryocautery has similar efficacy as long as treatment is limited to lesions less than two quadrants in size or of lower grade. Large, HSIL lesions treated with cryocautery are likely to recur 40% of the time, and cryocautery is not recommended for treatment of this group. Follow-up examination is important to detect the 10% to 15% of patients who develop recurrent dysplasia. ACOG has recommended that follow-up Pap smears be performed every 3 months for the first year after treatment. There is little information in the literature to clarify whether cytologic versus colposcopic evaluation is necessary at the time of these follow-up evaluations. A patient treated for cervical dysplasia should not have Pap smears performed at an interval of greater than 1 year for the rest of her life.

Prevention of Cervical Dysplasia

Cervical cancer and cervical dysplasia are sexually transmitted diseases. Probably the most effective treatment of HPV infection is prevention. First intercourse at less than 16 years of age or first intercourse less than a year after menarche greatly increases the relative risk of developing cervical cancer. Sex education programs have the potential to have a great impact on cervical cancer incidence if the age of first intercourse can be delayed and if numbers of sexual partners can be limited. Howard, working in inner-city Atlanta middle schools, demonstrated that *teen-peer* counseling programs, coupled with traditional sex education, delayed the age of first intercourse in a statistically significant number of eighth-graders. Delay of first intercourse from 15 years of age to 17 years of age reduces the relative risk of developing cervical cancer fivefold.

Safe sex practices have been popularized partly because of the HIV epidemic. Although condom use dramatically reduces risk of HIV transmission, the effect on HPV transmission is less pronounced. Use of condoms has been reported in two retrospective studies to result in a relative risk of HPV transmission of 0.2. Because HPV infects vulvar skin on the female and skin of the scrotum on the male, it is clear that even careful condom use cannot always prevent HPV transmission because of sexual contact with unprotected skin.

Male partners of women with dysplasia or cervical cancer should potentially be counseled regarding their high likelihood of carrying HPV. Although aggressive treatment of male HPV-associated lesions has been shown not to decrease recurrence risk in the female patient, appropriate counseling could potentially decrease the risk of spread to new sexual partners.

Management of Invasive Cervical Cancer

Cervical dysplasia and invasive cancer represent a continuous spectrum of disease. Once the abnormal cells penetrate the basement membrane into the underlying stroma, invasion is diagnosed, and the potential to spread locally or to metastasize develops. Conservative resection or ablative therapy is contraindicated once invasion is documented. The majority of invasive cervical cancers are of squamous histology, although 10% to 20% of cervical cancers are adenocarcinomas arising in the endocervix. In contrast to squamous cervical carcinoma in which HPV DNA is detectable in more than 90% of cases, HPV DNA is present in only 30% to 40% of cervical adenocarcinoma cases. Epidemiologic evaluation of cervical adenocarcinoma has identified other causative risk factors such as in utero DES exposure, Peutz-Jeghers syndrome, and possibly prolonged oral contraceptive or estrogen exposure. Cervical adenocarcinoma is treated the same as squamous cancer on a stage-for-stage basis. Many series show decreased survival in stage-matched adenocarcinoma patients compared to squamous carcinoma, although this observation is not universal.

Table 6–9. FIGO Staging for Cervix, Revised 1995

0	Carcinoma in situ
I	Carcinoma confined to the cervix (disregard extension to corpus)
Ia1	Measurable invasion <3 mm in depth and <7 mm in diameter
Ia2	Measurable invasion >3 and <5 mm in depth as well as <7 mm in diameter
Ib1	Lesion of >5 mm depth and/or >7 mm diameter, but £4 cm in diameter
Ib2	Lesion of >4 cm diameter
II	Tumor extends beyond the cervix but not to the pelvic wall. Tumor may involve vagina, but not the lower ⅓
IIa	No parametrial involvement
IIb	Parametrial involvement
III	Tumor extends to the pelvic wall or may involve the lower ⅓ of vagina
IIIa	No extension to pelvic wall
IIIb	Extension to pelvic wall. Includes all cases with hydronephrosis or nonfunctioning kidney
IV	Spread beyond the true pelvis or involvement of bladder or rectal mucosa
IVa	Spread to adjacent organs
IVb	Spread to distant organs

Patients should be staged to determine appropriate treatment and to counsel accurately regarding prognosis. The staging system for cervical cancer, summarized in Table 6–9, is defined by the International Federation of Gynecology and Obstetrics (FIGO) in conjunction with the World Health Organization (WHO). Stage is assigned based on clinical findings, including the bimanual pelvic and rectovaginal examination. Tests that may officially be used to stage include biopsy, colposcopy, intravenous pyelogram, chest x-ray, cystoscopy, and sigmoidoscopy. By international convention, tests that may not be used to stage officially include surgery, computed tomography or magnetic resonance imaging scans, and lymphangiograms. Tests are used selectively based on the clinical examination. For example, cystoscopy and sigmoidoscopy examinations are recommended when the clinical examination suggests a stage III or stage IV lesion but are not cost-effective because of low yield on stage I or stage II lesions. Similarly, computed tomography scan of the abdomen and pelvis is unlikely to detect lymphadenopathy for stage IB-1 lesions but is likely identify lymph node metastases in larger stage IB-2, stage II, and stage III lesions. Figure 6–13 outlines appropriate pretreatment testing and cancer therapy, based on initial clinical stage.

Treatment

Disease confined to the cervix is defined as stage I. The substage (i.e., IA-1, IA-2, IB-1, IB-2) is assigned based on depth of invasion in the cervix, which correlates well with likelihood of metastases as well as survival. Squamous carcinoma that invades less than or equal to 3 mm below the basement membrane is defined as *microinvasive*. The clinical significance of microinvasive cancer is that it is an empirically defined subset of stage I disease in which the risk of lymph node metastasis and recurrence is less than 1%. Because many women who develop cervical cancer are in their early reproductive years, it is helpful to define a group of patients with little risk of recurrence. If fertility is desired, these patients are treated with CKC and close follow-up. Women with microinvasion who no longer desire their fertility may be treated with simple hysterectomy via either the abdominal or vaginal approach. If invasion is deeper than 3 mm but still confined to the cervix (FIGO stage IA-2, IB-1, IB-2) or adjacent vagina (FIGO stage IIA), either surgery or radiation therapy may be used to treat the lesion. Appropriate surgery includes a radical hysterectomy with pelvic lymphadenectomy, which differs from a simple, or extrafascial, hysterectomy by including resection of all supporting ligaments of the uterus to the pelvic side wall in addition to removing the upper portion of the vagina. The increased operative time, blood loss, and morbidity of the radical hysterectomy are justified by the vastly lower recurrence risk in patients treated with radical hysterectomy (9%) versus simple hysterectomy alone (70%). Advantages of the surgical approach include preservation of

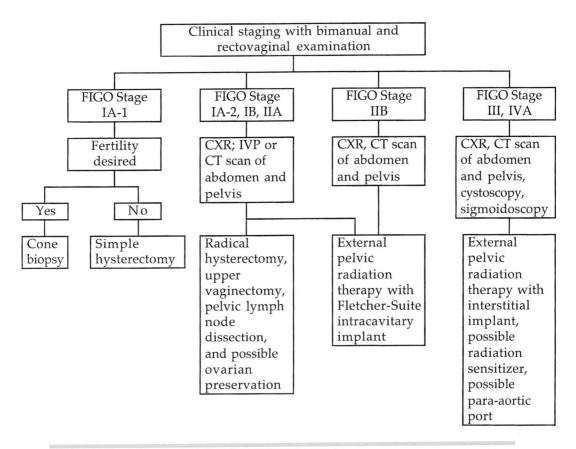

Figure 6–13. Flow chart for management of invasive cervical cancer. CXR = Chest x-ray; IVP = intravenous pyelogram; CT = computed tomography.

ovarian function and normal pliability of vaginal mucosa. The alternative approach for treatment of cancer confined to the cervix or adjacent vagina is radiation therapy. Radiation therapy for cervical cancer usually includes external beam treatments to the pelvis, administered in daily fractions for about 5 weeks, followed by one or two intracavitary implants that remain in place for 1 to 3 days each. Radiation therapy is appropriate for all stages of cervical cancer and is the standard of care in the United States for treatment of cervical cancers in stages II, III, and IVA. Treatment of widely metastatic disease (stage IVB) consists of individualized combinations of radiation and chemotherapy. The most active chemotherapy combinations include cisplatin, ifosfamide, and bleomycin, with objective response rates of up to 70% reported for nonradiated tumor sites. Unfortunately, chemotherapy is virtually never curative for metastatic disease. Surgery is indicated only for palliation in patients with metastatic cervical cancer. Recurrent cervical cancer that is confined to the pelvis is treated based on the original treatment method. For example, patients with recurrence who were treated initially with surgery may be treated with radiation therapy to the pelvis. Central pelvic recurrence in patients previously treated with radiation may be amenable to pelvic exenteration, an ultraradical surgical procedure that removes uterus, tubes, ovaries, vagina, bladder, and rectum. Reconstructive surgical techniques allow restoration of bladder, rectal, and vaginal function via continent urinary conduit formation, low rectal reanastomosis, and vaginoplasty.

Survival

Five-year survival of patients with micro-invasive squamous carcinoma of the cervix (stage IA-1) is 99%, even when conservative surgical therapy is used to preserve fertility. Patients with larger lesions still confined to the cervix (stage IA-2, IB-1, IB-2) have 90% likelihood of 5-year survival, whether treated with surgery or radiation. The subset of patients who are treated surgically and who have no evidence of lymph node metastases survive 5 years 96% of the time. Once disease extends beyond the cervix, 5-year survival falls to 65% for patients with stage II lesions, 45% for stage III lesions, and less than 10% for stage IV lesions. Recurrent disease in the pelvis that is treated with radiation results in long-term survival of up to 45% of patients. Pelvic exenteration for recurrences can potentially salvage up to 60% of patients in whom disease is confined to the central pelvis. Chemotherapy for metastatic recurrent cervical cancer results in objective responses only 10% to 15% of the time, and progression-free intervals are typically no longer than 1 year.

RECOMMENDED READINGS

Barron BA, Cahill MC, Richart RM. A statistical model of the natural history of cervical neoplastic disease: The duration of carcinoma in situ. Gynecol Oncol 1978; 6:196.

Barron BA, Richart RM. A statistical model of the natural history of cervical carcinoma based on a prospective study of 557 cases. J Natl Cancer Inst 1968; 41:1343.

Barron BA, Richart RM. A statistical model of the natural history of cervical carcinoma. II. Estimates of the transition time from dysplasia to carcinoma in situ. J Natl Cancer Inst 1970; 45:1025.

Bearman DM, MacMillan JP, Creasman WT. Papanicolaou smear history of patients developing cervical cancer: an assessment of screening protocols. Obstet Gynecol 1987; 69:151.

Benedet JL, Selke PA, Nickerson KG: Colposcopic evaluation of abnormal Papanicolaou smears in pregnancy. Am J Obstet Gynecol 1987; 157:932–937.

Cartier R. Practical Colposcopy (2nd ed.). Paris, Laboratorie Cartier 1984.

Cervical Cytology: Evaluation and Management of Abnormalities. American College of Obstetricians and Gynecologists Technical Bulletin, No. 183, August 1993.

Committee on Gynecologic Practice: Recommendations on Frequency of Pap Test Screening. American College of Obstetricians and Gynecologists Committee Opinion, No. 152, March 1995.

Hatch KD: Handbook of Colposcopy. Boston, Little Brown, 1989.

Hoskins WJ, Perez CA, Young RC: Principles and Practice of Gynecologic Oncology. Philadelphia, JB Lippincott, 1992.

Howard M, McCabe JB: Helping teenagers postpone sexual involvement. Fam Plann Perspect 1990; 22:21–26.

Kottmeier H. Evolution et traitment des épithéliomas. Rev Franç Gynécol 1961; 56:821.

Kurman RJ: Blaustein's Pathology of the Female Genital Tract, 4th ed. New York, Springer-Verlag, 1994.

Meisels A, Fortin R. Condylomatous lesions of the cervix and vagina. Acta Cytol 1976; 20:505.

Morrow CP, Curtin JP, Townsend DE: Synopsis of Gynecologic Oncology, 4th ed. New York, Churchill Livingstone, 1993.

Nasiell K, Nasiell M, Vaclavinkova V. Behavior of moderate cervical dysplasia during long-term follow-up. Obstet Gynecol 1983; 61:609–614.

Nasiell K, Roger V, Nasiell M. Behavior of mild cervical dysplasia during long-term follow-up. Obstet Gynecol 1986; 76:665.

Reagan JW, Hamonic MJ. The cellular pathology in carcinoma in situ; a cytohistopathological correlation. Cancer 1956; 9:385.

Shy K, Chu J, Mandelson M, et al: Papanicolaou smear screening interval and risk of cervical cancer. Obstet Gynecol 1989; 74:838.

Stenchever M: Congenital anomalies. In: Herbst AL, Mishell DR, Stenchever M, Droegemueller W, eds: Comprehensive Gynecology. Baltimore, Mosby, 1992.

Wright TC, Gagnon S, Ferenczy A, Richart RM. Excising CIN lesions by loop electrosurgical procedure. Contemporary Ob/Gyn, March 1991; 57.

CHAPTER 7

Contraception

Kamran S. Moghissi

The desire for family planning dates back to antiquity. In early times, a combination of disease, high mortality rate among newborns, abortion, infanticide, and frequent wars usually controlled population size. Within the individual families, measures to prevent conception, such as prolonged lactation, delayed marriage, coitus interruptus, or various substitutes for natural sexual intercourse, were developed. In addition, primitive societies often relied on the rites of medicine men or on diets, potions, or crude devices to prevent conception.

In today's society, despite the availability of effective and safe methods of contraception, a high proportion of pregnancies are unplanned and frequently unwanted. In the United States, it is estimated that 56% of 6.4 million pregnancies each year are unplanned. Available data indicate that of the 39 million in the United States who are at risk for unintended pregnancy, 90% use some form of contraception. The 10% of women who do not use contraception account for 53% of unintended pregnancies, half of which end in abortion. Younger women and teenagers are particularly at risk.

The degree of fertility varies with age. For some months or years after menarche, there is a relative degree of infer-

tility. The fertility rate is the highest between the ages of 20 and 30 and declines after the age of 35. In the first few weeks postpartum, pregnancy is unlikely. Similarly, the lactation period is associated with infertility. Neither the age-related infertility nor lactation, however, provides sufficient protection against unwanted pregnancies.

An ideal contraceptive has been defined as one that is safe, is highly effective, is inexpensive, is noncoitally related, and requires no motivation. Such a contraceptive is not yet available and probably will not be forthcoming in the foreseeable future. There is now available, however, an array of contraceptive preparations and devices to suit the needs of almost any population group. This chapter reviews the applications of these formulations and devices and discusses their respective risks and benefits.

ORAL CONTRACEPTIVES

Oral contraceptives (OCs) have been available since 1962 and are used by approximately 39% of women in the United States. The first-generation OCs contained large amounts of estrogen and progestogens and was associated with a number of undesirable side effects. Currently available OCs contain lower doses of estrogen, in the range of 20 to 35 μg of ethinyl estradiol, and reduced amount of progestins. Despite their lower doses, newer OCs approach 100% efficacy in preventing pregnancy. This estimate, however, may be substantially diminished by failure of compliance.

Formulation

Monophasic OCs deliver the same dose of estrogen and progestin throughout the cycle, whereas multiphasic OCs provide two or three different hormone doses throughout each cycle. The estrogen component in the majority of formulations available in the United States is ethinyl estradiol, a synthetic estrogen. Mestranol is used in a few others. Progestogen components consist of seven different types of steroids, including norethindrone; ethynodiol diacetate; norgestrel; and three new progestin preparations, norgestimate, desogestrel, and gestodene.[1] All these progestins are 19 nor steroids derived from testosterone.

Combination OCs are usually taken for 21 days out of every 28 days. In the 28-day regimen, the last seven pills are placebos. Progestin-only agents, known as minipills, contain only a low-dose progestin that is administered continuously.

Mechanism of Action

For all OCs, the primary mechanism of action is the inhibition of ovulation. This is achieved by a synergistic action of estrogens and progestins on the hypothalamic-pituitary centers to eliminate luteinizing hormone (LH) surge and suppress the secession of gonadotropins. In addition to ovulation suppression, contraceptive compounds affect several other target sites. These include the cervix, the endometrium, and the oviduct. Almost all synthetic oral or parenteral progestogens, alone or in combination with estrogen, diminish mucorrhea to some degree and alter many physical and chemical properties of cervical secretion and inhibit sperm migration through cervical mucus to varying degrees.

OCs also affect endometrial morphology. Under the influence of combined preparations, there is rapid progression of endometrium from proliferative phase to early secretory changes. By midcycle, a varying degree of mixed hormonal effect is observed. Thereafter, the endometrium shows regressive change and appears to be thin and inactive and unsuitable for implantation. Inhibitions of sperm migration through cervical mucus and endometrial changes are believed to provide additional efficacy for OC action should a breakthrough ovulation occur.

With continuous low-dose progestin therapy, most women exhibit suppression of midcycle LH and follicle-stimulating hormone (FSH). Corpora lutea, presumably indicating ovulation have been visualized in 85% of women treated with continuous daily minipills. Inhibition of sperm transport through cervical mucus and endometrial changes appear to be primarily responsible for contraceptive action of these agents.[2,3]

Risks and Benefits of Oral Contraceptives

Modern OCs are highly effective and safe. They are devoid of many side effects and complications associated with high-dose OCs of earlier years. Most common adverse effects of OCs occur during the first few months of use and may include nausea, weight changes, headache, spotting, and breakthrough bleeding. Nausea is related to the estrogenic component of the OC and is dose related. It is self-limiting and usually disappears after the first 3 months. Selection of a pill with reduced estrogen content usually alleviates nausea and other gastrointestinal problems.

Breakthrough spotting and bleeding is likely to occur within the first 3 to 6 months of use and is related to the dosage and type of progestogen. An important cause of breakthrough spotting and bleeding is the missed pill. Management of spotting and bleeding is best prevented by taking the pill faithfully at approximately the same time each day. It is seldom advisable to change to another formulation to obviate this side effect.

Several surveys have suggested that weight gain may be an important contributor to patient compliance. Appropriate management of diet and use of pills containing newer progestins are recommended to prevent excessive weight gain.

Headache is also experienced by some women and usually subsides within the first few months of use. Persistent headache may be an indication to switch to another OC preparation with lower estrogenic or lower progestogenic content. Severe headache or a history of migraine is considered to be a relative contraindication to OC use.

The most important risks of combined OCs are those related to cardiovascular disease and include thromboembolic diseases, myocardial infarction, stroke (thrombotic and hemorrhagic), and hypertension. Those risks assume greater magnitude among smokers and with pills containing high doses of estrogen component.[4,5]

Older epidemiologic studies indicated a dose-related effect of estrogen on the increased incidence of venous thrombosis in current OC users, an increased risk of myocardial infarction in women over age 35, and an association between the use of higher-dose OCs and neurovascular accidents in otherwise healthy young women. According to these retrospective studies, OC use increased the risk of thrombotic stroke threefold and that of hemorrhagic stroke twofold. Subsequent studies have demonstrated that increased risk of cardiovascular disease in OC users, particularly in older women, is related to the dosage of estrogen.[4,5] With the advent of low dose estrogen–containing OCs (20 to 35 μg ethinylestradiol), this risk is believed to be eliminated or be negligible.[5] Higher-dose OCs may also have an adverse influence on lipoprotein level. These alterations, however, are not observed with low-dose OCs.

Cancer Risks

OC use protects against endometrial and ovarian cancers.[7–9] There appears to be an increased risk of cervical dysplasia and carcinoma in situ, however, in women taking OCs. Invasive cervical cancer may be increased minimally after 5 years of use.[9,10] Because of this concern, OC users should have at least yearly pelvic

examination and Papanicolaou (Pap) smear. The relationship between breast cancer and OC use is more controversial. The results of a large number of epidemiologic studies indicate that in the middle of reproductive life (ages 25 to 39), the combination OCs have no effect on breast cancer risk. A few studies, however, suggest that a subgroup of young women who use OCs early and for a long time (>4 years) have a slightly increased risk of breast cancer before the age of 45.[9]

Benefits of Oral Contraceptives

Health benefits of OCs have been well documented. The most important health benefit of OCs is their high degree of efficacy in preventing pregnancy and its associated morbidity and mortality. Other noncontraceptive health benefits of OCs are shown in Table 7–1.[11,12] In addition to those benefits listed in Table 7–1, it is known that prolonged use of OCs is also effective in preventing other disease processes, such as the risk of first attack of rheumatoid arthritis, acne, hirsutism, and loss of bone mineral density. Considering the risk-to-benefit ratio of OCs, it is clear that the benefit of OCs far out

Table 7–1. Noncontraceptive Benefits of Oral Contraceptives

Pregnancy Mortality	Reduction in Risk (%)
Ectopic pregnancy	90
Cancer	
Ovary	40
Endometrium	40
Benign breast disease	40
Functional ovarian cysts	
Luteal	78
Follicular	49
Fibroids (5 years of combined oral contraceptives)	17
Pelvic inflammatory disease	50
Menorrhagia	50
Iron-deficiency anemia	50
Dysmenorrhea	40

From Drife JO: The Benefits and Risks of Oral Contraceptives. New York, Parthenon, 1993, pp 1–31.

weighs their potential risk. In addition to reducing the risk of endometrial and ovarian malignancies, OCs prevent many benign gynecologic conditions. Appropriate counseling of women regarding these issues goes a long way toward alleviating the fear of those women who have been influenced by inappropriate advice and adverse publicity.

Contraindications to Oral Contraceptives

Absolute contraindications to OCs are listed in Table 7–2. Table 7–3 lists relative contraindications for the use of these agents. Thus, clinical judgment and expertise are required when the use of OCs is considered in patients with a history of gestational diabetes, leiomyoma of uterus, elective surgery, and sickle cell disease. Appropriate counseling and possibly a consent form may serve to avoid future misunderstanding when the use of OCs is considered in patients with these disorders.

The use of OCs during pregnancy is contraindicated. There is no evidence, however, that OCs increase the risk of congenital anomalies if taken inadvertently during pregnancy. Combination OCs have been shown to diminish the quantity and alter the quality of lactation in postpartum women. Therefore, they should not be used in postpartum lactating women. Progestogen-only contraception orally (minipills) or parenterally does not interfere with lactation.

Table 7–2. Absolute Contraindications to the Use of Oral Contraceptives

Thrombophlebitis and thromboembolic disorders or a past history of these conditions
Known or suspected breast cancer
Undiagnosed abnormal vaginal bleeding
Known or suspected pregnancy
Suspected estrogen-dependent neoplasia
Marked impairment of liver function
Smoker over the age 35

Table 7–3. Relative Contraindications to the Use of Oral Contraceptives

Migraine headache
Hypertension
Epilepsy
Gallbladder disease

Selection of Appropriate Oral Contraceptives

A wide variety of OC formulations (Table 7–4) is available today that permits the clinician to tailor therapy to individual patients. In selecting the most suitable preparation, the clinician should take into consideration the needs and characteristics of the patient as well as relying on his or her own expertise.

For the first-time user, acceptance of OC therapy is of utmost importance to insure compliance and continuation. It is therefore recommended to prescribe a preparation with minimal side effects. Common troublesome problems, such as gastrointestinal symptoms, breakthrough bleeding, spotting, and breast tenderness, should be discussed with the patient and appropriate steps taken to address these side effects.

Progestin-Only Contraceptives (Minipills)

Since 1966, it has been recognized that several progestational steroids, ingested continuously in small doses, exert a potent antifertility effect and are free of certain systemic and metabolic side effects characteristics of the estrogen-containing oral agents. In the mid-1960s and early 1970s, several progestin-only contraceptive pills were developed, but only two of these were actually marketed and are available to date in the United States. Table 7–5 lists the so-called minipills available worldwide. Minipill OCs exert their antifertility action in several ways: (1) alteration of physical and chemical properties of cervical mucus along with inhibition of sperm transport, (2) subtle disturbances of hypothalamic-pituitary

Table 7-4.   Oral Contraceptives Available in the United States

Estrogen Type and Dose (µg)	Progestin and Dose (mg)	Trade Name (Manufacturer)
Ethinyl estradiol 30	Desogestrel 0.15	Desogen (Organon), Ortho-Cept (Ortho Pharmaceutical)
Ethinyl estradiol 35	Norgestimate 0.25	Ortho-Cyclen (Ortho Pharmaceutical)
Ethinyl estradiol 35	Norgestimate 0.18/0.215/0.25	Ortho Tri-Cyclen
Ethinyl estradiol 20	Norethindrone acetate 1.0	Loestrin 1/20 (Parke-Davis)
Mestranol 50	Norethindrone 1.0	Norinyl 1 + 50 (Searle), Ortho-Novum 1/50 (Ortho-Pharmaceutical), Norethin 1/50 M (Schiapparelli Searle)
Ethinyl estradiol, 30/40/30	Levonorgestrel 0.05/0.075/0.125	Triphasil (Wyeth-Ayerst), Tri-Levlen (Berlex)
Ethinyl estradiol 30	Levonorgestrel 0.15	Nordette (Wyeth-Ayerst), Levlen (Berlex)
Ethinyl estradiol 30	Norgestrel 0.3	Lo/Ovral (Wyeth-Ayerst)
Ethinyl estradiol 30	Norethindrone acetate 1.5	Loestrin 1.5/30 (Parke-Davis)
Ethinyl estradiol 35	Norethindrone 0.4	Ovcon 35 (Mead Johnson Laboratories)
Ethinyl estradiol 35	Norethindrone 0.5	Brevicon (Searle), Modicon (Ortho Pharmaceutical), Jenest (Organon)
Ethinyl estradiol 35	Norethindrone 0.5/1.0	Ortho-Novum 10/11 (Ortho Pharmaceutical)
Ethinyl estradiol 35	Norethindrone 0.5/1.0/0.5	Tri-Norinyl (Searle)
Ethinyl estradiol 35	Norethindrone 0.5/0.75/1.0	Ortho-Novum 7/7/7 (Ortho Pharmaceutical)
Ethinyl estradiol 35	Norethindrone 1.0	Norinyl 1 + 35 (Searle), Ortho-Novum 1/35 (Ortho Pharmaceutical), Norethin 1/35 E (Schiapparelli Searle)
Ethinyl estradiol 35	Ethynodiol diacetate 1.0	Demulen 1/35 (Searle)
Ethinyl estradiol 50	Norethindrone 1.0	Ovcon 50 (Meade Johnson Laboratories)
Ethinyl estradiol 50	Norethindrone acetate 1.0	Norlestrin 1/50 (Parke-Davis)
Ethinyl estradiol 50	Norethindrone acetate 2.5	Norlestrin 2.5/50 (Parke-Davis)
Ethinyl estradiol 50	Norgestrel 0.5	Ovral (Wyeth-Ayerst)
Ethinyl estradiol 50	Ethynodiol diacetate 1.0	Demulen 1/50 (Searle)
	Norethindrone 0.35	Micronor (Ortho Pharmaceutical), Nor-QD (Searle)
	dl-Norgestrel 0.075	Ovrette (Wyeth)

function characterized by suppression or modification of the midcycle FSH and LH, (3) inhibition of ovulation in some cases and changes in the function of morphologically normal corpus luteum, and (4) endometrial changes preventing implantation.[3]

Minipills are taken daily and continuously beginning on the first day of the menstrual cycle. Their failure rate ranges from 1.1 to 9.6 per 100 women in the first year of use. The average failure rate is about 3.1 per 100 women per year in younger women and 0.3 per 100 women per year in women over 40.

The major side effect of minipills is irregularity of vaginal bleeding, which is the result of unpredictable effect of these preparations on ovulation and possibly endometrial development. Approximately 40% of women receiving minipills have normal ovulatory cycles; 40% short, irregular cycles; and 20% acyclic pattern of anovulatory cycle. This is the major reason for discontinuation of these contraceptives despite their safety record otherwise.

Women on minipills are more likely to develop functional follicular cysts of the ovary. These cysts, however, resolve spontaneously. Progestin-only contraceptive pills are particularly useful for

Table 7-5. Progestin-Only Oral Contraceptives (Minipills)

Progestin	Dose (μg)	Trade Name
Norethindrone	350	Micronor*, Nor-O.D.*, Norad
Norgestrel	75	Ovrette*, Norgest
Levonorgestrel	35	Microval, Norgeston, Microlut
Lynestrenol	500	Exluton
Ethynodiol diacetate	500	Femulen

*Available in the United States.

postpartum use because they do not interfere with lactation.

INJECTABLES AND IMPLANTS

Injectables and implants provide effective and continuous contraception for prolonged periods, extending from several months to several years. Depo-medroxyprogesterone acetate (DMPA) is the only injectable contraception available in the United States. DMPA, a 17-acetoxy-progesterone, is similar in structure to naturally occurring progesterone. It is administered by deep gluteal or deltoid intramuscular injection in a dose of 150 mg every 3 months. It is recommended that the injection site not be massaged to ensure slow release of the drug. DMPA should be administered within 5 days of the onset of menses to ensure that the patient is not pregnant and that ovulation is inhibited to provide immediate contraception. DMPA acts primarily by inhibiting ovulation. There is also some effect on the endometrium and minor changes on cervical mucus.[13,14] During DMPA use, the ovary continues to secrete estradiol in amounts similar to early follicular phase of a normal cycle. Clinically, therefore, signs and symptoms of estrogen deficiency do not develop in women using DMPA. Safety and efficacy of DMPA have been established by its use in more than 90 countries by at least 30 million women. Most women using DMPA become amenorrheic. Breakthrough and unpredictable bleeding may occur during the first few months of use. Irregular bleeding, however, is usually not heavy and eventually ceases with continuous use. DMPA may safely be used during the postpartum period because it does not interfere with lactation. The return of fertility is delayed in women using DMPA. Approximately 70% of otherwise fertile women, however, are expected to conceive within the first 12 months following discontinuation and the remaining group within 24 months. Early concerns about the potential for increased risk of breast cancer with DMPA have been largely refuted. The multicenter World Health Organization (WHO) Collaborative Study showed no significant increase in the overall relative risk of breast cancer in ever-users of DMPA.[15,16] In women under age 35, short-term exposure to DMPA was associated with a slight increase in relative risk (1.4) of the same magnitude as that for OCs. Use of DMPA is not associated with clinically significant changes in coagulation parameters.[13,14] Minimal changes in serum lipids and lipoproteins have been observed in some studies. As with all progestins, evidence of impaired glucose tolerance is sometimes seen in users of DMPA. Thus, women with a history of diabetes should be carefully monitored while using any hormonal contraceptive. On the positive side, a WHO study found that the use of DMPA was associated with a major (80%) reduction in the risk of endometrial cancer with no significant impact on the risk of epithelial ovarian cancer or squamous cervical cancer.

Norplant

Development of long-acting contraceptive implants releasing progestogens has been in progress for many years. Only two implants, however, both releasing levonorgestrel, have so far been released for general clinical use. Norplant is the only contraceptive implant available in the United States. It consists of a set of six capsules, each 34 mm in length and 2.4 mm in diameter.[17] The set contains a total of 216 mg of crystallized levonorgestrel. One third of the drug load is released in 5 years, the currently approved lifetime of the implant. Silicone rubber provides the encapsulating rate metering membrane through which levonorgestrel diffuses into the body.

Norplant implants are inserted sequentially beneath the dermal layer of the arm through a 2- to 3-mm incision after a local anesthetic has been applied. No. 10 gauge trocar deposits the capsules in a superficial plane 5 to 6 mm above the incision. The recommended site of placement is in the inner aspect of the upper arm, contralateral to the handedness of the woman, well above the elbow.

Levonorgestrel is detectable in blood within 2 hours of placement. Maximum drug concentrations of 1000 to 2000 pg/mL are found at 8 to 24 hours. Drug release and concentrations are maximal in the first month of use when a set of six capsules releases approximately 85 mg/day of levonorgestrel. Release is 25 to 30 mg/day at 60 months.

Norplant is a highly effective contraceptive with a failure rate below those of OCs. In large population studies, the pregnancy rate was 0.02 pregnancies per 100 women-years of use. Norplant exerts its contraceptive action in several ways. Ovulation is inhibited in many cycles. If ovulation occurs, low levels of progesterone render the woman infertile. A marked alteration of cervical mucus renders it impenetrable to spermatozoa. There is also change of endometrial morphology.

Use of Norplant is associated with marked changes of menstrual bleeding patterns.[17,18] Most women, particularly those of lighter weight, tend to experience oligomenorrhea or amenorrhea, whereas women who weigh 60 kg or higher are likely to experience irregular bleeding. Much of these episodes of bleeding or spotting occur during the first year of use, when 70% to 80% of women may experience disruption of normal menstrual pattern. By the fifth year of use, approximately 62% of users have regular cycles, whereas 38% continue to have irregular cycles. Irregular bleeding and spotting is, in fact, the major reason for discontinuation of this form of contraception.[18]

Candid comprehensive counseling about all aspects of Norplant implants before insertion and appropriate support and reassurance during use are essential and go a long way toward the acceptance of this form of contraception. In the event of prolonged bleeding, a short course of ethinyl estradiol (20 to 50 μg four times a day for 10 to 20 days) or ibuprofen (400 to 800 mg three times a day for 5 days) may be used. Menstrual blood loss is eventually decreased with continuous use, and most women experience modest increase in hemoglobin.[18]

Other side effects include headache, acne or other skin problems, and changes of weight and of mood. Despite these minor side effects, Norplant is highly acceptable for prolonged contraceptive use and as an alternative to sterilization for those women who wish to maintain their reproductive function.

POSTCOITAL (EMERGENCY) CONTRACEPTION

These contraceptive methods are recommended when unprotected coitus has occurred and may result in an unwanted pregnancy. They should be considered and offered in all cases of rape.

The initial regimen included the use of large doses of estrogen, such as conjugated estrogen 15 mg twice a day for 5 days or 50 mg intravenously on each of 2 consecutive days. Alternatively, ethinyl estradiol 2.5 mg twice a day may be used for 5 days.[19] More recently, the administration of a combination OC (Ovral, 2 tablets initially and 12 hours later) has been found to be better tolerated and equally effective.[20] The mechanism of action is believed to be due to rapid endometrial changes that prevent implantation. The failure rate is reported to be approximately 1% with high doses of estrogen and 2% with combination OCs.[19,20] For best results, these formulations should be given as soon as possible after coitus and no later than 72 hours. Because of the potential harmful effect of these agents, the presence of an existing pregnancy should be excluded by a sensitive assay. Furthermore, the patient should be offered therapeutic abortion if the method fails. The use of high-dose estrogen is frequently associated with nausea and sometimes vomiting. Combination OCs are less likely to cause nausea and vomiting.

Another method of postcoital contraception is the insertion of a copper intrauterine device (IUD) (TCu-380) up to 5 days following unprotected intercourse. The reported failure rate is low (0.1%). This method clearly interferes with implantation and is not recommended for nulliparous women or those at risk for pelvic infection.[19]

INTRAUTERINE DEVICES

The forerunners of modern IUDs were already in use in 1800s. The modern IUDs were introduced in the early 1960s. These devices were made of plastic (polyethylene) impregnated with barium sulfate for ready identification by x-ray. They performed well and were devoid of major complications. The Dalkon Shield was introduced in 1970. Because of its defective construction and a multifilamented tail allowing a pathway for bacteria to ascend into the uterine cavity, the use of this device was found to be associated with a high rate of pelvic infection. The Dalkon Shield was removed from use in 1980. The risk of pelvic infection resulting from the Dalkon Shield brought about a general decline in the use of all IUDs, even those that were believed to be perfectly safe.

A major innovation in IUD technology was the discovery that the copper had spermicidal activity and acted on the endometrium in such a way as to create a hostile environment for sperm survival.

Types

The Lippes loop and other plastic IUDs are still used throughout the world but are no longer available in the United States. There are only two types of IUDs available in the United States, a copper IUD and a progesterone-releasing IUD.

An early type of copper IUD, the Copper 7, was extensively used throughout the world, but its sale was discontinued in 1986 in the United States because of the increasing cost of litigation.

The modern IUDs have more copper, which increases their efficiency and life span. Currently, only one copper IUD, TCu-380A (Paragard), is available in the United States. This device has a T-shaped configuration and is made of a

polyethylene for holding 380 mm^3 of exposed surface area of copper. The pure electrolytic copper wire wound around the stem weighs 176 mg, and copper sleeves on the horizontal arms weigh 66.5 mg. A polyethylene monofilament is tied through the ball of the stem, providing two white threads for detection and removal.[21]

The contraceptive action of copper IUDs, similar to all IUDs, is by their action on the uterine cavity creating a sterile inflammatory environment that is spermicidal. Ovulation is not affected, but there may be a cytotoxic effect on ova. Additionally the copper IUDs release free copper and copper salts, which exert biochemical and morphologic action on the endometrium as well as being spermicidal.[22]

The progestogen released from the progestin-releasing IUDs also acts directly on the endometrium and brings about decidual and atrophic changes of the glands. Thus, these IUDs have adverse effects on sperm survival and capacitation and inhibit implantation as well as sperm migration through cervical mucus.

Contraceptive Efficacy

The TCu-380A is approved for use for 10 years. The Progestasert (progesterone-releasing IUD) must be replaced every year. In large clinical studies, the cumulative pregnancy rates associated with TCu-380A IUD have been reported to be between 0.5% and 1.6%. Cumulative ectopic pregnancy rates were 0.1%. IUDs do not increase the risk of ectopic pregnancy and may offer some protection.[23] In selecting appropriate candidates for IUDs, the needs of the individual patients must be considered. IUDs are appropriate for parous women who are at low risk of sexually transmitted diseases; have no history of pelvic inflammatory disease; and are in a stable, mutually monogamous relationship.[23]

IUDs are contraindicated in women with a uterine size or shape incompatible with IUD use and those with medical conditions such as valvular heart disease or suppression of immune system known or suspected pregnancy, known or suspected pelvic inflammatory disease, undiagnosed vaginal bleeding, or those at high risk for sexually transmitted diseases. Additionally, copper IUDs should not be used in patients with Wilson's disease.

IUDs can be safely inserted during the menstrual cycle, after delivery, or after abortion. To reduce the rate of expulsion, it is suggested that copper IUDs be inserted between 4 and 8 weeks' postpartum. Insertion during menstruation is somewhat easier and preferred by many physicians. In every case, the insertion technique recommended by the manufacturer should be observed.

Side effects and complications of IUDs include increased cramping and menstrual flow, pelvic infection, uterine perforation, and displacement and expulsion. Cramping and menorrhagia are usually responsive to nonsteroidal anti-inflammatory drugs. If perforation or displacement is suspected, ultrasound of the pelvis should be performed to determine the proper location of the IUD. Mild pelvic infection in IUD wearers may be treated with appropriate antibiotic therapy. Persistent or severe infection, however, should be vigorously treated and the IUD removed.

To remove the IUD, the cervix should be exposed by a vaginal speculum and the string of the IUD grasped with a dressing ring forceps. The string is then pulled with a firm traction until the device is extracted.

BARRIER CONTRACEPTIVES

Barrier contraceptives are among the oldest and most widely used methods of birth control. Throughout history, a variety of barrier techniques have been devised to prevent deposition of semen in the vagina, to interfere with survival of spermatozoa in the vagina, or to interfere with their migration to the upper reproductive tract of the woman. There has been a resurgence of interest in barrier contraceptives because of their ability to prevent sexually transmitted diseases. Modern barrier methods and their efficacy relative to fertility control are listed in Table 7–6. Barrier contraceptives are safe and have the great advantage of protecting against sexually transmitted diseases and pelvic inflammatory diseases, including gonorrhea, chlamydia, herpes simplex, cytomegalovirus, human papillomavirus, and human immunodeficiency virus (HIV). Other benefits consist of lack of any effect on menstrual cycle and systemic and metabolic processes. The disadvantages of these techniques include a higher pregnancy rate relative to hormonal contraceptives and IUDs, their being coitally related, and their requiring the motivation to use them consistently and correctly. There is also an increased risk of toxic shock syndrome and occasional allergic reaction to spermicidal chemicals or rubber.

Vaginal Diaphragm

The vaginal diaphragm was one of the earliest contraceptives used by women in the United States and throughout the developed countries. The efficacy of the diaphragm depends on two key factors: correct selection of the type and size for

Table 7–6. Barrier Contraceptives (Failure Rate)

Method	Effectiveness (%)	Use Effectiveness (%)
Diaphragm and spermicide	6	18
Spermicides alone	3	21
Cervical cap	6	18
Sponge		
Parous women	9	28
Nulliparous women	6	18
Condom	2	12
Female condom	5	25
No method	85	85

individual women and proper usage (see Table 7–6).[24,25]

Diaphragms are shallow rubber cups with a metal rim. They are inserted in the upper of the vagina in such a way as to cover the cervix. The rim must fit snugly, behind the symphysis pubis and posterior cul de sac behind the cervix. They act as a mechanical barrier that provides a receptacle for spermicidal agents. Diaphragms range in size from 50 to 105 mm in diameter with 2.5 to 5 mm gradation. Three types of diaphragms are currently available: the coil spring, flat spring, and arching spring. Each one is designed for use in a specific situation.

The coil spring diaphragm is commonly used when the vagina is of normal size and shape with a deep arch behind the symphysis pubis and there is no uterine displacement. The flat spring is best suited when there is a shallow arch behind the symphysis pubis with an anteflexed uterus. The arching spring type is selected for women with poor vaginal muscle tone, moderate prolapse, or anteflexion or retroversion of the uterus. Diaphragms must be fitted and the correct size selected by the use of fitting rings. Diaphragms should be covered with spermicidal preparation before use and left in the vagina for at least 8 hours after intercourse. If repeated coital activities are attempted, additional spermicidal creams should be inserted without removing the diaphragm before each intercourse. The patient must also be taught how to insert the diaphragm correctly and maintain it. Most diaphragm failures occur as a result of incorrect insertion or nonuse. Diaphragms should be changed at least yearly. After each pregnancy, the patient should be refitted for her diaphragm when postpartum changes have subsided.

Female Condom

The female condom is a thin, soft, loose-fitting pouch made of polyurethane plastic with two flexible rings at either end. One ring helps to hold the device in place inside the vagina over the cervix while the other ring rests outside the vagina. The female condom covers the inside of the vagina, cervix, and perineum and may be construed as a combination of diaphragm and condom. The device acts as a barrier to prevent pregnancy and sexually transmitted diseases. The failure rate of female condom, according to data provided by the Food and Drug Administration, is 25% after 6 months of clinical trials with a pregnancy rate of 12.4% with average use.[26,27] When data were reanalyzed, it was estimated that with perfect use the estimated failure rate was only 5.1%.[27] Protection against sexually transmitted diseases also depends on correct and consistent use. With perfect use, it is estimated that the device could afford 94% protection against HIV.

Cervical Cap

The cervical cap was used extensively in Europe before its reintroduction in the United States. A reason for its lack of popularity is difficulty of insertion and removal. The cervical cap is similar to the diaphragm in structure but is made of much more rigid plastic and has to be inserted deeper in the vagina in a fashion to fit snugly around the cervix without touching the cervical os. Most women can be fitted with caps measuring 24, 30, or 36 mm in diameter.

The cervical cap has several advantages over the diaphragm. Cervical caps can be left in place up to 36 hours. Also, they may be used by women with cystocele, rectocele, and uterine prolapse. They should not be used, however, in women who have an abnormally long or short cervix or those with cervicitis, cervical erosion, or lacerations. Similar to the diaphragm, caps should be properly fitted to the patient and the patient appropriately instructed in its insertion and removal. Cervical caps are removed by pulling the rim away from the cervix to break the seal. Cervical caps have about the same degree of efficacy as the diaphragm (see Table 7–6).

Contraceptive Sponge

The vaginal contraceptive sponge was a dimpled disk made of polyurethane impregnated with nonoxynol 9, a spermicide that is released from the sponge for 24 hours. The sponge was thoroughly moistened with water before insertion to activate the spermicide. It provided continuous protection for up to 24 hours. In most studies, the failure rate of the sponge is lower than that of foam and jellies but higher than diaphragm.[28] Side effects include vaginal irritation and allergic reaction in about 4% of users. This product is no longer in production and is not available.

Spermicides

A large number of vaginal spermicidal preparations are currently in use. They can be categorized in five general groups: jellies, creams, aerosol foams, suppositories, and foaming tablets or films. These products contain a relatively inert base material that acts to block the passage of sperm physically and simultaneously serves as a carrier for an effective spermicide. The majority of these preparations contain nonoxynol 9, a surfactant, as an active spermicide. More than 170 types of vaginal spermicidal products are being used throughout the world. In the United States, they are available without prescription.

Vaginal spermicides must be used at the time of anticipated sexual intercourse. This is advantageous for women who have infrequent sexual relations but represents a disadvantage for women with frequent sexual activity because it requires the motivation to use them consistently. Additionally, some couples dislike the required preparation in the middle of lovemaking and the messiness of some of the products.

The contraceptive failures of these agents ranges from less than 1% to almost 30% in the first year of use, depending on the population studied and to some extent the product used. A 20% failure rate during the first year of use is frequently reported (see Table 7–6).[24]

Vaginal spermicides provide protection against sexually transmitted diseases. There is no evidence, however, that these products can prevent HIV infection. Vaginal spermicides are safe, and their use has not been associated with any major side effect. Approximately 1% to 5% of users may exhibit minor allergic reactions (both female and male), which resolve readily with discontinuation of the suspected product.

Condoms

The condom is by far the most used contraceptive product worldwide. In 1990, it was estimated that 6 billion condoms were used worldwide. The great advantage of condom is that if used continuously and correctly, it effectively prevents pregnancy as well as sexually transmitted diseases, including HIV (see Table 7–6). To achieve these goals, however, condoms must be affordable and readily available. Almost all condoms are made of latex with a thickness of 0.3 to 0.8 mm that prevents sperm, which are 0.003 mm in diameter, from penetrating them. The organisms that cause HIV or sexually transmitted diseases are also unable to penetrate latex condoms. About 1% of condoms sold are made of natural skin (intestine).

Because spermicides also provide protection against both pregnancy and sexually transmitted diseases, condoms and spermicides used together offer greater protection than either method used alone. A large array of condoms has been developed to suit individual tastes and include those that are straight or tapered, smooth or ribbed, colored or clear, lubricated or nonlubricated, and with or without spermicide impregnation.

A concern expressed by some couples is the alleged reduction in penile sensitivity that accompanies condom use. This may be, however, more a matter of perception than reality. Condoms must be placed on the penis before it touches a partner. The tip of the condom should extend beyond the end of the penis to provide a reservoir for semen collection. Oil-based lubricant (e.g., Vaseline) should not be used because they weaken the condom. If there is evidence of spillage or breakage, a spermicidal agent should be quickly inserted in the vagina. Condoms should never be used more than once.

Table 7–7. Median Times and Range of Ovulation Relative to Hormonal Events

Hormone	Median Time (h)	Ranges (h)
LH surge	16	8–40
Estradiol peak	24	17–32
Progesterone rise	8	−12.5 to +16

PERIODIC ABSTINENCE

Periodic abstinence or natural family planning is used by couples who, because of their religious or moral belief, find hormonal or barrier contraceptives unacceptable. These methods are based on the period of viability of the sperm in the female reproductive tract (estimated to be 2 to 7 days) and the life span of the ovum (1 to 3 days). The central issue in devising an effective method of natural family planning is accurate timing of ovulation, which shows considerable variation in different female populations (Table 7–7).

The method requires a serious commitment from both partners and is more effective in women who have regular menstrual cycles. For best results, women considering these methods should receive appropriate training before use and practice them correctly and consistently. The current methods of natural family planning are based on the concept of fertility awareness—the woman's ability to identify on a day-to-day basis certain physiologic changes that depend on hormonal changes associated with ovulation. These methods include calendar method, basal body temperature method, ovulation or cervical mucus method, and symptothermal method.[29] Among these, the two latter have proven to be more reliable and are commonly practiced.

Ovulation (Cervical Mucus) Method

The ovulation method was devised and popularized by Billings[29] and is based on periovulatory changes of cervical mucus characteristics that have been shown to reflect closely hormonal events. To use the ovulation method, the woman has to learn to recognize the sequence of changes in the quantity and quality of her mucus and the associated sensation of the vulva. These changes consist of:

1. Dry days, extending over several days, during which there is no mucus secretion; correspond to early follicular phase.
2. End of dry sensation; indicates that the production of cervical mucus has started. This infertile type of mucus is characterized by being tacky, crumbly, and white or yellow.
3. Preovulatory or fertile period; characterized by the appearance of clear, thin, glistening, lubricative mucus similar to raw egg white. The last day of lubricative mucus is called the *peak day.* The peak day indicates the day of maximum fertility and coincides with ovulation.
4. Postovulation days; during which the mucus becomes thick, tacky, scanty, and opaque.

Symptothermal Method

This method combines the cervical mucus method with the shift of basal body temperature. Additionally, other symptoms and signs of ovulation, such as midcycle pain or bleeding and breast fullness and tenderness may be used. These methods of natural family planning incorporate several markers of peripheral changes associated with cyclic hormonal changes in ovulatory women.

Efficacy

In multicenter studies conducted by world health organizations among those who learned the method, the pregnancy rate was 22.5 per 100 women year.[30] Almost all failures, however, could be attributed to a conscious departure from the method. Abstinence was necessary for 17 days in each cycle. For those who followed the method strictly, the actual method failure during the first year was only 3.1%, but imperfect use resulted in a pregnancy rate of 86.4%. Thus, if used correctly and consistently, natural family planning method is highly effective, but imperfect use results in unacceptable pregnancy rates.

The cervical mucus method has also been compared to the symptothermal method. The two methods were found to be comparable with pregnancy rates of 20% to 24%.[31] Once again, most pregnancies resulted from imperfect use.

HOW TO SELECT A CONTRACEPTIVE

Appropriate selection of a contraceptive for a couple depends on their preference, age, medical condition, parity, and other factors. OCs are highly effective and safe and may be used at any age, unless there is a specific medical contraindication for their use. They should not be used by smokers after the age of 35. Steroidal injectables and implants are preferred for those who lack motivation and discipline to take OCs and plan a relatively long period of fertility control. IUDs are ideal contraceptives for parous women in a monogamous relationship. Barrier contraceptives are suitable for almost any couple at any age. They are particularly indicated for couples at risk of sexually transmitted diseases. Specifically the use of condoms should be encouraged for all couples in a casual sexual relationship or those with multiple sexual partners. Female or male sterilization should be recommended to those couples who have an absolute medical contraindication to pregnancy or have completed their family and are no longer interested in their future fertility.

CONCLUSION

Even though the ideal contraceptive, as yet, does not exist, a large number of contraceptive methods are available to suit almost every population and any couple. They include oral hormonal preparations, injectable and implant formulations, IUDs, barrier methods, and natural family planning. Physicians should be prepared to inform their patients about these methods and, in agreement with the couples, select the best method that is most appropriate for them. Above all, no pregnancy should be conceived if not desired.

REFERENCES

1. Speroff L, DeCherney A: Evaluation of a new generation of oral contraceptives. Obstet Gynecol 81:1034, 1993.
2. Goldziehier JW: Hormonal Contraception: Pills, Injections and Implants, EMIS, 3rd ed. Canada, London, Ontario, 1994.
3. Moghissi KS, Evans TN, eds: Microdose progestogens for contraception in regulation of human fertility. Detroit, Wayne State University Press, 1976, pp 57–84.
4. Bottinger LE, Boman G, Eklund G, et al: Oral contraceptives and thromboembolic disease. Effects of lowering estrogen content. Lancet 1:1097, 1980.
5. Gerstman BB, Piper JM, Tomita DK, et al: Oral estrogen dose and the risk of deep venous thromboembolic disease. Am J Epidemiol 133:32, 1991.
6. Centers for Disease Control: Combination oral contraceptives and the risk of endometrial cancer. JAMA 257:796, 1987.
7. Centers for Disease Control: The reduction in risk of ovarian cancer associated with oral contraceptive use. N Engl J Med 316:650, 1987.
8. Mishell DR: Noncontraceptive benefits of oral steroidal contraceptives. Am J Obstet Gynecol 142:819, 1982.
9. Schlesselman JJ: Cancer of the breast and reproductive tract in relation to use of oral contraceptives. Contraception 40:1, 1989.
10. Vessey MP: Oral contraception and cancer. *In* Filshie M, Guillebaud J, eds: Contraception: Science and Practice. London, Butterworths, 1989, pp 52–68.
11. Ross RK, Pike MC, Vessey MP, et al: Risk factors for uterine fibroids: Reduced risk associated with oral contraceptives. Br Med J 293:359, 1986.
12. Drife JO: The Benefits and Risks of Oral Contraceptives. New York, Parthenon, 1993, pp 1–31.
13. Kaunitz AM, Mishell DR: Progestin only contraceptives, current perspectives, and future directions. Dialogues in Contraception 4:1, 1994.
14. Ginsburg K, Moghissi KS: Alternative delivery system for contraceptive progestogens. Fertil Steril 49(suppl 2):165, 1988.
15. WHO Collaborative Study of Neoplasia and Steroid Contraceptives: Breast

cancer and depomedroxyprogesterone acetate: A multi-national study. Lancet 338:833, 1991.

16. WHO Collaborative Study of Neoplasia and Steroid Contraceptives: Depomedroxyprogesterone acetate (DMPA) and risk of endometrial cancer. Int J Cancer 49:186, 1991.

17. Sivin I: Contraception with Norplant implant. Human Reprod 9:1818–1826, 1994.

18. Darney PD, Klaisle CM: Management of menstrual changes in Norplant implant recipient. Dialogues in Contraception 4:6–8, 1994.

19. Fasoli M, Parazzini F, Cacchetti G, LaVecchia C: Postcoital contraception: An overview of published studies. Contraception 39:459, 1989.

20. Yuzpe AA, Smith RP, Rademaker AW: A multicenter clinical investigation employing ethinyl estradiol combined with dl-norgestrel as a postcoital contraceptive agent. Fertil Steril 7:508, 1982.

21. Mosher WD: Contraception practice in the United States, 1982–1988. Fam Plann Perspect 22:198, 1990.

22. Alvarez F, Brachi V, Fernandez E, et al: New insights on the mode of action of intrauterine contraceptive devices in women. Fertil Steril 49:768, 1988.

23. World Health Organization: The TCu-380A, TCu220C, multiload 250 and Nova T IUD's at 3.5 and 7 years of use-results from three randomized multicenter trials. Contraception 42:141, 1990.

24. Connell EB: Vaginal contraception. In Mishell DR, ed: Advances in Fertility Research, Vol 1. New York, Raven Press, 1982, pp 19–38.

25. World Health Organization: A prospective multicenter trial of the ovulation method of natural family planning: II. The effectiveness phase. Fertil Steril 36:591, 1981.

26. Shervington DO: Female condom becomes available nationwide. Contraception Report 5:11–13, 1995.

27. Trussell J, Sturgen K, Strickler J, et al: Comparative contraceptive efficacy of female condom and other barrier methods. Fam Plann Perspect 26:66–72, 1994.

28. McIntyre SL, Higgins JE: Parity and use effectiveness with the contraceptive sponge. Am J Obstet Gynecol 155:796, 1986.

29. Bonnas J: Natural family planning including breast feeding. In Mishell DR, ed: Advances in Fertility Research, Vol I. New York, Raven Press, 1982, pp 1–18.

30. Wade ME, McCarthy P, Braurnstein GD, et al: A randomized prospective study of the use effectiveness of two methods of natural family planning. Am J Obstet Gynecol 141:368, 1981.

31. Medina JE, Cifuentes A, Abernathy JR, et al: Comparative evaluation of two methods of natural family planning in Columbia. Am J Obstet Gynecol 138:1142, 1980.

CHAPTER 8

Chronic Pelvic Pain and Dysmenorrhea

Gary H. Lipscomb

Frank W. Ling

Complaints of pelvic pain or pelvic discomfort are not infrequently encountered by practitioners providing primary care to women. Although most such pain is resolved in a timely fashion, some patients continue to have pain despite all attempts at diagnosis and treatment. Pain that persists for greater than 6 months' duration is defined as chronic pain and, although rarely life-threatening, is potentially debilitating. By its nature, chronic pelvic pain often causes frustration for both the physician and the patient. This chapter presents a logical, methodical approach to the workup and treatment of the patient with chronic pelvic pain.

Traditionally the gynecologic approach to chronic pelvic pain has focused on the female reproductive tract organs as the sole source of pain. This excessively narrowed approach, sometimes referred to as *gynevision,* may fail to recognize other common contributors to pelvic pain (e.g., gastrointestinal tract, urinary tract, or psychological factors). Such an approach tends to encourage more of a surgical approach in which organic pathology of the reproductive tract is a top priority. This overly simplistic view serves neither the patient nor the physician. A more holistic, multidisciplinary approach, centered around the idiosyncratic needs of the individual patient, offers a more logical methodology for dealing with this difficult clinical syndrome.

This chapter focuses on the workup and treatment of chronic pelvic pain and includes various aspects of the multidisciplinary approach necessary to carry out a complete management scheme of some of the more difficult to treat subtypes. Regardless of whether an individual physician chooses to incorporate any or all of the recommendations made, ultimately, it is the patient who may benefit as she is taught to cope with and manage her pain better. Curing all patients with chronic pelvic pain is an ideal goal. Realistically, however, the physician should recognize that some patients are best helped by management of pain, with a goal of minimally disrupting her lifestyle and enabling her to carry on her normal daily activities and maintain her self-image.

EVALUATION OF THE PATIENT WITH CHRONIC PELVIC PAIN

A complete history is essential for proper evaluation of chronic lower abdominal or pelvic pain. The patient should be questioned about the character of her pain as well as its duration, frequency of occurrence, location, and any radiation patterns. Any exacerbating or alleviating factors should be determined. It should also be noted whether the severity of pain is stable or has become better or worse with time. The relationship, if any, of the pain to the menstrual cycle, sexual activity, bladder and bowel function, and emotional state may prove critical.

Particular attention should be focused on past surgical procedures or presumptive episodes of pelvic inflammatory disease (PID). The patient's psychological response to her pain and its effect on her lifestyle, family, and friends should also be determined if possible. The patient should be questioned about any prior treatment, both medically or self-administered, and its effect on the pain.

The classic gynecologic approach of dividing the pain into cyclic and noncyclic categories may help to determine whether there is a menstrual cycle–related origin of the pain. Table 8–1 and 8–2 list the differential diagnoses of chronic pelvic pain and provide a generally accurate starting point for categorizing pelvic pain causes. The two lists are not mutually ex-

Table 8–1. Differential Diagnosis of Chronic Pelvic Pain

Predominantly Noncyclic
Pelvic inflammatory disease
Pelvic adhesions
Displacement of the uterus
Symptomatic pelvic relaxation
Chronic pelvic pain without organic
  abnormalities
Musculoskeletal disorders
Urinary tract disorders
Gastrointestinal tract disorders
Psychogenic/psychological factors

Predominantly Cyclic
Mittelschmerz
Primary dysmenorrhea
Secondary dysmenorrhea
  Endometriosis
  Adenomyosis
  Endometritis
  Cervic stenosis
  Intrauterine device
  Leiomyoma
Premenstrual syndrome

Table 8–2. Treatment of Chronic Pelvic Pain

General measures
  Multidisciplinary management
  NSAIDs
  Psychological support
  Antipsychotics
Irritable bowel syndrome
  Bulk-forming agents
Musculoskeletal
  Multidisciplinary management
  Physical therapy
  Trigger point injections
  NSAIDs
Urinary tract
  Urethral syndrome
    Voiding schedule
    Suppressive antibiotics
    Urethral dilatation
    Anxiolytics
    Surgical therapy
  Interstitial cystitis
    Hydrodistention
    Dimethyl sulfoxide
    Voiding schedule
    Surgical therapy
Primary dysmenorrhea
  NSAIDs
  Oral contraceptive pill
Secondary dysmenorrhea
  NSAIDs
  Oral contraceptive pill
  Specific therapy for cause
Surgical
  Diagnostic laparoscopy
  Adhesiolysis
  Uterine suspension
  Uterosacral nerve ablation
  Presacral neurectomy
  Hysterectomy

NSAIDs = Nonsteroidal anti-inflammatory drugs.

clusive because conditions that generally produce cyclic pain may occasionally present with noncyclic pain and vice versa. The physician must also be wary of nonmenstrual-related pain that may be exacerbated by the menstrual cycle (i.e., dysmenorrhea must be differentiated from pelvic pain that is constant throughout the month but is exacerbated at the time of the menstrual cycle).

If the pain does appear to be cyclic or menstrual related, a detailed menstrual history should be obtained. This should include the time of menarche, cycle regularity and length, and number of days of bleeding as well as some quantification of blood loss. It should be determined whether this pain has been present since menarche or is a relatively new phenomenon.

Once the history is obtained, this information should be used to direct the physical examination further. Although a complete physical examination is essential, particular attention should be paid to certain aspects of the physical examination. The patient's posture and walk should be noted. Generally poor posture, slouching, and standing with the weight on one leg may suggest a possible musculoskeletal cause. A gentle abdominal examination searching for masses and areas of tenderness should be performed. Special attention to superficial palpation is critical in identifying musculoskeletal pain. If a painful area is encountered, the patient should be questioned whether or not this pain reproduces the complaint for which she is being evaluated. Pain produced by palpation that increases or remains constant during voluntary tightening of the abdominal musculature is usually of abdominal wall rather than visceral origin. This maneuver can be easily accomplished by asking the patient to elevate her head from the examination table or by elevating both legs from the table while the examiner applies gentle pressure to the painful area. A brief neurologic examination with attention to lower extremity reflexes should be performed. Abnormal reflexes or pain on straight leg raises may indicate a possible herniated disk and signal the need for a more extensive neurologic evaluation.

Before the bimanual examination, gentle palpation of the introitus, sometimes with a moistened cotton-tip swab, can aid in identifying vulvar vestibulitis, a variant of pelvic pain that often presents as new-onset entrance dyspareunia. A one-handed pelvic examination (monomanual) should precede the traditional bimanual examination to aid in differentiating pain that is caused by the abdominal wall as opposed to pain whose cause is within the pelvis. Gentle palpation of the relaxed levator muscles, with the index finger directed posteriorly, helps diagnose levator spasm. The patient should also be asked to contract these muscles during palpation with the index finger to identify muscular pain

further. Then the same finger is rotated anteriorly to palpate the urethra and bladder base gently. Cervical motion tenderness and vaginal fornix pain are also evaluated before the bimanual examination by performing a complete internal evaluation using the vaginal hand. The physician can thus avoid mislabeling lower abdominal muscular pain elicited with a bimanual examination as some other pelvic pathologic conditions, such as adhesions from PID.

During the bimanual examination, uterine size, mobility, and tenderness should be noted. Specific notation should be made whether the uterus itself is tender and the source of the complaints of pain. This is a pivotal concern if hysterectomy is subsequently considered. Similar information should be obtained regarding both adnexa. Rectovaginal examination is necessary to evaluate adequately any induration or nodularity of the uterosacral ligaments owing to endometriosis.

Nongynecologic causes of chronic pelvic pain should always be thoroughly evaluated and ruled out before proceeding with any surgical therapy. Of particular concern should be possible contributions of the gastrointestinal tract (e.g., irritable bowel syndrome), urogynecologic causes (e.g., chronic urethritis, interstitial cystitis), and musculoskeletal factors.

PREDOMINANTLY CYCLIC CAUSES OF PELVIC PAIN

It is estimated that 30% to 50% of women of childbearing age suffer from cyclic pelvic pain. In 10% to 15% of these women, symptoms are severe enough to interfere with normal activities. Although the cyclic nature of the pain implies a causal relationship with the female reproductive system, care must be taken to differentiate true menstrual-related symptoms from symptoms aggravated by the body changes occurring during the menstrual cycle. The practitioner also must differentiate cyclic pain unrelated to the menstrual cycle from true dysmenorrhea.

Dysmenorrhea is broadly divided into two categories: primary and secondary. In contrast to many other diagnoses (e.g., infertility or amenorrhea), the terms *pri-*

mary and *secondary* do not imply a temporal meaning but instead relate to causality. In secondary dysmenorrhea, a readily identifiable cause, such as fibroids or endometriosis, is found, whereas in primary dysmenorrhea, there is no identifiable cause.

Primary dysmenorrhea to some degree has been experienced by most menstrual women at some time in their lives. The pain is characteristically sharp or cramplike and generally occurs in the first 3 days of menstruation. The pain is generally suprapubic but may radiate to the back, inner thighs, or deep pelvis. Nausea, with or without vomiting, and diarrhea also may occur. Dyspareunia, even during menstruation, is uncommon and should suggest other pathology. The diagnosis of primary dysmenorrhea is one of exclusion (i.e., there should be no other noted abnormalities on history or physical examination that might suggest the cause of the dysmenorrhea).

Patients with secondary dysmenorrhea often have other symptoms, in addition to cyclic pain, that may suggest the underlying cause. Heavy menstrual flow with dysmenorrhea suggests a diagnosis of uterine leiomyomata, adenomyosis, or endometrial polyps. Likewise, cyclic pain in a patient with primary amenorrhea suggests outflow obstruction. Gastrointestinal, urinary, or musculoskeletal complaints should raise the possibility of a nongynecologic process. Diagnosis and management of these entities are further discussed in the section on primarily noncyclic disorders.

In addition to the physical examination previously discussed, the examiner should pay particular attention to the size, mobility, and tenderness of the uterus and adnexa. A mildly enlarged, boggy, tender, symmetric uterus suggests adenomyosis or perhaps fibroids. A markedly enlarged or asymmetrically enlarged uterus is more consistent with fibroids. A poorly mobile uterus may indicate fibrosis owing to endometriosis. Any nodularity or induration of the uterosacral ligaments, which would also suggest endometriosis, should be further assessed with a rectal examination.

Laboratory studies are of limited use in the evaluation of patients with dysmenorrhea. Blood counts for assessing blood loss in patients with excessive bleeding or sedimentation rates to identify a chronic inflammatory process are occasionally helpful.

Ultrasound and other radiologic modalities rarely provide additional helpful information except in cases in which the physical examination was either inadequate or suspicious but not conclusive of a particular condition. In fact, these imaging techniques often may further confuse the diagnosis by identifying a small physiologic ovarian cyst or other benign process. This misleading information may then result in additional unnecessary tests and occasionally even unnecessary surgery. Diagnostic laparoscopy is usually reserved for patients in whom additional pathology is suspected based on the history and physical examination or for patients who respond poorly to nonsteroidal agents and oral contraceptive pills (OCPs).

Because the underlying pathophysiology in patients with primary dysmenorrhea relates to prostaglandins, the mainstay of treatment is nonsteroidal anti-inflammatory drugs (NSAIDs). Generally the similarities between the NSAIDs are such that the practitioner need be familiar with only one or two agents. Although the chemical structures of the NSAIDs are so similar that one would not expect marked clinical differences in response between different NSAIDs, patients who have poor or partial response to one NSAID may respond well to a different agent. Apparently subtle differences in the site or mechanism of action are responsible for this phenomenon.

Hormonal agents are frequently prescribed for dysmenorrhea. The most common of the hormonal agents is the OCP. OCPs are widely used for relief of primary dysmenorrhea in patients not desiring pregnancy. No one pill has been shown to be superior to another in this regard; thus, physicians should use the OCP with which they are most familiar for this purpose. Although OCPs are generally prescribed on a 28-day cycle (21 days of hormone followed by 7 hormone-free days), they can be used continuously (no hormone-free days) in an attempt to produce amenorrhea if patients still have dysmenorrhea during withdrawal bleeding. Unfortunately, breakthrough bleeding is common and often limits the use of this regimen. Medroxyprogesterone acetate (Depo-Provera) may also be used to induce hypomenorrhea or amenorrhea in these patients. Only 50% of patients, however, can be expected to become totally amenorrheic in the first year of use. Likewise, gonadotropin-releasing hormone (Gn-RH) agonists have been used to obtain amenorrhea, but their use is limited by the high cost of therapy and association with bone loss when long-term use is contemplated. Their use for dysmenorrhea should probably be reserved for therapy of symptomatic endometriosis.

Although all of the above-mentioned modalities for treatment of primary dysmenorrhea may also be used as treatment for secondary dysmenorrhea, results are frequently less than satisfactory. Only specific therapy for the cause of secondary dysmenorrhea ultimately gives satisfactory results.

PREDOMINANTLY NONCYCLIC CAUSES OF PELVIC PAIN

Gastrointestinal Causes

It has been estimated that up to 60% of referrals for chronic pelvic pain may be attributed to a gastrointestinal origin, particularly irritable bowel syndrome. Because of the visceral innervation of the bowel, it is often difficult to differentiate lower abdominal pain of gynecologic origin from that of gastrointestinal origin. Unfortunately, in women, the lower abdominal pain is not infrequently interpreted as pelvic pain by both the patient and the physician.

A careful history may reveal details that suggest a gastrointestinal cause. Bowel habits are a particularly useful source of information. Abdominal pain associated with irritable bowel syndrome characteristically improves following a bowel movement and is often worse with eating. There also may be a sense of rectal fullness or incomplete rectal evacuation. Hard pelletlike stools in the rectum are also suggestive of irritable bowel syndrome. Exacerbation of pain during times of stress is a common finding. Correlation of pain with food intake should

be discussed. Patients with infrequent bowel movements associated with pain during or preceding evacuation may have only chronic constipation; however, patients with diarrhea should be evaluated for intrinsic bowel disease as a possible underlying cause. Although dyspareunia is frequently gynecologic in origin, many women with irritable bowel also have dyspareunia.

The physical examination is similar to that previously described and should always include a rectal examination and examination of the pelvic floor. Tenderness localized over the sigmoid colon in the absence of inflammatory signs is frequently present in patients with irritable bowel syndrome, whereas a tender mass in the left lower quadrant in a febrile patient suggests diverticulitis.

Although the history and physical examination is the most effective method to rule out acute and most chronic conditions, the differential diagnosis of irritable bowel syndrome includes inflammatory bowel disease as well as malignancy. Thus, a thorough workup to exclude these conditions is appropriate. Laboratory tests may include a complete blood count and stool for occult blood and white cells. A plain film of the abdomen may reveal radiologic evidence of acute or chronic disease. Likewise, ultrasound may detect gallstones, ascites, or the presence of an intra-abdominal mass. In selected patients, flexible sigmoidoscopy, colonoscopy, or barium enema may be helpful and appropriate.

Although there is no known detectable structural or biochemical abnormality associated with irritable bowel syndrome, activation of hypersensitive receptors in the bowel wall because of physiologic distention or contraction may be responsible for the pain. Studies also suggest that the conscious threshold for perception of visceral sensation in the form of pain is altered in patients with irritable bowel syndrome. In addition, a large number of women with this syndrome have been shown to have coexisting psychopathology, such as somatization disorders, anxiety disorders, and depression as well as other psychological syndromes.

Current medical treatment for irritable bowel syndrome is generally unsatisfactory, with 30% to 70% of patients with continued symptoms even after long-term treatment. Treatment primarily consists of reassurance, education, stress reduction, bulk-forming agents, anxiolytics, and low-dose tricyclic antidepressants, with bulk-forming agents being the single most effective therapy. Anticholinergics are generally ineffective. In many instances, multidisciplinary pain management is appropriate for these patients, just as it is for any patient with chronic pelvic pain.

Urinary Tract Causes of Pelvic Pain

Pain originating from the urinary tract may be difficult to differentiate from gynecologic sources, owing to their common embryologic origin. Thus, the urinary tract should always be considered in the differential diagnosis of pelvic pain, particularly when the standard gynecologic evaluation is inconclusive. Symptoms of urgency, frequency, and dysuria may indicate an acute or chronic urinary tract problem. Likewise, recurrent episodes of urinary tract infection with negative urine cultures should raise the suspicion of a chronic inflammatory process of noninfectious origin. A history of hesitancy or incomplete emptying may indicate a disorder of the urethra or bladder neck. Postcoital voiding difficulties are strongly associated with urethral syndrome secondary to chronic urethritis. Likewise, dyspareunia is common with urethral syndrome.

In many instances in which there is a suspicion of urinary dysfunction, a 24-hour voiding diary can be helpful in providing insight into the frequency of voiding, episodes of leakage, and amount of fluid intake. For example, frequency at night may relate to sensory problems of the bladder and urethra, whereas constant voiding throughout the day may suggest limited bladder capacity because of an intrinsic bladder condition.

The physical examination should always include a cursory neurologic examination of the lower extremities and perineal area. The tone and sensation of the pelvic floor musculature should be ascertained during the pelvic examination. Excessive tone or tenderness of the levator ani musculature may indicate an underlying urethral or bladder disorder (e.g., levator ani spasm has been suggested as one of the causes of pain in patients with interstitial cystitis). In these patients, gentle palpation of the urethra, bladder trigone, and base frequently identifies a specific source of pain.

Cystourethroscopy should be considered in all women with chronic pelvic pain of suspected urologic origin. The urethra and the bladder mucosa can be inspected and any evidence of chronic infection or the presence of structural deformities such as diverticula or tumors visualized. Although cystourethroscopy is normally performed in the office setting without anesthesia, for painful conditions such as interstitial cystitis, cystourethroscopy may require general anesthesia. In these cases, it should be performed in a hospital or outpatient surgical setting. Findings of erythema and exudate in patients with pelvic pain and irritative urinary symptoms without other bladder pathology are consistent with urethral syndrome as a result of chronic urethritis. In the patient without any demonstrable findings but with significant symptoms, urethral spasm should be considered. In patients with suspected interstitial cystitis, the bladder is filled, allowed to remain distended for 1 minute, emptied, and then refilled. Patients with interstitial cystitis develop characteristic submucosal hemorrhages and petechiae after this *double-fill cystoscopy*.

As might be expected in a condition for which no specific cause is known, no one specific therapy is uniformly successful for patients with urethral syndrome. One treatment that can be initiated in all cases, however, is modification of voiding habits. Patients are taught to tighten and relax their pelvic floor musculature to gain control of the voluntary or learned spastic behavior of the urethral sphincter. Additionally the use of a regular voiding schedule through bladder retraining drills aids the patient's ability to control the urge and need to void.

In patients with suspected chronic urethritis, the use of low-dose antibiotic therapy with trimethoprim/sulfamethoxazole or nitrofurantoin for bedtime suppression is appropriate. Normally a

3- to 6-month trial is used. Urethral dilatation is an often used therapy for urethral syndrome. The mechanism of action is unclear but may be due to opening of obstructed and inflamed periurethral glands. Summitt, reporting on a group of patients initially presenting with complaints of pelvic pain and dyspareunia, showed that therapy with long-term suppressive antibiotics and serial urethral dilatation resulted in marked improvement or resolution in all of these patients. All had reduced pain and were subsequently able to resume sexual activity without discomfort.

Other treatments for urethral syndrome that have been used with variable success include anxiolytics, psychotherapy, periurethral steroid injections, and internal urethrotomy. Because these patients present with a confusing or changing clinical picture, consultation with a urologist or urogynecologist may be extremely helpful in diagnosing and treating this syndrome.

Treatment for interstitial cystitis is aimed at treating the inflammation or correcting the bladder wall permeability. Hydrodistention performed at the time of diagnosis may itself be therapeutic. Similarly, behavior modification using increasing voiding intervals can produce similar results. Tricyclic antidepressants have been used to provide sedative effects as well as pain relief through peripheral neuroblockade and central stimulation. Dimethyl sulfoxide as an intravesical instillation is one of the more frequently used medical therapies. Surgical therapy has been used but should be considered a last resort.

Musculoskeletal Causes of Chronic Pelvic Pain

The musculoskeletal system is perhaps the most common source of non-gynecologic chronic pelvic pain. Unfortunately the musculoskeletal evaluation is also the most frequently overlooked component of the comprehensive evaluation of the patient with chronic pelvic pain. Some factors that may indicate a musculoskeletal source of pain include poor posture, scoliosis, unilateral standing habits, marked lumbar lordosis, leg length discrepancy, abnormal gait, abdominal wall trigger points or tenderness, history of low back trauma, and a previous normal laparoscopy.

The typical bimanual pelvic examination can be a poor discriminator as to the cause of pelvic pain because it is a simultaneous evaluation of the abdominal wall, the vaginal wall, and the tissues in between. For example, in the bimanual evaluation of the anteverted uterus, the two examining hands palpate the abdominal wall, including skin, subcutaneous tissue, fascia, and muscle; the uterus; the bladder; and the vaginal wall. The initial use of the monomanual pelvic examination previously described helps avoid mislabeling abdominal wall and levator muscle pain as uterine/adnexal pain. Careful palpation of the rectus muscles both in a relaxed and in a tensed state often elicits the patient's pain. The lateral borders of the abdominal rectus muscles as well as their insertion site into the symphysis pubis are particularly common sites of tenderness.

Slocumb has suggested that hypersensitive areas of the abdominal wall (trigger points) are the most common cause of pelvic pain. These trigger points are hyperirritable areas that are tender when compressed and may also generate referred pain and tenderness. Trigger points typically start after some type of muscle strain and can often be found within a taut band of skeletal muscle. Trigger points can respond dramatically to specific trigger point therapy. In his classic study, Slocumb used trigger point injections of local anesthetic agents to treat 122 patients who presented with chronic pelvic pain. Greater than 50% of patients in this study became pain-free. Only 13 had surgery, and all patients who received only injections of the abdominal wall were reported to have a successful response. Those with vaginal trigger points had an 84.6% response rate to their injections.

In the patient with demonstrable trigger points, injection with local anesthetic may be a useful therapeutic and diagnostic aid. The use of a 1- to 1.5-inch 22-gauge needle is recommended for superficial musculature. Although smaller-gauge needles cause less discomfort on skin penetration, they have the disadvantage of being less able to disrupt a trigger point mechanically as well as reducing the clinician's sensitivity in detecting passage through the various tissue planes. Smaller needles may also be too flexible, thus sliding around taut muscle bands and masking the tactile clues that a clinician may use.

When injecting a trigger point, an aseptic technique should be used. The patient should also be forewarned that she may feel a muscle twitch or flash of referred pain during the insertion. The palpating finger should maintain tension on the skin as various injection tracts are made. If a trigger point is not identified directly, the injection may be less effective but still useful diagnostically. Successful injection results in a loss of tenderness and, if originally present, relaxation of the tight band of muscle. The patient should also be able to note a symptomatic difference when palpating the area.

Although any of the local anesthetic agents may be used for trigger point injections, bupivacaine 0.25% is the authors' agent of choice. Volumes of 10 mL or less are commonly adequate to produce a clear diagnostic test. Interestingly the pain relief often extends far longer than would be predicted by the normal duration of action of the drug. This time frame is frequently longer with subsequent injections and may reflect recovery of normal muscle and nerve function.

Relief of the pain after trigger point injection helps the patient to understand that her pain is at least partially musculoskeletal and not necessarily from gynecologic causes such as ovarian cysts, endometriosis, or infection. When used in this fashion, trigger point injections can clearly be diagnostic and, as shown by Slocumb, can be therapeutic, either alone or in a series of injections. Because relief of pain from one source may uncover pain from other causes, trigger point injections should be viewed as helpful adjuvants in an overall management plan.

Physical therapy, when included in a multidisciplinary approach, has been successful in managing patients with chronic pelvic pain owing to musculoskeletal pain. Referral to a physical therapist for further evaluation or more intensive physical therapy instruction than can be provided by the practitioner is frequently helpful in these patients. In cases in which such referral is unavailable or not practical, the use of NSAIDs, muscle relaxants, and heat application may be effective. Initial use of these agents on a scheduled rather than an as-needed basis for the first 1 to 2 weeks of treatment is recommended. These medications may also be used in conjunction with physical therapy.

PSYCHIATRIC FACTORS IN PELVIC PAIN

All patients who have chronic pelvic pain undergo adaptive responses to the pain. What might otherwise be perceived as an abnormal response to pain may, based on the duration of symptoms, be normal. With passage of time, the patient goes through a *normal* series of significantly altered emotional states in response to chronic pain, starting at what is often an unknown baseline. Initially the patient has high expectations, but with the passage of time frustration and despair predominate with the patient giving up on improvement. "Doctor shopping," hostility, and eventually clinical depression occur as the patient passes through these stages. The physician needs to interpret the patient's words and actions with these emotional changes in perspective.

For patients with chronic pain, the exercise of trying to differentiate mental from physical pain is not useful because *mental* factors such as clinical depression, anxiety, and anger are clearly part of the patient's perception of discomfort. In this regard, patients with chronic pelvic pain are not unique from patients with other types of chronic pain. The patient's response to pain is affected by such varied factors as cultural value on pain tolerance or display of emotion; the patient's perception of the risk involved with the pain; and work, social, financial, and idiosyncratic considerations.

As with any other disease process, psychiatric illness may be totally unrelated to the chronic pain or a contributory factor that must be dealt with for patient improvement. It is beyond the scope of this chapter to discuss diagnosis and management of major psychiatric illness such as manic-depressive disorders or schizophrenia. Patients with these disorders are often best managed in close collaboration with mental health professionals. Because it is impossible to separate totally the relationship of mind and body on chronic pelvic pain, however, some common psychiatric issues frequently encountered in the patient with chronic pelvic pain are briefly discussed.

One particular psychiatric disorder frequently encountered in chronic pelvic pain patients is somatization. In patients with this disorder, emotional problems may become manifest as physical complaints. In these patients, their emotional state may adversely affect their adaptation to a mild but persistent pain. There are multiple physical complaints for which there is no identifiable organic basis. Psychological and psychiatric intervention, in a nonthreatening way, may be of therapeutic benefit. In general, these patients need ongoing supportive care (i.e., no cure is anticipated). Principles of management of somatizing patients are based on their ongoing need for sanctioned caretaking and their tendency to express problems of the mind in the language of the body. These principles can also be modified for the treatment of the syndrome of chronic pain in general. These principles are summarized as follows:

1. See the patient at regular intervals to avoid the need to use symptoms as a "ticket of admission" to the medical system.
2. Accept the patient's need to be considered ill. The patient should be told even if symptoms improve, the illness will probably always be present. Promise understanding and support but not complete relief because this can be as much a threat as a reward in some patients. Emphasizing management rather than cure can help the patient gain a more realistic view of her condition.
3. Do not make physician contacts contingent on physical complaints.

If the patient knows that the patient-physician relationship will continue even if the patient feels well, the use of symptoms as a means of ensuring access to the physician will decrease.
4. Do not prolong contacts with the patient in response to increased symptoms. A specific visit length does not encourage the patient to have more symptoms to see the physician more.
5. Allow the patient to structure the content of the discussions. Open-ended questions such as "how are you feeling" are usually sufficient to allow the patient this option.
6. Minimize secondary gain. If the patient is being paid for the illness, improvement is likely to be financially as well as emotionally threatening. The family should be helped to avoid reorganizing their lives around the patient's illness and be encouraged to increase gradually their demands that the patient function more effectively as a family member regardless of how she is feeling.
7. Teach the patient to express emotions in words. When the patient describes a situation in which a strong emotion such as anger should have been experienced but pain or some other physical sensation was felt instead, ask "were you angry, too?" If the patient responds that anger did not cause the pain, point out that anger and pain can be two different states that may or may not have anything to do with each other, but both are important to physicians who wish to treat the whole patient.
8. Control strong reaction to the patient. Patients who covertly refuse to cooperate often arouse strong feeling in the physician, often resulting in hostility or argumentative behavior by the physician. Doing so tells the patient not to return unless symptoms become worse or to behave with excessive hostility or solitude.
9. Remain alert for intercurrent medical illness. Changes in the patient's

symptoms that cannot be explained by new stress or unavailability may mean that the patient is expressing a new medical problem in characteristic ways that make it appear to be more of the original functional complaint.

SEXUAL ABUSE HISTORY

Many patients with chronic pain have or have had abusive family relationships, either as children or in adulthood. Sexual victimization, in particular, has been linked to later development of chronic pelvic pain. This complicates both the evaluation and the treatment of women with chronic pelvic pain. For example, the use of antidepressant medications appears to be less efficacious in women who have a history of sexual victimization. These patients may also be less able to develop a close relationship with their physicians, a situation that may make long-term therapeutic attempts less effective. Because of the greater risk of other psychiatric illness such as anxiety and mood disorders, these patients may not easily fall within the purview of those physicians typically seeing these patients as first-line physicians. The most important factor for the clinician and the patient is that the physician be made aware of sexual trauma. The initial evaluation of patients who have chronic pelvic pain should include a gentle inquiry as to current or past sexual or physical abuse. For example, "have you ever been touched against your will, either as a child or an adult?" is one possible entry statement. Recognition of this factor may help frame future discussions and therapeutic interventions, including supportive listening, use of community resources, referral to support groups, and treatment with antidepressants.

ROLE OF ANTIDEPRESSANTS IN CHRONIC PELVIC PAIN

The use of antidepressants in the patient with difficulty coping with chronic pain or with the emotional demands that the illness may cause in the family unit may prove beneficial. A clinical trial of these agents given at bedtime often results in an increased quality of sleep as well as an overall improvement in adjustment to the patient's illness. Tricyclic antidepressants also may provide pain relief through peripheral neuroblockade and central stimulation in addition to their other actions. In a meta-analytic review of 39 controlled antidepressant trials, Onghena and Van Houdenhove found that the average chronic pain patient who received an antidepressant had less pain than 74% of the chronic pain patients who received a placebo.

Amitriptyline, an antidepressant with sedative effects, is a good choice when such agents are needed in the treatment of chronic pain. It should not be used in patients on monoamine oxidase inhibitors or with cardiovascular disorders, particularly arrhythmias. Common side effects are related to its anticholinergic effects and include urinary retention, dry mouth, and constipation. Serious side effects include myocardial infarction, cardiac arrhythmias, and bone marrow depression. Dosages start at 25 mg at bedtime and can be increased to 150 mg if needed. Other antidepressants such as nortriptyline, imipramine, and fluoxetine have also been used successfully. Nortriptyline may be started, using 25 mg at bedtime and increasing by 25 mg every 3 to 4 days thereafter, as tolerated, with a maximum dosage of 100 mg/day. Fluoxetine may be given 20 mg/day. Sertraline may be given at a dosage of 50 mg/day.

ROLE OF SURGICAL MANAGEMENT IN CHRONIC PELVIC PAIN

Surgery is often a logical extension of a thorough diagnostic and therapeutic management scheme in patients who have chronic pelvic pain. In particular, diagnostic laparoscopy remains the best procedure when a diagnostic dilemma exists. For the nonsurgically trained clinician, this requires referral to a specialist in this area. Often for the nonsurgically trained clinician to make appropriate referrals, some knowledge of the procedures themselves is necessary. Therefore, surgical options frequently used in the treatment of chronic pelvic pain are briefly reviewed.

Diagnostic Laparoscopy

Diagnostic laparoscopy has four roles in the management of the pelvic pain patient: (1) Patient reassurance, (2) documentation of adhesive disease, (3) elimination of diagnostic errors, and (4) histologic documentation.

Diagnostic laparoscopy can result in a therapeutic response in patients who may be anxious about neoplasia, infection, or other pelvic cause for their pain. Thus, physicians should not minimize the importance of patient reassurance and other nonsurgical intervention in the management of patients with chronic pelvic pain. This reassurance is potentially aided by the use of videotaping or photographs taken at the time of surgery.

Documentation of pelvic adhesions is necessary if therapeutic surgery is contemplated. Overall, the patient's history and physical examination has been shown to be a poor predictor as to which patient will or will not have pelvic adhesions. An abnormal pelvic examination with two abnormal findings, however, has been shown to predict the presence of pelvic adhesions in 74% of patients. These data show that all patients presenting with chronic pelvic pain do not necessarily need diagnostic laparoscopy regardless of history or physical findings; moreover, in the absence of history or physical findings, patients with chronic pelvic pain may sometimes best be served initially by nonoperative therapy.

Diagnostic laparoscopy does eliminate presumptive treatment of suspected pathology by providing direct visualization of pelvic structures. The presence and extent of significant pathology, such as endometriosis, pelvic infection, or adhesions, can be documented both for baseline comparative purposes and for proper selection of therapy. Approximately 30% of chronic pelvic pain patients, however, can be expected to have normal findings. In these patients, reassurance could potentially be therapeutic.

In no group of patients is histologic documentation more important than in those patients with suspected endometriosis. Evidence indicates that many endometrial implants may not fit the classic description of black or blue lesions. Because many conditions can simulate endometriosis, biopsy specimens should be liberally taken of classic lesions as well as any abnormal appearing areas of peritoneum. It is certainly not unusual at the time of laparoscopy for patients with a history of PID to be found instead to have endometriosis as a cause of their pain.

Adhesiolysis

Surgical lysis of adhesions whether via the laparoscope or by laparotomy would, at first glance, appear to be the logical therapy for patients who have documented adhesive disease from PID. Unfortunately, there is no documented evidence that adhesions are always a cause of such pelvic pain. As previously indicated, only a small percentage of patients with chronic pelvic pain have documented adhesive disease. Other studies have shown a comparable incidence of adhesions in both chronic pelvic pain patients and control patients. Nevertheless, in a study by Chan of 100 patients followed for a minimum for 6 months, adhesiolysis produced complete or partial pain relief in 65% of patients, whereas 20.9% said the pain was unchanged and 11.6% had more severe pain. This type of information is useful when counseling patients who are considering adhesiolysis. They should be informed that (1) adhesions are present but may not be the cause of pain, (2) they may not obtain relief with the procedure or the pain may become worse, and (3) adhesions may reform and result in further pain.

Uterine Suspension

Although unusual, uterine retrodisplacement may be associated with pelvic pain. The mere presence of retrodisplacement is not an indication for suspension because up to one third of all women may have a retroverted uterus. Typically, symptoms associated with uterine retroversion include a pressure sensation of the pelvis or low back or both. In addition, deep thrust or *bump* dyspareunia is a common symptom. *No surgical therapy for symptomatic retrodisplacement should be undertaken without a successful trial of pessary.* Such a trial entails placement of a pessary such as a Smith-Hodge to antevert the uterus. Uterine anteversion should relieve the pain if due to retrodisplacement. Removal of the pessary should result in return of pain.

In the older patient who does not desire future childbearing, vaginal hysterectomy is appropriate. In the younger patient, uterine suspension may be considered. The modified Gilliam suspension in which the round ligaments are drawn through an opening near the internal inguinal ring and sutured to the fascia is an excellent and classic choice for suspension. A more modern approach is laparoscopically to draw the round ligament up to the abdominal wall through second and third puncture sites and suture them to the rectus sheath.

Uterosacral Nerve Ablation and Presacral Neurectomy

Uterosacral nerve ablation appears to have only a limited role in the management of chronic pelvic pain. Uterosacral nerve ablation transects the afferent pain fibers within the uterosacral ligaments. Lichten reported significant relief of dysmenorrhea in 60% of patients refractory to OCPs and NSAIDs with laparoscopic uterosacral nerve ablation.

In the authors' opinion, uterosacral nerve ablation offers a secondary line of therapy for dysmenorrhea only. It can be performed at the time of diagnostic laparoscopy in those patients who do not respond to medical therapy. Potential long-term complications have not been evaluated and potentially include loss of cervical support and creation of large denuded areas posterior to the uterus, which may lead to adhesion formation in the area of the tubes and ovaries. The proximity of the ureters is also of concern to the gynecologic surgeon. It should be noted that the procedure should be reserved for dysmenorrhea only and not chronic pelvic pain. Considering that adhesions from PID are most likely in the adnexal area, the role of laparoscopic uterosacral nerve ablation should be quite limited.

Presacral neurectomy has also been advocated by some authors for patients with central pelvic pain. Current indications for presacral neurectomy are for relief of dysmenorrhea, deep thrust dyspareunia, sacral backache, and chronic recurrent pain in the center of the pelvis. In patients with chronic pelvic pain, Lee and colleagues reported a group of 50 patients undergoing presacral neurectomies for failed medical therapy for chronic pelvic pain, including dysmenorrhea and selected cases of dyspareunia. They found a 73% success rate in relieving dysmenorrhea, 77% in relieving dyspareunia, and 63% in relieving pelvic pain. The addition of bilateral uterosacral ligament did not increase the success rate. There was an 18% lateral pain recurrence but no recurrence of dysmenorrhea. The authors recommend that presacral neurectomy be reserved only for cases that fail all other conservation measures.

Hysterectomy

Although hysterectomy is usually reserved for those patients who do not obtain pain relief from medical or conservative surgical therapy, chronic pain is the third most common indication for hysterectomy. A study at the University of Tennessee, Memphis, evaluated the long-term outcome of 99 women who underwent hysterectomy for pelvic pain of at least 6 months' duration. All of these patients had symptoms and physical examination findings suggestive of disease confined to the uterus. Those patients with previously documented extrauterine disease or uterine weight exceeding 200 g were excluded from this review. Twenty-two patients had persistent pelvic pain even after hysterectomy, five describing their pain as being worse than before surgery. Information such as this regarding the likelihood of postoperative pain relief should be shared with all patients considering undergoing hysterectomy for pelvic pain of presumed uterine origin. Although a 75% cure rate may be appealing to some patients, others may prefer to explore other nonsurgical approaches when given these odds.

SUMMARY

The basic approach to the patient with chronic pelvic pain as practiced at the University of Tennessee, Memphis, has been described. Using this approach allows the practicing physician to evaluate and manage realistically or refer appropriately most patients with chronic pelvic pain. The key to management of patients who have chronic pelvic pain is to use all available diagnostic and therapeutic modalities to identify the source(s) and direct therapy. By having at least a working knowledge of the various diagnostic and therapeutic modalities available to the patient, the individual clinician can better aid the patient in her understanding of chronic pelvic pain generally and her own pelvic pain specifically.

RECOMMENDED READINGS

Chan C, Wood C: Pelvic adhesiolysis: The assessment of symptom relief by 100 patients. Aust NZ Obstet Gynaecol 25:295, 1985.

Fernandes M, Seebode J: Urologic causes of pelvic pain in the female. *In* Weiss G, ed: Clinical Consultations in Obstetrics and Gynecology. Philadelphia, WB Saunders, 1991, pp 46–53.

Lee R, Stone K, Magelssen D: Presacral neurectomy for chronic pelvic pain. Obstet Gynecol 68:517, 1986.

Milburn A, Reiter RC, Rhomberg AT: Multidisciplinary approach to chronic pelvic pain. Obstet Gynecol North Am 20:643, 1993.

Onghena P, Van Houdenhove BV: Antidepressant-induced analgesia in chronic nonmalignant pain: A meta-analysis of 39 placebo controlled studies. Pain 49:205, 1992.

Powell EM, Wattenburg CA: Treatment of urethritis in the female: With a clinical and pathological study. J Urol 72:392, 1954.

Rubelowski J, Machiedo G: Gastrointestinal causes of pelvic pain. *In* Weiss G, ed: Clinical Consultations in Obstetrics and Gynecology. Philadelphia, WB Saunders, 1991, pp 41–45.

Slocumb J: Neurologic factors in chronic pelvic pain: Trigger points and the abdominal pelvic pain syndrome. Am J Obstet Gynecol 149:536, 1984.

Summitt R, Ling F: Urethral syndrome presenting as chronic pelvic pain. J Psychol Obstet Gynecol 12:77, 1991.

Walling MK, Reiter RC, O'Hare MW, et al: Abuse history and chronic pain in women: I and II. Prevalences of sexual and physical abuse. Obstet Gynecol 84:193, 1994.

CHAPTER 9

Pelvic Mass

Shawn A. Menefee

Thomas Elkins

Every provider who sees women in his or her practice realizes that pelvic masses are common and difficult problems to evaluate. A pelvic mass can range from a simple physiologic ovarian cyst to an advanced ovarian malignancy. The provider must understand that a pelvic mass is not necessarily an adnexal mass or an ovarian cancer. The conditions that can present as a pelvic mass are quite vast and can involve a wide range of organ systems. These facts often make the evaluation of a pelvic mass a concerning problem for the primary care provider. This chapter discusses the differential diagnosis of pelvic masses in broad terms, including gynecologic and nongynecologic causes, and develops basic guidelines in evaluation and treatment that health care providers can follow when encountering this condition. It is often best to divide the patients into age groups to understand the underlying condition best and the best route of evaluation and therapy. In each age group, the concern with benign and malignant conditions is different; however, some conditions may be present in each age group. This chapter primarily discusses the gynecologic origin of pelvic masses and stresses that nongynecologic conditions must always be considered, especially in the very young and postmenopausal ages. The most troublesome problem in the evaluation and treatment of pelvic masses by the primary care provider is the misdiagnosis of conditions that may be life-threatening, such as an ectopic pregnancy that subsequently ruptures or a prolonged delay in diagnosis of a gynecologic malignancy. The basic considerations involved in a pelvic mass evaluation are outlined. The guidelines for emergent and routine referral and some controversial tests and management plans that the primary care provider may use in evaluating and treating pelvic masses are discussed later in the chapter. This chapter does not provide a detailed review of tumor types, pathology, or surgical management of these pelvic masses.

NEWBORNS AND CHILDREN

The primary care provider often has the advantage of caring for a patient beginning at birth and extending through the patient's life. In caring for these patients, an abdominal or pelvic mass may be encountered on routine physical examination. The presence of a pelvic mass in the newborn is most commonly related to estrogen stimulation that is provided by the

Table 9–1. Differential Diagnosis of a Pelvic Mass in Newborns and Children

Newborns
  Functional ovarian cyst
Children
  Ovarian
    Teratoma
    Dysgerminoma
  Wilms' tumor
  Neuroblastomas
  Lymphoma
  Burkitt's tumor
  Gastrointestinal
  Musculoskeletal

mother while the child is in utero resulting in the development of a follicular cyst on the fetal ovaries (Table 9–1). These cysts may be diagnosed in utero by fetal ultrasound or as an asymptomatic abdominal mass secondary to the shallow pelvis of the neonate and displacement upward of the cyst into the abdomen. These cysts generally regress after the first few months of life. The appearance of pelvic masses is rare in childhood until puberty. If abdominopelvic masses are encountered in children, they are usually related to Wilms' tumor or neuroblastomas.[1] Ovarian tumors are the most common genital neoplasm that occurs during childhood; however, overall ovarian tumors account for only about 1% of childhood tumors, and fortunately most are benign. The occurrence of an adnexal mass is rare in this age group; however, when found in this age group, the neoplasm is usually a dysgerminoma or teratoma.[2–5]

The evaluation and treatment of the neonate with a large follicular cyst, which is secondary to in utero stimulation by maternal gonadotropins or persistent hypothalamic pituitary activity, involve a detailed physical examination followed by abdominal ultrasound to assess the characteristics of the mass. The ultrasound usually reveals a simple ovarian follicular cyst. Because these cysts usually regress in 3 to 6 months, observation is an appropriate means of treatment. When observation is recommended for the simple cyst, the symptoms of ovarian torsion should be explained to the persons responsible for caring for the new-

born. If the simple cyst is persistent, ultrasound-guided cyst drainage may be performed.

In children, abdominopelvic masses usually are nongynecologic in origin. In this age group, genital neoplasms are a rare occurrence; however, the most common genital neoplasm is ovarian in origin and must be considered in the differential diagnosis. Even though the majority of these ovarian neoplasms are benign, the 35% malignancy rate requires referral to an appropriate specialist.[2–5,20] The symptoms of ovarian neoplasms in children may be nonspecific, including nausea, vomiting, chronic abdominal pain, fullness, and urinary complaints related to the size of the tumor. It may be noted by the child's caregiver or physician as an increase in abdominal girth or as an asymptomatic mass because of the abdominal location of the adnexa in children. The ovarian neoplasm may be of germ cell origin and produce estrogen or testosterone resulting in precocious development or masculinization. An adnexal mass may also present as acute severe pain related to torsion, perforation, or infarction that may resemble appendicitis. Intermittent severe abdominal pain may represent intermittent torsion of even a normal adnexa, which can progress into a pelvic mass with congestion followed by infarction. The evaluation must include an abdominal palpation with rectoabdominal examination. In the patient with severe abdominal pain, immediate referral is needed after the history and physical examination is performed by the primary care provider. In those patients with a stable adnexal mass, it is appropriate to perform a pelvic ultrasound for assessment. A timely referral is required to a qualified specialist who may desire alternative imaging in children. The use of tumor markers in this age group does not affect preoperative management and is usually reserved for postoperative follow-up; thus, serum tumor markers need not be obtained by the primary care provider before referral.

ADOLESCENTS

The beginning of menarche to age 20 is an age group in which pelvic masses be-

Table 9–2. Differential Diagnosis of Pelvic Mass in Adolescent Girls

Obstructive genital lesion
    Imperforate hymen
    Blinded uterine horn
Ovarian
    Functional
    Germ cell tumors
    Other ovarian neoplasm
Tubal
    Paratubal cyst
    Ectopic gestation
    Tubo-ovarian abscess
    Pyosalpinx
Uterine
    Cornual ectopic gestation
    Leiomyoma
    Pregnancy including molar gestation
Gastrointestinal
    Appendiceal abscess

gin to become a more commonly encountered problem. The differential diagnosis at this time becomes more varied for several reasons, including the menstrual cycle, the functioning ovary, and the possibility of pregnancy (Table 9–2). With the onset of the menarche, the mechanical obstruction of the genital tract may first become apparent when associated with a pelvic mass because of hematocolpos, hematometra, or a dilated uterine horn. With the onset of ovulation, the functional ovary begins to produce physiologic ovarian cysts that may become symptomatic throughout the reproductive years in some women. Benign and malignant neoplasms, however, even though a rare occurrence in this age group, must be considered in the differential diagnosis. In addition to producing physiologic ovarian cysts, the functional ovary allows the adolescent to become fertile, which can result in pregnancy. Pregnancy in either intrauterine and extrauterine location is a major cause for a pelvic mass in this age group. Lastly, with the onset of sexual relationships for some in this age group, pelvic infection and salpingitis may progress to pyosalpinx or a tubo-ovarian abscess. The sequelae of these pelvic infections are more commonly seen in the reproductive-age group discussed next. When evaluating an adolescent with an infectious pelvic mass, the occurrence of appendiceal abscess must be considered in the differential diagnosis. Adolescents often present with symptomatic pelvic masses because they are usually otherwise healthy and do not seek care on a regular basis.

The basic evaluation of patients in this age group includes a complete history and physical examination. This evaluation should include a menstrual history, including the presence of dysmenorrhea. The congenital obstructive lesion often presents with absent menstrual cycles but cyclic lower abdominal pain. The physical examination enables the primary care physician to identify the hematocolpos secondary to an imperforate hymen. A blind uterine horn presents with cyclic menstrual bleeding; however, the patient also has severe cyclic pelvic pain and a pelvic mass on examination. These patients should be referred for gynecologic care in a timely manner after assessing the hemodynamic status of the patient. With congenital reproductive tract abnormalities, approximately one third of the patients also have urinary tract abnormalities, including pelvic kidney, renal agenesis, horseshoe kidney, or abnormality in the collecting ducts; thus, some advocate intravenous pyleogram to assess the urinary tract.

Pelvic masses are most commonly the result of physiologic ovarian cysts and are frequently treated by the primary care provider. This is related to a physiologic ovulatory response that can range from being asymptomatic to requiring surgical management related to rupture of hemorrhagic cyst or torsion of the adnexa. Even though a large percentage of adolescent pelvic masses are physiologic ovulatory cysts, adnexal masses in this age group may be neoplastic in origin. The majority of these neoplasms are benign cystic teratomas; however, malignant tumors, usually of the germ cell type, are also encountered in this age group.[2–5] This fact requires that these patients have a complete evaluation, including a gynecologic examination, pregnancy testing, and complete blood count if indicated by the clinical condition. The majority of adnexal masses, however, are due to functional ovarian cysts, which may be followed and treated symptomatically with nonsteroidal anti-inflammatory drugs if the size of the cyst is less than 5 cm and the patient has no evidence of an acute abdomen. The addition of oral contraceptives does not affect the resolution of the current ovarian cyst but allows suppression of future ovulation and prevents future symptomatic ovarian cysts if so desired by the patient. Thus, in this group, ultrasound is not required as long as a follow-up examination is performed in 4 to 6 weeks. Patients with cysts greater than 5 cm or not resolving over 4 to 6 weeks should have a pelvic ultrasound. The use of vaginal and abdominal ultrasound can often help characterize the adnexal mass. An abdominal radiograph may also be helpful in diagnosis of teratoma with its calcification and fat pad. Patients with severe pain, persistent cyst, or cyst greater than 10 cm should be referred to a gynecologist. In addition, any adolescent patient with pelvic mass and masculinization should have a timely referral. Although most adnexal masses in this age group are benign, it is important for the primary care provider to make the diagnosis early to improve the prognosis for malignant lesions and decrease the possibility of adnexal torsion and possible loss of the adnexa.

The other possible causes of pelvic masses in this age group are often related to pregnancy or infection. The need for urine pregnancy testing in adolescents with a pelvic mass cannot be stressed enough because it allows the physician to recognize the potential life-threatening condition of an extrauterine pregnancy, especially in this age group in which patients often deny and avoid treatment for the pregnancy.[7] Thus, any adolescent with a pelvic mass or fullness should have a urine pregnancy test to rule out pregnancy. In patients who also have abdominal pain with a positive urine pregnancy test and normal size uterus, a pelvic ultrasound should be obtained with quantitative human chorionic gonadotropin (hCG) assay. When obtaining hCG levels, the primary care provider needs to be aware of the levels that can alert the physician to difficulties with the pregnancy. In the acute setting, the hCG level should be correlated with the ultrasound findings. With a vaginal ultrasound, the hCG level at which the ultrasound should reveal evidence of an intrauterine pregnancy is between 1000 and 1500 IU/L.[8] With abdominal ultrasound evidence of an intrauterine pregnancy should be observed at an hCG level of 6500 IU/L or greater.[43] If ectopic gestation is suspected or discovered, gynecologic consultation should be obtained at that time. If the uterus is found to be enlarged to 10 weeks' size or larger, the presence of fetal heart tones can assure fetal viability, and thus hCG and ultrasound may not be needed.

For the patient who presents for evaluation with a pelvic mass associated with signs of infection, the primary care provider must consider pyosalpinx and a tubo-ovarian abscess as well as an appendiceal abscess. It is important to obtain a complete blood count, cervical cultures, and screen for other sexual transmitted diseases as part of the initial evaluation. These patients require hospitalization for intravenous antibiotics to treat the salpingitis aggressively in hopes of decreasing the severity of tubal damage and preventing sequela of pelvic inflammatory disease. With inadequate treatment or progression of the pelvic infection, a tubo-ovarian abscess may develop in the pelvis resulting in a palpable pelvic mass usually with elevation of white blood cell count, fever, and abdominal pain. If there is a question of appendicitis, appendiceal abscess, or ruptured tubo-ovarian abscess, these patients need immediate referral to the appropriate surgical team (Table 9–3).

Table 9–3. Surgical Emergency

Ruptured ectopic gestation
  Tubal
  Cornual
  Abdominal
Torsion of the adnexal
Ruptured tubo-ovarian abscess
Ruptured hemorrhagic ovarian cyst (hemodynamically comprised)

Table 9-4. Nongynecologic Causes
of Pelvic Masses

Gastrointestinal
   Cecal carcinoma
   Crohn's at terminal ileum
   Sigmoid colon diverticulitis
   Appendiceal abscess
   Rectosigmoidal carcinoma
Urinary tract
   Urologic neoplasm
   Pelvic kidney
Retroperitoneal tumors
   Lymphoma
   Anterior meningocele
   Neurogenic tumors
      Neurofibromas
   Soft tissue neuromas
   Retroperitoneal cyst
Vascular
   Iliac aneurysm
   Arteriovenous fistula
Peritoneum
   Peritoneal cysts
Metastatic
   Gastrointestinal primary
   Breast

Adapted from Isaacs JH: Nongynecologic conditions encountered by the gynecologic surgeon. *In* Thompson JD, Rock JA, eds: Te Linde's Operative Gynecology. Philadelphia, JB Lippincott, 1992, pp 1049–1063.

REPRODUCTIVE-AGE WOMEN (20 TO 45 YEARS)

In the reproductive-age woman, the cause of a pelvic mass begins to expand quite rapidly. Nongynecologic causes of a pelvic mass must be considered in this age group (Table 9–4). In this group of women, however, a pelvic mass usually arises from the genital tract (Table 9–5). As previously discussed with the adolescent patient, the primary care provider must always consider pregnancy as a cause of a pelvic mass because an extrauterine pregnancy can be a life-threatening condition if not considered in all potentially fertile women.[7] Thus, an ectopic gestation must be considered in those pregnant patients with an adnexal fullness or mass and must be ruled out by an appropriate evaluation. The adnexa (the ovary and fallopian tube) is commonly involved in conditions that present as a pelvic mass. The ovary may be the site of an ovarian cyst, primary and metastatic neoplasm, or an endometrioma. In the reproductive-age group, the most common adnexal mass is a physiologic ovarian cyst, with the most common neoplasm being a benign cystic teratoma. Several conditions involving the fallopian tube can result in a pelvic mass as well. Most commonly, this is related to a paratubal cyst or the sequela of previous salpingitis with the occlusion of the fallopian tube resulting in a pyosalpinx, hydrosalpinx, or tubo-ovarian abscess. Lastly a pelvic mass can be more commonly related to the uterus and cervix, including the leiomyomatous uterus and cancer of the uterus and cervix. The evaluation and treatment of these genital causes of a pelvic mass in the reproductive woman are discussed.

The evaluation and treatment of an intrauterine pregnancy, ectopic pregnancy, or functional ovarian cysts does not differ from that for the adolescent age group. When expectant management does not result in resolution of the mass, symptoms exceed over 6 weeks, or symptoms have become severe, the woman should be referred to a gynecologist for a consultation. Patients with worsening symptoms and patients with multiple or complex cysts should be referred for further evaluation. Percutaneous needle aspiration for functional ovarian cyst has been recommended by some and is discussed later.

Table 9-5. Differential Diagnosis of a Pelvic
Mass in Reproductive-Age Women

Uterine
   Leiomyoma
   Cornual ectopic
   Pregnancy including molar gestation
Cervical
   Neoplasm
Tubal
   Paratubal cyst
   Ectopic gestation
   Tubo-ovarian abscess
   Pyosalpinx
   Hydrosalpinx
Ovarian
   Functional
   Neoplastic
   Endometrioma

The fallopian tube can cause of pelvic mass in this age group. A paratubal cyst usually presents as an asymptomatic unilocular cyst found on ultrasound or becomes symptomatic if it undergoes torsion. The sequela of previous salpingitis with occlusion of the tube resulting in pyosalpinx, hydrosalpinx or tubo-ovarian abscess may present as a pelvic mass as well. Tubo-ovarian abscesses have been reported to occur in up to one third of women hospitalized with salpingitis.[10] Tubo-ovarian abscess is one of the most common causes of pelvic masses in reproductive-age women, and it is the most common intra-abdominal abscess in premenopausal women.[11] The patient with a tubo-ovarian abscess typically presents with abdominal or pelvic pain that is associated with elevated temperature. Physical examination reveals lower abdominal or pelvic tenderness often with peritoneal signs. The patient with a tubo-ovarian abscess may have severe abdominal tenderness, and it is often difficult to palpate a mass on bimanual examination. Thus, a pelvic ultrasound should be obtained on all patients when a tubo-ovarian abscess is suspected. The laboratory tests that are helpful include complete blood count, sexually transmitted disease screening with cervical cultures or probes, human immunodeficiency virus, rapid plasma reagin, blood cultures, and sedimentation rate. Antibiotic therapy is successful in most women.[12–15] Even with these excellent rates of cure in the acute phase, the primary care provider must keep in mind that many of these patients subsequently require surgical intervention, and thus early consultation with a gynecologist is helpful. Surgical intervention is required for suspected rupture, appendicitis, and failure to respond to antibiotic therapy. Percutaneous drainage of tubo-ovarian abscesses is discussed later.

The other adnexal masses in the reproductive years may involve any known ovarian tumor, including metastatic tumors. The most common neoplastic ovarian mass is the benign cystic teratoma.[9] Even though the presence of adnexal malignancy is rare in this age group, ovarian cancer must be considered in patients with suspicious histories, physical examination, or radiographic findings. Endometriosis can present as an endometrioma of the ovary. Patients often have symptoms of endometriosis.

A pelvic mass related to the uterus and cervix is more common in the reproductive-age woman. The evaluation of the uterus and cervix is an essential component in the evaluation of a pelvic mass in this group of women. In the United States, leiomyomas are found in 10% of white women and 30% to 40% of African-American women over the age of 35.[16] In any of the varied locations of myomas, degeneration, infarction, and infection can occur with these neoplasms and be associated with a pelvic mass, significant lower abdominal and pelvic pain, and abnormal bleeding. Uterine leiomyomas are usually asymptomatic. The asymptomatic enlargement of the uterus does not require surgical therapy. Myomas can be subserosal, intramural, submucosal, pedunculated, and within the leaves of the broad ligament. The myomatous uterus, however, can grow to a significant size in the absence of menorrhagia resulting in symptoms related to its size, including pain, pressure, increasing abdominal girth, and bladder and bowel complaints. A pedunculated myoma or a broad ligament myoma may present as a solid adnexal mass on examination. Lastly, uterine and cervical malignancies start to occur in this age group and must be considered in the differential diagnosis.

A pelvic mass related to a leiomyomatous uterus can be followed by an experienced physician. The patient may have numerous symptoms related to the size of the leiomyoma or may be asymptomatic. In the patient with a symptomatic leiomyomatous uterus, a conservative or definitive myomyectomy or hysterectomy may be the best treatment plan. In these cases the patient should be referred to a gynecologist for possible surgery. An endometrial biopsy should be performed on those patients with an enlarged uterus, abnormal uterine bleeding, or prolonged anovulation. In those patients with asymptomatic leiomyomatous uterus or those desiring expectant management, it is often prudent to obtain an ultrasound to confirm the diagnosis. As stated earlier, endometrial biopsy may also be of benefit in certain patients who desire expectant management along with a complete blood count to ensure that the uterine blood loss is not being underestimated by the patient. In addition, if the patient is anemic, the primary care provider can place her on iron therapy if the anemia is related to blood loss. The use of gonadotropin-releasing hormone agonists in the treatment of the leiomyomatous uterus has two indications: The first purpose is to reduce menorrhagia and improve the anemia, and the second is to decrease the size of the leiomyoma to assist the surgeon with myomectomy or vaginal hysterectomy. This is best managed in conjunction with or by a gynecologist. Likewise, a pelvic mass associated with a cervical lesion should be managed in a similar fashion by the primary care provider including cervical biopsy if the provider is experienced in the biopsy of potential cervical malignancy. Because primary care providers often care for reproductive-age women on a regular basis, annual cytologic examination of the cervix should be performed as preventive care.

PERIMENOPAUSAL AND POSTMENOPAUSAL WOMEN (OLDER THAN 45 YEARS)

In this age group, the presence of pelvic mass must be considered more carefully because neoplasms from both the genital and other organ systems occur more frequently (Table 9–6). Ovarian cancer affects 1 in every 70 women in their lifetime, with two thirds of these cancers being advanced stage III or IV at diagnosis, and ovarian cancer causes more deaths than any other genital tract cancer. The majority of these cases, 80%, involve women over the age of 50.[17-19] Obviously a physician should be concerned whenever a pelvic mass is discovered in a postmenopausal woman. In addition, gastrointestinal tract diverticuli and cancer must be considered in every patient with a pelvic mass, especially those in the perimenopausal and postmenopausal age group. Primary tumors from the genitourinary, musculoskeletal, and lymphatic tract are also more common in this group of patients. Metastatic tumors to

Table 9–6. Differential Diagnosis of a Pelvic Mass in Perimenopausal and Postmenopausal Women

Uterine
Leiomyoma
Neoplasm
Cervical
Neoplasm
Fallopian tube
Paratubal cyst
Neoplasm
Ovarian
Neoplasm
Benign
Malignant

the ovaries include gastrointestinal and breast cancers.

The benign genital conditions seen in the reproductive-age group are seen in this age group, such as uterine myomas and endometriosis, but less frequently require surgical therapy. In the postmenopausal age group, leiomyomatous uterus has been reported to have an incidence of 30% in white women and 40% to 50% in African-American women.[16] These neoplasms are hormone dependent and usually shrink following menopause. Uterine myomas and endometriosis, commonly found in the reproductive-age group, can be considered in the differential diagnosis; however, the malignant uterine tumors, including adenocarcinoma, sarcomas, and mixed mesodermal tumors, are most commonly present in this age group. These uterine tumors must be considered in the postmenopausal patient with enlarging uterine mass. Sarcomatous elements within the uterus may present as a rapidly enlarging mass often associated with pain and tenderness. Likewise, adnexal masses occurring in the postmenopausal age group can be benign, but the likelihood of malignancy increases with age.

The evaluation and treatment in the perimenopausal and postmenopausal age groups must include a thorough evaluation of other organ systems. The health care provider must inquire about gastrointestinal complaints and history of breast mass or lesions. If the history or physical examination points toward another organ system, appropriate screening tests must be performed, including mammogram, barium enema, or colonoscopy/flexible sigmoidoscopy.

The evaluation of gynecologic origin of a pelvic mass must again be complete, with a malignancy from the vagina, cervix, uterus, fallopian tube, and ovaries all being possible in this age group. A history of any previous gynecologic surgery or tumors needs to be discussed as well as obtaining operative and pathologic records if possible because many patients do not know the details of previous illnesses. The date of last gynecologic examination allows the physician to determine if the mass is rapidly growing or not. Any visible abnormality of the vulva, vagina, or cervix should be biopsied and sent for pathologic study. A cytologic smear may be obtained from the cervix or vaginal cuff if not screened recently. The pelvic mass associated with postmenopausal bleeding or menstrual irregularities should be evaluated with endometrial biopsy. A negative endometrial biopsy for hyperplasia or cancer with an enlarged uterus, however, should not delay referral with the possibility of sarcoma, which is usually not obtained on endometrial biopsy because of the intramural location. As stated previously, the presence of leiomyoma in the postmenopausal woman is not an indication for surgery as long as the uterus is not enlarging. An enlarging postmenopausal myoma is suspicious for a sarcoma and should be referred for evaluation and surgical removal.

A pelvic mass present on pelvic examination with a normal cervix and uterus suggests the fallopian tubes and ovaries as a possible source for the adnexal mass. The fallopian tube as a source of pelvic mass is uncommon in the postmenopausal age group, with infectious and pregnancy causes not present. Fallopian tube carcinoma is rare accounting for less than 1% of all genital cancers.[21] The classic presentation is watery cervical discharge, pain, and menorrhagia with a pelvic mass. It should be treated similar to ovarian cancer with referral to a gynecologic oncologist.

The primary concern of an adnexal mass is ovarian cancer. The history should include questions about abdominal discomfort, increased abdominal girth, and previous surgical therapy along with other general questions. The physical examination, similar to all gynecologic examinations with pelvic mass, should include rectovaginal examination with testing for occult blood. Ultrasound is helpful in evaluating the adnexal mass. Factors that increase the likelihood of an ovarian malignancy include size greater than 10 cm, ascites, and bilaterality.[22] A CA-125 tumor marker should be ordered in the postmenopausal patient with a pelvic mass. There may be a role for conservative management in postmenopausal cystic adnexal structures that are unilateral, unilocular with no septation or ascites, and less than 3 to 5 cm, with follow-up examination and ultrasound every 10 to 12 weeks.[22-25] It is best for the primary care provider, however, to refer the postmenopausal patient with an adnexal mass as described previously for evaluation by a gynecologist.

CONTROVERSIAL ISSUES

Cyst Aspiration

As stated earlier, a large percentage of pelvic and adnexal masses are related to physiologic ovarian cyst. The possibility of cyst aspiration to relieve pain related to these cysts has been considered with numerous reports in the literature.[26-29] The aspiration of ovarian cysts and pelvic fluid collection (tubo-ovarian abscess, pelvic abscess, and endometrioma) has also been described in the literature. Aspiration of cysts may be enhanced with computed tomography (CT) and ultrasound.

The role of cyst aspiration is controversial. Malignant cells may be spread if an ovarian cancer is drained by aspiration. Cyst rupture intraoperatively has not been shown to affect the prognosis even though it does change the stage. The possibility of spillage exists without the ability to irrigate and remove any gross spillage as the surgeon can do at laparotomy or laparoscopic surgery. This fact is concerning to all that treat ovarian cancer.[30] Tubo-ovarian abscess or pelvic abscess drainage may result in spillage of purulent material resulting in peritonitis and thus resembling ruptures of intra-abdominal abscess that may result in sepsis and may require surgical therapy. Hemorrhage may occur if vascular damage occurs or the cyst bleeds.

Most primary care providers do not have adequate experience with ultrasound to perform ultrasound-guided aspirations themselves; thus, they must rely on an interventional radiologist or gynecologist to assist or perform this procedure. One should understand the risks and benefits to this controversial procedure before requesting it as treatment. The ultrasound-guided cyst aspiration should definitely not be performed on the following patients: premenarcheal or postmenopausal patients with the exception being the newborn with persistent simple cyst or suspicious cyst by ultrasound. The use of ultrasound must be standardized when describing adnexal masses. Sassone and colleagues[31] described a grading scale with transvaginal ultrasound to determine the likelihood of benign or malignant neoplasms. This scale allows physicians to observe safely or perform needle aspiration on benign ovarian cysts and refer quickly those suspicious for malignancy (Table 9–7).

The aspiration of ovarian cysts may be considered in the adolescent and reproductive-age groups with simple unilocular ovarian cysts without evidence of ascites or excrescence and size less than 5 cm in diameter. It must be remembered that the majority of ovarian cysts are functional and resolve in 4 to 6 weeks.

Table 9–7. Adnexal Mass: Indications for Surgery

Ovarian cystic structure >5 cm that has been followed 6–8 wk without regression
Any solid ovarian lesion
  Any ovarian lesion with papillary vegetation on the cyst wall
Any adnexal mass >10 cm in diameter
Ascites
Palpable adnexal mass in a premenarcheal or postmenopausal patient
Torsion or rupture suspected

From DiSaia PJ, Creasman WT: The adnexal mass and early ovarian cancer. *In* DiSaia PJ, Creasman WT, eds: Clinical Gynecologic Oncology. St. Louis, Mosby-Year Book, 1993, p 304.

Those that do not resolve are more likely to represent endometriomas or benign serous or mucinous tumors that may be better evaluated and treated via laparoscopy or laparotomy.

Several investigations demonstrated CT-guided or ultrasound-guided percutaneous drainage of tubo-ovarian abscess to be safe, effective therapy with clinical improvement and avoidance of surgery in 77% to 93%.[32–35] The use of percutaneous drainage may consist of drainage only or aspiration with insertion of catheters for drainage. If one is considering percutaneous drainage, the abscess must be well defined and localized with a safe access route. Unilocular abscesses have higher success rates and lower complication rates when compared with more complex multiloculated abscesses.[36] The use of percutaneous drainage of pelvic abscesses, including the tubo-ovarian abscess, is best managed by a gynecologist or a radiologist experienced in aspiration. In certain patients, especially those who are poor surgical candidates, the use of percutaneous drainage may be helpful because it can be performed under local anesthesia only in most cases.

Tumor Markers

A screening test for ovarian cancer is needed desperately with a large majority of ovarian cancers presenting as stage III or IV cancers with poor prognosis. The CA-125 is the only tumor marker currently approved by the Food and Drug Administration in the United States for assessing women with ovarian cancer. It is approved for only one indication, as an alternative to second-look operation. The CA-125 has been used as a screening test for ovarian cancer in high-risk patients; however, it is not recognized as a cost-effective screening tool. The CA-125 is the antigenic determinant of a high molecular glycoprotein that is recognized by a monoclonal antibody raised to an ovarian cancer cell line as an immunogen.[37] Other tumor markers for ovarian cancers have been introduced to be used as a screening tool alone and in combination; however, these markers seem to be more of a research tool at this time. Standard tumor markers may be elevated in other tumor types, including alpha$_1$-feto protein with germ cell ovarian neoplasm, hCG with embryonal carcinoma of the ovary or molar gestation, and estrogen and testosterone with stromal cell tumors produced by specific ovarian neoplasms. The CA-125 seems to have good utility detecting nonmucinous epithelial cancers of the ovary, the most common ovarian tumor in the perimenopausal and postmenopausal age group.[37–40]

The major disadvantage to CA-125 is the lack of sensitivity because many conditions result in elevated levels, including pregnancy, myomas, endometriosis, adenomyosis, and pelvic inflammatory disease. Nongynecologic conditions include cirrhosis; colonic, pancreatic, and breast tumors; and any condition that irritates the peritoneum. Nonmalignant conditions occur in the reproductive-age group and limit the use of CA-125. CA-125 levels may not be elevated even with some nonmucinous ovarian neoplasms in stage I and II disease.[41] The use of CA-125 may be appropriate in the postmenopausal patient with a pelvic mass who is being referred to a gynecologist or gynecologic oncologist. Currently the use of CA-125 as a screening tool is not recommended.

Imaging of the Pelvic Mass

In the past, the major tool for the diagnosis of a pelvic mass involved a gynecologic physical examination and clinical history. The physical examination can help characterize the pelvic mass and often allow the experienced examiner to determine the location and origin of the mass in the pelvis. Even experienced examiners, however, may be surprised at the operative findings. The use of an ultrasound examination is more precise in detecting ovarian tumors than pelvic examination.[28] The use of imaging with a pelvic mass has allowed the gynecologic health care provider to assess the character of these masses, often resulting in safe expectant management of the pelvic mass. The use of ultrasound in evaluation of pelvic masses often allows characterization and location of the mass.

Ultrasound for ovarian cancer has been considered in the past. As with all screening tests, numerous factors must be considered in determining the reliability and advantages for use, and this discussion is beyond the scope of this chapter. The major considerations in the use of pelvic ultrasound for screening involve the following factors: the low incidence of ovarian cancer in the general population, the cost of the screening, and how abnormal ovaries that do not appear malignant on ultrasound would be managed. The use of abdominal and vaginal ultrasound is helpful in characterizing pelvic masses. The authors recommend ultrasound as a screening tool for ovarian masses.

REFERENCES

1. Stenchever MA: Significant symptoms and signs in different age groups. *In* Herbst AL, Mishell DR, Stenchever MA, Droegemueller W, eds: Comprehensive Gynecology. St. Louis, Mosby, 1992, p 176.
2. Asadourian LA, Taylor HB: Dysgerminomas: An analysis of 105 cases. Obstet Gynecol 1969; 33:370–379.
3. Caruso PA, Marsh MR, Minkowitz S, Karten G: An intense clinical pathologic study of 305 teratomas of the ovary. Cancer 1971; 27:343.
4. Costin ME, Kennedy RJL: Ovarian tumors in infants and children. Am J Dis Child 1948; 76:127.
5. Mueller CW, Thompkins P, Lapp WA: Dysgerminona of the ovary: An analysis of 427 cases. Am J Obstet Gynecol 1950; 60:153.
6. Speroff L, Glass RH, Kase NG: Amenorrhea. *In* Speroff L, Glass RH, Kase NG, eds: Clinical Gynecologic Endocrinology and Infertility. Baltimore, Williams & Wilkins, 1994, p 420.
7. Ansbacher R, Mills EM, Thrush JC, Stevenson LO: Ectopic pregnancy and maternal mortality in Michigan. Am J Gynecol Health III 1989; 4:118–123.
8. Keith SC, London SN, Weitzman GA, et al: Serial transvaginal ultrasound scans and beta-human chorionic gonadotropin levels in early singleton and multiple pregnancies. Fertil Steril 1993; 59:1007.
9. Peterson WF, et al: Benign cystic teratoma of the ovary: A clinico-statistical study of 1007 cases with a review of the literature. Am J Obstet Gynecol 1955; 70:568.

10. Sweet RL, Gibbs RS: Pelvic infection and abscess. *In* Sweet RL, Gibbs RS eds: Infectious Diseases of the Female Genital Tract. Baltimore, Williams & Wilkins, 1990, p 90.

11. Wiesenfeld HC, Sweet RL: Progress in the management of tuboovarian abscess. Clin Obstet Gynecol 1993; 36:433–444.

12. Landers DV, Wolner-Hanssen P, Paavonen J, et al: Combination antimicrobial therapy in the treatment of acute pelvic inflammatory disease. Am J Obstet Gynecol 1991; 164:849.

13. Walters MD, Gibbs RS: A randomized comparison of gentamicin-clindamycin and cefoxitin-doxycycline in the treatment of acute pelvic inflammatory disease. Obstet Gynecol 1990; 75:867.

14. Soper DE, Despres B: A comparison of two antibiotic regimens for treatment of pelvic inflammatory disease. Obstet Gynecol 1988; 72:7.

15. Sweet RL, Schachter J, Landers DV, et al: Treatment of hospitalized patients with acute pelvic inflammatory disease: Comparison of cefotetan plus doxycycline and cefoxitin plus doxycycline. Am J Obstet Gynecol 1988; 158:736.

16. DiSaia PJ, Creasman WT: The adnexal mass and early ovarian cancer. *In* DiSaia PJ, Creasman WT, eds: Clinical Gynecologic Oncology. St. Louis, Mosby-Year Book, 1993, pp 302–332.

17. Boring CC, Squires TS, Tong T: Cancer statistics, 1991. CA 1991; 41:19.

18. Culter SJ, Young JL, eds: Third National Cancer Survey: Incidence Data. Washington, DC, National Cancer Institute Monogr 41, U.S. Department of Health, Education, and Welfare publication (NIH) 75–77, 1975.

19. Petterson F, ed: Annual Report on the Results of Treatment in Gynecologic Cancer. International Federation of Gynecology and Obstetrics. Stockholm, 1990, p 20.

20. Breen JL, Maxon WS: Ovarian tumors in children and adolescents. Clin Obstet Gynecol 1977; 20:671.

21. DiSaia PJ, Creasman WT: The adnexal mass and early ovarian cancer. *In* DiSaia PJ, Creasman WT, eds: Clinical Gynecologic Oncology. St. Louis, Mosby-Year Book, 1993, p 484.

22. Rulin MC, Prestin AL: Adnexal masses in postmenopausal women. Obstet Gynecol 1987; 70:578–581.

23. Hall DA, McCarthy KA: The significance of the postmenopausal simple adnexal cyst. J Ultrasound Med 1986; 5:503–505.

24. Goldstein SR, Subramanyam B, Snyder JR, et al: The postmenopausal cystic adnexal mass: The potential role of ultrasound in conservative management. Obstet Gynecol 1989; 73:8–10.

25. Goldstein SR: Conservative management of small postmenopausal cystic masses. Clin Obstet Gynecol 1993; 36:395–401.

26. Dordoni D, Zaglio S, Zucca S, Favalli G: The role of sonographically guided aspiration in the clinical management of ovarian cysts. J Ultrasound Med 1993; 12:27–31.

27. Weinraub Z, Avrech O, Fuchs C, et al: Transvaginal aspiration of ovarian cysts: Prognosis based on outcome over a 12 month period. J Ultrasound Med 1994; 13:275–279.

28. Caspi B, Zalel Y, Lurie S, et al: Ultrasound-guided aspiration for relief of pain generated by simple ovarian cysts. Gynecol Obstet Invest 1993; 35:121–122.

29. Lee CL, Lai YM, Chang SY, et al: The management of ovarian cysts by sonoguided transvaginal cyst aspiration. J Clin Ultrasound 1993; 21:511–514.

30. Trimbos JB, Hacker NF: The case against aspirating ovarian cysts. Cancer 1993; 72:828–830.

31. Sassone AM, Timor-Tritsch IE, Artner A, et al: Transvaginal sonographic characterization of ovarian disease: Evaluation of a new scoring system to predict ovarian malignancy. Obstet Gynecol 1991; 78:70–76.

32. Tyrrel RT, Murphy FB, Bernardino ME: Tubo-ovarian abscesses: CT-guided percutaneous drainage. Radiology 1990; 175:87.

33. Worthen NJ, Gunning JE: Percutaneous drainage of pelvic abscess: Management of the tubo-ovarian abscess. J Ultrasound Med 1986; 5:551.

34. Casda G, van Sonnenberg E, D'Agostino HB, et al: Percutaneous drainage of tubo-ovarian abscesses. Radiology 1992; 182:399.

35. Shulamn A, Maymor R, Shapiro A, et al: Percutaneous catheter drainage of tubo-ovarian abscesses. Obstet Gynecol 1992; 80:555.

36. Fabiszewski NL, Sumkin JH, Johns CM: Contemporary radiographic percutaneous abscess drainage in the pelvis. Clin Obstet Gynecol 1993; 36:445–456.

37. Bast RC Jr, Klug TJ, St John E, et al: A radioimmunoassay using a monoclonal antibody to monitor the course of epithelial ovarian cancer. N Engl J Med 1983; 309:883.

38. Mann WJ, Pastner B, Cohen H, et al: Preoperative evaluation of serum CA 125 levels in patients with surgical stage I invasive ovarian adenocarcinoma. J Natl Cancer Inst 1988; 80:208.

39. Romero R, Schwartz PE: Alpha fetaprotein determinations in the management of endodermal sinus tumors and mixed germ cell tumors of the ovary. Am J Obstet Gynecol 1981; 141:126.

40. Schwartz PE, Chambers SK, Chamber JT, et al: Ovarian germ cell malignancies: The Yale University experiences. Gynecol Oncol 1992; 45:26.

41. Mann WJ, Bast RC Jr, Knapp RC, et al: Preoperative evaluation of serum CA 125 levels in patients with primary epithelial ovarian cancer. Obstet Gynecol 1986; 67:414.

42. Andolf E: Ultrasound screening in women at risk for ovarian cancer. Clin Obstet Gynecol 1993; 36:423–432.

43. Kadar N, Caldwell BV, Romereo R: A method of screening for ectopic pregnancy and its indications. Obstet Gynecol 1981; 58:162.

CHAPTER 10

Abnormal Vaginal Bleeding

Richard E. Leach

Menstrual disorders are among the most common disorders treated by gynecologists constituting 10% to 35% of patient encounters. Hypermenorrhea or menorrhagia, which is excessive bleeding both in amount and duration of flow, is reported to occur in 2% to 4% of women.[1] It is important to have a disciplined and systematic approach to the evaluation and treatment of abnormal bleeding. This chapter provides a rational and deliberate scheme in caring for women with menstrual abnormalities.

The characteristics of the normal menstrual cycle have been clearly defined. The mean interval between menstrual cycles is 28 days and is considered abnormal if the frequency of menses is less than or equal to 21 days (polymenorrhea) or greater than 35 days (oligomenorrhea). The mean duration of menstrual flow is 4 days. If the duration of flow is greater than 7 days or the mean blood loss exceeds 80 ml, the woman is considered to have menorrhagia.[2] It is difficult to estimate menstrual volume; however, a clinically useful estimate of excessive bleeding is suggested when a woman is saturating a sanitary napkin hourly over a several-hour period. Hypomenorrhea is defined as decreased menstrual flow at regular intervals. Metrorrhagia is uterine bleeding at regular intervals and menometrorrhagia is frequent irregular heavy uterine bleeding. Uterine bleeding may be categorized into three groups: (1) organic, (2) systemic, and (3) dysfunctional (Table 10–1 and 10–2).

By definition, dysfunctional uterine bleeding (DUB) is a diagnosis of exclusion when no organic or systemic cause can be identified. It is clearly important that sufficient consideration of organic and systemic causes be made before the diagnosis of DUB is made.

EVALUATION

History and Physical Examination

Early in the evaluation, it is helpful to evaluate the causes of abnormal uterine bleeding as related to age. For example, in a woman of childbearing age, pregnancy or related complications, infection, and contraceptive methods are the most common associated conditions. For the perimenopausal woman, organic lesions such as leiomyoma and polyps occur frequently as well as ovarian dysfunction. Lastly, postmenopausal women frequently have irregular bleeding because of hormone replacement therapy, but the

Table 10-1. Organic Causes of Abnormal Vaginal Bleeding Classified by Anatomic Site

Site	Diagnosis
Vulva/vagina	Vulvitis, vaginitis
	Atrophic changes
	Coitus
	Tumor
	Foreign body
Cervix	Cervicitis
	Ectropion
	Polyp, carcinoma
	Ectopic pregnancy
	Endometriosis
Uterus	Pregnancy
	Fibroids
	Polyps
	Endometritis
	Hyperplasia, carcinoma
	Adenomyosis
	Intrauterine device
Adnexa	Ectopic pregnancy
	Ovarian tumors
	Salpingo-oophoritis
	Endometriosis

potential for endometrial hyperplasia and carcinoma must always be kept in mind.

The initial assessment of the patient should elicit a clear understanding of the bleeding pattern and volume. Is the bleeding cyclic but excessive (menorrhagia), or acyclic with variable amount

Table 10-2. Systemic Causes of Abnormal Vaginal Bleeding

Endocrinopathy
Hypothalamic/psychogenic
Polycystic ovary syndrome
Hyperprolactinemia
Thyroid dysfunction
Adrenal dysfunction

Systemic Diseases
Blood dyscrasia
  Thrombocytopenic purpura
  Von Willebrand's disease
  Leukemia
Hepatic disease
Renal disease
Iatrogenic causes
  Anticoagulants, hormone therapy, contraception, NSAIDs

NSAIDs = Nonsteroidal anti-inflammatory drugs.

(metrorrhagia), or a combination of both (menometrorrhagia)? An acute episode of active bleeding in a woman with otherwise regular menstrual cycles is typical for organic causes such as pregnancy complications or uterine leiomyomas. Postcoital bleeding is often associated with cervical infection, ectropion, cervical polyps, or neoplasia. Vaginal bleeding of a more chronic nature, especially in someone with a history of irregular menses with months of amenorrhea, suggests anovulatory breakthrough bleeding or DUB. These relationships should be used to guide the physician in consideration of the differential diagnosis, not the basis of making a diagnosis and instituting therapy without further evaluation. The history of a prior ectopic pregnancy increases the risk of a repeat ectopic pregnancy from a baseline of 2% to 12% to 15% after one and greater than 25% for two prior episodes.[3] The history of three or more spontaneous abortions by definition confirms the diagnosis of habitual abortion and warrants further evaluation. The recent delivery of a third-trimester infant associated with abnormal vaginal bleeding should provoke the evaluation of retained placenta, laceration, endometritis, and gestational trophoblastic disease. The history of abnormal Papanicolaou (PAP) smear warrants consideration of cervicitis or cervical neoplasia. Associated symptoms with vaginal bleeding should be identified, including fever, suggesting pelvic infection and pain, associated with pregnancy complications, infection, endometriosis, adenomyosis, or persistent corpus luteum. Questioning should focus on signs of bleeding dyscrasias, including ecchymosis, petechiae, and gingival bleeding. Bleeding disorders caused by leukemia, von Willebrand's disease, and thrombocytopenia are responsible for approximately 25% of teenagers complaining of severe menorrhagia.[4] Acquired thrombocytopenia, either autoimmune or drug induced, and leukemia can cause abnormal vaginal bleeding in later years. Inquiries into symptoms of hypothyroidism are necessary because it is found in 22% of women with severe menorrhagia.[5] Exogenous hormone therapy, intrauterine device, anticoagulants, and phenothiazine use should be determined.

The physical examination should begin with measuring temperature to rule out fever and blood pressure and pulse in the supine and standing position to rule out orthostatic changes associated with hypovolemia. Examine the conjunctiva and capillary filling pressure in the nail bed for signs of anemia. A general survey of signs of hypothyroidism including increased hair coarseness, decreased skin thickness, pretibial edema, and diminished reflexes should be performed. The abdominal examination should determine the presence of hepatosplenomegaly associated with bleeding dyscrasias and hepatomegaly seen with disorders of the liver. An enlarged uterus or an ovarian mass may be palpable. The groin should be palpated for evidence of lymphadenopathy associated with vulvar infection or malignancy. Extragenital causes of bleeding in the perineum should be identified first. The urethra is examined to identify a curuncle and inflamed diverticuli, and the anus is examined for hemorrhoids, polyps, and masses. If no obvious bleeding is identified in the vagina, guaiac testing of the rectum for occult blood should be performed.

Pelvic examination is necessary to identify the source of vaginal bleeding accurately. A speculum examination can identify a foreign object such as a forgotten tampon or condom. When gross vaginal and cervical malignancies are encountered, they should be biopsied. Occasionally, biopsy of a malignancy can cause florid hemorrhage often seen in the late stages of disease. A vaginal laceration can be identified. The cervix should be observed for the presence of bleeding originating from above the os or from its surface, identifying a uterine versus a cervical source. The presence of polyps or friable surface can be easily identified and treated. A Pap smear should be performed if the cervix appears to be the source of bleeding and cervical cultures if an exudate is suggestive of chlamydia and gonorrhea. The bimanual examination identifies enlarged pelvic structures and the presence of tenderness. Uterine enlargement may represent a gravid or fibroid uterus, endometrial cancer, or adenomyosis. Adnexal tenderness or enlargement may be associated with ectopic pregnancy, pelvic inflammatory disease,

and ovarian or fallopian tube neoplasms. Ovarian granulosa cell tumors and thecomas are functioning ovarian tumors that cause uterine bleeding by excessive estrogen secretion. A child with prepubertal uterine bleeding requires immediate evaluation by a trained specialist.

Laboratory Evaluation

After a thorough history and physical examination is completed, a laboratory evaluation is begun (Table 10–3; Figure 10–1). All women during their reproductive years require a sensitive serum human chorionic gonadotropin (hCG) to rule out a complication of pregnancy. If the woman is pregnant, further evaluation for normalcy and location is warranted. A complete blood count gives information about the degree of anemia if present. Red cell indices of microcytic/hypochromic anemia reflect chronic blood loss, whereas normocytic/normochromic anemia implies acute hemorrhage. White cell count showing a leukocytosis with a left shift suggests an infectious cause of the vaginal bleeding. The complete blood count also rules out leukemia and thrombocytopenia.

If the history or physical examination suggests a bleeding abnormality, a prothrombin time, partial thromboplastin

---

Table 10–3. Diagnostic Tests and Procedures Used in the Evaluation of Abnormal Vaginal Bleeding

Serum human chorionic gonadotropin
Complete blood count with differential analysis

Ovulatory signs and symptoms
Diagnostic hysteroscopy
Endometrial biopsy

Pelvic mass
Transvaginal with or without transabdominal
  ultrasound

Bleeding Disorder
Prothrombin time
Partial thromboplastin time
Bleeding time

Hypothyroidism
Serum thyroid-stimulating hormone

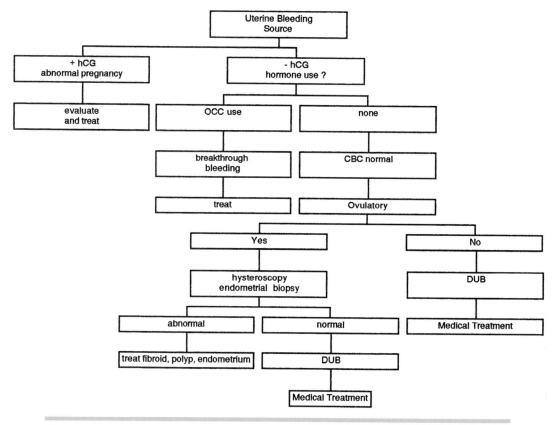

Figure 10-1. Diagnostic scheme used in the evaluation of abnormal vaginal bleeding. hCG = Human chorionic gonadotropin; OC = oral contraceptive; CBC = complete blood count; DUB = dysfunctional uterine bleeding.

time, and bleeding time are ordered. Similarly a history or physical finding suggestive of hypothyroidism should prompt measurement of thyroid-stimulating hormone. If a pelvic mass, including uterine enlargement, is identified on pelvic examination, a transvaginal and abdominal ultrasound is performed to identify and characterize the pelvic mass. If an ovarian cyst is identified, further evaluation and management for ovarian mass are warranted. If a fibroid uterus is diagnosed, further evaluation and management of fibroid uterus as a cause of vaginal bleeding are recommended. This may include hysteroscopic evaluation of the uterine cavity to identify submucosal myomas or polyps as the cause of bleeding if present. Hysteroscopy is recommended for those patients who are ovulatory or in whom medical therapy has failed. Diagnostic hysteroscopy, commonly performed in the office setting, is useful in identifying organic causes of vaginal bleeding. Following hysteroscopy, an endometrial biopsy provides tissue diagnosis to differentiate proliferative from secretory endometrium and varying degrees of hyperplasia from carcinoma. Premenopausal patients who are at risk for endometrial cancer, including those who have chronic anovulatory syndrome and intermittent amenorrhea associated with obesity, should also have an endometrial biopsy. Women with postmenopausal bleeding on no hormone replacement therapy and women on hormone replacement therapy with unexplained bleeding require tissue diagnosis by endometrial biopsy or dilatation and curettage (D&C). At this point, in the evaluation, organic and systemic causes of vaginal bleeding have been ruled out. If no abnormalities have been identified, the diagnosis of DUB can be made and treatment begun.

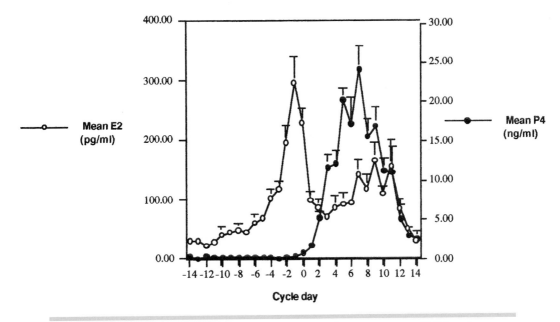

Figure 10–2. Pattern of serum estradiol (E2) and progesterone (P4) levels across the menstrual cycle. Day 0 represents the day of the LH surge, and remaining days are reported as ± from this reference point.

ENDOCRINOLOGY OF THE MENSTRUAL CYCLE

Before therapeutic options are discussed, a brief overview of current understanding of the endocrinology of the menstrual cycle and how anovulation results in histologic changes of the endometrium resulting in abnormal uterine bleeding is presented. Anovulatory menstrual cycles occur more commonly at the extremes of a woman's reproductive life, when irregular menstrual bleeding more commonly occurs. Greater than 50% of cases of DUB occur during the 30s and 40s, and 20% occur during adolescence.[6] During puberty, maturation of the hypothalamic-pituitary-ovarian axis results in differential gonadotropin-releasing hormone pulse amplitude and frequency, which results in varied follicle-stimulating hormone (FSH) and luteinizing hormone (LH) secretion. Nearly 50% to 80% of menstrual cycles are anovulatory during the year following menarche.[7] The dynamic FSH and LH pulse amplitude and frequency results in differential ovarian steroid secretion from the developing follicle over time.[8] FSH stimulation of the granulosa cells of the

dominant follicle results in the gradual increase in estradiol secretion (Fig. 10–2).[9] Progressively increased estradiol levels, in turn, among other actions, stimulate endometrial growth. The timing and level of the midcycle LH surge (day 0; see Fig. 10–2) induce several known functions, including (1) the escape of the oocyte from the diplotene stage to complete the first meiotic division, (2) the initiation of the proteolytic cascade responsible for stigma formation and ultimate extrusion of the oocyte,[10] and (3) the stimulation of granulosa cell secretion of progesterone.[11] Progesterone secretion from the corpus luteum is increased nearly 10-fold during the midluteal phase and declines thereafter unless pregnancy occurs.

The endometrial mucosa can be divided into two layers, the functionalis and the basalis. The functionalis corresponds to the upper two thirds and thickens under the steroid hormone influences previously described.[12] During the proliferative phase of the endometrium, corresponding to the ovarian follicular phase, the functionalis shows specific histologic changes in response to increasing estradiol. After ovulation, continued secretion of estradiol and progesterone results in histologic changes termed the *secretory phase*. These changes are most evident in the glandular epithelium and stromal cells during the first and second half of the secretory phase. The glandular epithelium is aligned in an orderly fashion within the subnuclear vacuole location. The supranuclear cytoplasm increases in volume with apocrine secretion into the lumen around day 20 in an ideal cycle of 28 days. Stromal changes include edema and predecidualization. Withdrawal of estradiol and progesterone from resorption of the corpus luteum results in necrosis of the functionalis followed by menstruation. The basalis comprises the lower one third of the endometrium and interdigitates with the myometrium. The basalis is responsible for the regeneration of the functionalis, which is initiated in the cornual regions of the uterus after menstruation.

Unopposed estradiol induces an increase in endometrial volume and specific histologic changes within the endometrium, including fragmented proliferative glands with phagocytized nuclear debris and fibrin deposition within thin-walled vessels. This pattern is heterogeneous throughout the endometrium and is responsible for dyssynchronous menstruation (or estrogen breakthrough bleeding) from different regions of the uterus. During the perimenopause, ovarian senescence results in alteration of the ovulatory process, and the estrogen-predominant state causes estrogen breakthrough bleeding to occur.

TREATMENT

As a general principle, once organic or systemic disorders have been identified, treatment should be focused on those conditions. It is important to keep in mind, however, that organic or systemic disorders identified may not be the cause of the abnormal bleeding, and continued follow-up is necessary. For example, a large subserosal or pedunculated leiomyoma may be noted on pelvic examination or ultrasound. By location, this may not be the cause of the menorrhagia the woman may be experiencing. If there are

Table 10–4. Hormonal and Nonhormonal Medicines Useful in the Nonsurgical Treatment of Abnormal Vaginal Bleeding

Hormone Preparation	Dose
Oral contraceptives (35 μg estrogen)	Acute: 4 tablets/d in divided doses for 7 d Chronic: continuous as recommended by package insert
Oral conjugated estrogen	Acute: 10 mg/d in divided doses for 24 h. Add progestin for 7 d Chronic: 0.625 mg/d. Add progestin for 12 d each month
Parenteral conjugated estrogen	Acute: 25 mg intravenously every 4–6 hr for 3 total dose. Add progestin or consider oral contraceptives
Progestin	Medroxyprogesterone acetate 10 mg/d for 10 d Norethindrone 5–10 mg/d for 10 d Norethindrone acetate 2.5–5 mg/d for 10 d Megestrol acetate 40 mg twice daily for 10 d
Nonsteroidal antiinflammatory	Start 1 wk before onset of menses and continue throughout menses

no organic or systemic disorders identified or if they have been treated or believed not to be responsible for the abnormal bleeding, one may confirm the diagnosis of dysfunctional uterine bleeding.

Medical Treatment

The treatment of DUB depends on the severity and duration of bleeding. In mild cases in which anemia is not present, hormonal management with oral contraceptives is sufficient to induce regular menses (Table 10–4).[13–19] When bleeding is acute, higher doses of oral contraceptives can be used for short-term therapy. Similarly, estrogen preparations and progestin can be cycled or given continuously in patients near the perimenopause. Cyclic progestins alone can be given for shorter intervals to synchronize endometrial development and induce menses after their withdrawal, especially in perimenarchal patients. Estrogen may need to be added if resumption of bleeding occurs because of the atrophic actions of progestins alone on the endometrium. The use of oral contraceptives in this situation, if no contraindications exist, is a convenient formulation to provide both steroids, especially to reproductive-age patients. Progestins alone are not typically effective for stopping acute, heavy uterine bleeding.

A trial of nonsteroidal anti-inflammatory drugs (NSAIDs) may prove effective, especially in those 15% of patients who are diagnosed with DUB and are ovulatory.[17–19] One report identified women with menorrhagia who had higher levels of prostaglandin E_2 and prostacyclin and decreased levels of prostaglandin E_2 and thromboxane.[17] This imbalance promotes a decrease in platelet aggregation and vasoconstriction consistent with a bleeding tendency.

Surgical Treatment

In women with DUB refractory to expectant or medical treatment, surgical options include D&C, endometrial ablation, and hysterectomy. Each has its relative benefits and risks that can be tailored to the particular needs and wishes of each patient. D&C has been used as a diagnostic tool with short-term therapeutic efficacy. The limited value of D&C to treat DUB primarily is due to the finding that 65% of patients have a recurrence of bleeding by 3 months.[20] This procedure, however, is useful in emergent situations to control hemorrhage with failed hormonal therapy or while it is being instituted.

Hysterectomy is the second most common gynecologic operation performed today, with approximately 750,000 reported cases each year. Approximately one third are performed for DUB.[21] The primary indication for hysterectomy is severe DUB that is refractory to medical treatment. Coulter and associates[29] found that of patients referred for evaluation and treatment of menstrual disorders, 50% underwent D&C and 50% underwent hysterectomy within 5 years of referral. Preoperative endometrial sampling is necessary to exclude gynecologic malignancy.

Endometrial ablation is a surgical alternative to hysterectomy in patients with severe DUB refractory to medical treatment with significant surgical risks or in patients who desire to retain their uterus. Goldrath and colleagues[22] first described successful endometrial ablation with a neodymium:yttrium-aluminum-garnet (Nd:YAG) laser in 1981. The later application of the urologic resectoscope using unipolar electrocautery to ablate the endometrium was reported yielding similar results.[23]

The preoperative evaluation, as with hysterectomy, includes an endometrial biopsy to rule out endometrial malignancy. The success of amenorrhea or eumenorrhea is dependent on ablating the endometrium when it is atrophic. Several preoperative hormonal treatments have been used to attain endometrial atrophy. Danazol 800 mg/day for 25 days before the procedure achieved amenorrhea or limited spotting in 97% of the 335 patients treated.[24] The gonadotropin-releasing hormone agonist leuprolide acetate induces hypoestrogenemia approximately 2 weeks after a single depot injection resulting in satisfactory rates of amenorrhea when given 4 weeks before surgery.[25] Decreasing endometrial thickness, with suction curettage immediately preoperatively, results in similar success to preoperative hormonal therapy.[26] The complications associated with endometrial ablation include uterine perforation and injury to adjacent organs, hemorrhage, and infection. A concern regarding the use of endometrial ablation in DUB is the uncertainty of an occult malignancy of the endometrium in remaining tissue. A case report of endometrial cancer was diagnosed after resection despite appropriate preoperative hysteroscopy and curettage.[27] The success of endometrial ablation in experienced hands ranges from 85% to 90%.[22,28] One study that compared success rates between ablations performed by electrosurgery versus laser vaporization showed no difference with improvement in bleeding at 4 years in 85% of patients.

CONCLUSION

The care of women with abnormal vaginal bleeding first begins with a thorough history and physical examination. Identifying organic and systemic causes of bleeding guides the physician to specific therapy. With the diagnosis of DUB, a systematic approach to therapy is instituted depending on the severity and chronicity of the bleeding patterns and desires of the patient. In those situations with acute heavy bleeding, medical treatment with high-dose estrogen, either orally or parenterally, is effective. If bleeding is refractory to this approach, a D&C is performed, which provides both short-term relief of symptoms and tissue for diagnosis. Instituting long-term hormonal therapy is necessary to prevent recurrences. The regimen selected depends on the particular needs of the patient. Therapy with the combination of estrogen and progestin, either separately or in oral contraceptive formulation, is effective in perimenopausal and reproductive-age women. Progestin-only therapy is particularly useful in perimenarchal patients. NSAIDs are effective in the treatment of menorrhagia and may be added to hormonal therapy. In those patients who do not respond to medical therapy, surgical options, including endometrial ablation and hysterectomy, may be offered.

REFERENCES

1. Mishell D Jr, Fisher H, Haynes P, et al: Menorrhagia—a symposium. J Reprod Med 1984; 29(suppl):763–782.
2. Hallberg L, Hagdahl A, Nilsson L, Rybo G: Menstrual blood loss—a population study. Acta Obstet Gynaecol Scand 1966; 45:320.
3. Leach R, Ory S: Modern management of ectopic pregnancy. J Reprod Med 1990; 70:45–52.
4. Claessens E, Cowell C: Acute adolescent menorrhagia. Am J Obstet Gynecol 1984; 139:277–280.
5. Wilensky D, Greisman B: Early hypothyroidism in patients with menor-

6. rhagia. Am J Obstet Gynecol 1989; 160:673–677.
6. March CM: Dysfunctional uterine bleeding. In Mishell DR, Davajan V, Lobo RA, eds: Infertility, Contraception and Reproductive Endocrinology. Boston, Blackwell Scientific Publications, 1991.
7. Namnoun A, Carpenter S: Abnormal uterine bleeding in the adolescent. Adolesc Med 1994; 5:157–170.
8. Knobil E: The neuroendocrine control of the menstrual cycle. Rec Prog Horm Res 1980; 36:36–53.
9. Leach R, Randolph J, Ginsburg K, et al: Hormone levels across the menstrual cycle in women with unexplained infertility: Data from the National Center for Infertility Research at Michigan. Proceedings of 51st Annual Meeting American Society of Reproductive Medicine, Seattle, 1995, P-139, S157.
10. Strickland S, Beers W: Studies on the role of plasminogen activator in ovulation: In vitro response of granulosa cells to gonadotropins, cyclic nucleotides, and prostaglandins. J Biol Chem 1976; 251:5694–5702.
11. Filicori M: Maintenance of the corpus luteum of the menstrual cycle: Hypothalamic-pituitary-ovarian axis. Semin Reprod Endocrinol 1990; 8:115–121.
12. Hansard L, Walmer D: Descriptive histology: The gold standard for clinically evaluating the endometrium. Infert Reprod Clin North Am 1995; 6:281–292.
13. American College of Obstetrics and Gynecology: Dysfunctional uterine bleeding. ACOG Technical Bulletin, No. 134, 1989.
14. Boyd ME: Dysfunctional uterine bleeding. Can J Surg 1986; 29:305–307.
15. Davis AJ: Abnormal bleeding in the adolescent patient. Clin Pract Gynecol 1989; 3:120–130.
16. DeVore GR, Owens O, Kase N: Use of intravenous Premarin in the treatment of dysfunctional uterine bleeding: A double-blind, randomized control study. Obstet Gynecol 1982; 59:285.
17. Long CA, Gast MJ: Menorrhagia. Obstet Gynecol Clin North Am 1990; 17:343–359.
18. Chamberlain G, Freeman R, Price F, et al: A comparative study of ethamyslate and mefenamic acid in dysfunctional uterine bleeding. Br J Obstet Gynaecol 1991; 98:707–711.
19. Milsom I, Anderson K, Andersch B, et al: A comparison of flurobiprofen, tranexamic acid, and a levonorgestrel-re-

leasing intrauterine contraceptive device in the treatment of idiopathic menorrhagia. Am J Obstet Gynecol 1991; 164:979–983.

20. Haynes P, Hodgson H, Anderson A: Measurement of blood loss in patients complaining of menorrhagia. Br J Obstet Gynaecol 1977; 84:763–768.

21. Pokras R, Hufnagel V: Hysterectomies in the United States, 1965–1984. DHHS Publication, #87-1753. Atlanta, Centers for Disease Control, National Center for Health Statistics, 1987.

22. Goldrath M, Fuller T, Segal S: Laser photovaporization of the endometrium for the treatment of menorrhagia. Am J Obstet Gynecol 1981; 140:14–19.

23. DeCherney A, Polan M: Hysteroscopic management of intrauterine lesions and intractable uterine bleeding. Obstet Gynecol 1983; 61:392–397.

24. Goldrath M: Use of Danazol in hysteroscopic surgery for menorrhagia. J Reprod Med 1990; 35:91–93.

25. Brooks P, Serden S: Preparation of the endometrium for ablation with a single dose of leuprolide acetate depot. J Reprod Med 1991; 36:477–478.

26. Lefler H, Sullivan G, Hulka J: Modified endometrial ablation: Electrocoagulation with vasopressin and suction curettage preparation. Obstet Gynecol 1991; 77:949–953.

27. Dwyer N, Stirrat G: Early endometrial cancer: Early incidental finding after endometrial resection: A case report. Br J Obstet Gynaecol 1991; 98:733–734.

28. Philips D: A comparison of endometrial ablation using the Nd:YAG laser or electrosurgical techniques. J Am Assoc Gynecol Laparosc 1994; 1:235–238.

29. Coulter A, Bradlow J, Agass M, et al: Outcomes of referrals to gynecology outpatient clinics for menstrual problems: An audit of general practice records. Br J Obstet Gynaecol 1991; 98:789–796.

CHAPTER 11

Evaluation and Management of Amenorrhea

Charla M. Blacker

Amenorrhea is defined as the absence or cessation of menstrual bleeding and is the symptom of a variety of pathophysiologic disorders. The criteria used for evaluation of amenorrhea include: (1) no period by age 14 in the absence of growth or development of secondary sexual characteristics such as breasts, pubic hair, or axillary hair; (2) no period by age 16 regardless of the presence of normal growth and development with the appearance of secondary sexual characteristics; or (3) the absence of periods for 6 months or for a length of time equivalent to a total of at least three of the previous cycle intervals in a woman who has previously menstruated. Clinical judgment must be used in the evaluation of amenorrhea because strict adherence to these criteria may cause needless delay in evaluation. It is not necessary to delay evaluation of a young girl with obvious Turner's stigmata, and delayed evaluation is inappropriate for an otherwise normal teen with vaginal outflow obstruction. It is appropriate to initiate evaluation when a patient's concern or that of her parents brings her to the office.

There have been several schemes proposed for the classification of amenorrhea. Primary amenorrhea has been defined as the absence of menses, whereas secondary amenorrhea is the absence of menses in a woman with previous menstrual function. This classification system is not always practical because almost half of those women suffering from primary amenorrhea have similar causes to those women with secondary amenorrhea.[1] Another system for the classification of amenorrhea is cause oriented. The cause of amenorrhea is diagnosed as of hypothalamic, pituitary, ovarian, or lower genital origin, and a specific diagnosis is sought in each case. Although approximately one third of amenorrheic women are diagnosed with normogonadotropic-anovulatory amenorrhea, approximately two thirds of women are hypoestrogenic, owing to either hypothalamic-pituitary hypofunction or end-organ failure. Another practical scheme for classification uses the response to a progestational challenge. A withdrawal bleed in response to progestogen administration indicates the presence of estrogen production and a patent outflow tract. Subsequent measurement of gonadotropin levels yields information about the pituitary-ovarian status. This system is utilized in this discussion of amenorrhea.

PHYSIOLOGY OF NORMAL MENSTRUAL FUNCTION

Normal menstrual function requires a series of closely orchestrated events and integrated systems, which ultimately results in the menstrual discharge. The arcuate nucleus in the medial basal hypothalamus must release the decapeptide gonadotropin-releasing hormone (GnRH) in a pulsatile fashion. GnRH is secreted into the portal blood system approximately every 90 minutes in the follicular phase of a normal menstrual cycle and approximately every 4 hours throughout the luteal phase. In response to the GnRH pulses, the anterior pituitary hormones luteinizing hormone (LH) and follicle-stimulating hormone (FSH) are released. Thus, the medial basal hypothalamus controls pituitary secretion. Multiple signals affect the hypothalamus, including the central nervous system and thyroid gland, and can alter GnRH pulsatility. Abnormal GnRH pulse patterns result in alterations in LH and FSH frequently associated with anovulatory cycles.

Under the stimulation of FSH, a follicle is recruited within the ovary and undergoes growth and development. Increasing numbers of granulosa cells manufacture and release estradiol into the circulation, producing a profound growth response in the endometrium. Through intense mitotic activity, the residual endometrium of the basalis layer grows several millimeters thick. Estradiol also inhibits FSH release and stimulates the midcycle LH surge. The LH surge leads to final follicular maturation events, the resumption of meiosis in the oocyte, and ovulation. Ovulation occurs approximately 36 hours after initiation of the LH surge.

Rising progesterone levels in the periovulatory period stimulate a concomitant FSH surge, which prepares the follicle for the steroidogenic events of the luteal phase. The follicle undergoes a rapid transition to the corpus luteum, whose major secretory hormone is progesterone. Progesterone induces maturational changes within the endometrium, preparing it for implantation. The endometrial glands become tortuous and convoluted and secrete glycogen. The stroma becomes edematous with subsequent decidualization. Progesterone modulates the GnRH pulse generator, resulting in high-amplitude but infrequent LH pulses throughout the luteal phase. This luteal secretion pattern of LH leads to continued progesterone secretion from the corpus luteum. With the demise of the corpus luteum, progesterone production falls, allowing escape of the hypothalamic pulse generator and a return to the rapid pattern of the follicular phase. Falling progesterone levels also have a profound effect on the endometrium, resulting in rhythmic contractions of the spiral arteries within the endometrium. Alternate ischemia and engorgement result in the eventual sloughing of the endometrium, the beginning of the next menstrual cycle. For the menstrual flow to reach the outside, an intact outflow tract is prerequisite. Thus, there is a complex cascade of events required to produce menstruation, and failure of a single element disrupts menstrual function.

EVALUATION OF AMENORRHEA

The first step in the evaluation of amenorrhea (Fig. 11–1) is a careful history and physical examination. Many physical clues are apparent even before initiation of the pelvic examination. For example, mature breast development requires a history of estrogen exposure, which, in turn, requires at least a previously intact hypothalamic-pituitary-gonadal axis. Conversely the absence of mature breast development indicates an absence of estrogen exposure, often the result of hypothalamic/pituitary or gonadal disease. Another etiologic clue is obtained

Figure 11–1. Algorithm for evaluation of the amenorrhea patient. DHEAS = Dehydroepiandrosterone sulfate; TSH = thyroid-stimulating hormone; MPA = medroxyprogesterone acetate; FSH = Follicle-stimulating hormone; LH = luteinizing hormone.

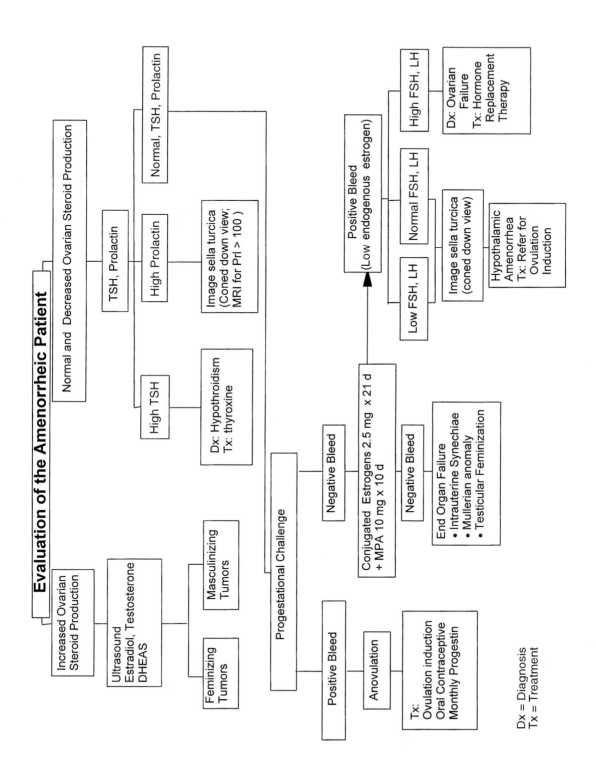

Evaluation of the Amenorrheic Patient

Increased Ovarian Steroid Production

Ultrasound
Estradiol, Testosterone
DHEAS

- Feminizing Tumors
- Masculinizing Tumors

Normal and Decreased Ovarian Steroid Production

TSH, Prolactin

- High TSH
  - Dx: Hypothroidism
  - Tx: thyroxine
- High Prolactin
  - Image sella turcica (Coned down view; MRI for Prl > 100)
- Normal, TSH, Prolactin

Progestational Challenge

- Positive Bleed
  - Anovulation
    - Tx: Ovulation induction, Oral Contraceptive, Monthly Progestin
- Negative Bleed
  - Conjugated Estrogens 2.5 mg x 21 d + MPA 10 mg x 10 d
    - Negative Bleed
      - End Organ Failure
        - Intrauterine Synechiae
        - Mullerian anomaly
        - Testicular Feminization
    - Positive Bleed (Low endogenous estrogen)
      - Low FSH, LH
      - Normal FSH, LH
        - Image sella turcica (coned down view)
        - Hypothalamic Amenorrhea Tx: Refer for Ovulation Induction
      - High FSH, LH
        - Dx: Ovarian Failure Tx: Hormone Replacement Therapy

Dx = Diagnosis
Tx = Treatment

Table 11–1.   Causes of Amenorrhea

Central nervous system (general)	Male pseudohermaphroditism
Infection	Androgen insensitivity
Neoplasm	Androgen biosynthetic defects
Congenital anomalies	Estrogen biosynthetic defects
Hypothalamic	Systemic diseases
Infection (e.g., tuberculosis,	Crohn's disease
syphilis)	Hepatic failure
Inflammatory	Systemic lupus erythematosus
Neoplasm	Glomerulonephritis
Syndrome	Thyroid disease
Kallmann's	Hypothyroidism
Frölich's	Hyperthyroidism
Laurence-Moon-Biedl	Adrenal diseases
Tumor	Cushing's syndrome
Congenital anomaly	Congenital adrenal hyperplasia
Idiopathic hypogonadotropic	Adrenal androgen tumor
hypogonadism	Chronic anovulation
Constitutional delay	Polycystic ovarian syndrome
Pituitary	Exogenous androgen exposure
Neoplasm	Nutritional
Adenoma	Generalized malnutrition
Idiopathic-congenital hypo-	Acute weight fluctuations
pituitarism	Psychiatric
Inflammatory (i.e., sarcoidosis)	Anorexia nervosa
Infiltrative	Psychosis
Space-occupying lesions	Exercise induced
Empty sella	Stress induced
Arterial aneurysm	
Gonadal	
Gonadal dysgenesis	
Premature ovarian failure	
Insensitive ovary	
Gonadal agenesis	
Ovarian tumor	

by noting the patient's body habitus. Anorexia is often diagnosed when patients present for evaluation of menstrual abnormalities. Short stature (<5 feet tall) in a girl older than 14 years should lead one to suspect a sex chromosome anomaly or hypopituitarism as the cause of delayed menarche.

Historical information regarding growth and development should be obtained before the physical examination. A well-kept pediatric growth chart can be invaluable; in its absence, historical clues about the growth spurt and normal growth patterns may be helpful. Hypothyroidism and systemic illness often present with initially normal growth patterns succeeded by a "falling off of the curve." Chronic illnesses associated with primary or secondary amenorrhea are listed in Table 11–1. Information should be obtained about pubertal development. Has breast and pubic hair development begun, and, if so, how far has it advanced? Familial history regarding pubertal development should be noted, with special reference to parents and siblings.[2]

As part of the physical examination, accurate height, weight, and arm span should be recorded. Breast and pubic hair development should be graded according to the Marshall-Tanner staging criteria.[3] Presence of galactorrhea should be noted at breast examination; galactorrhea is an important clinical sign, whether it is spontaneous or present only with careful expression by the examiner. Common anomalies associated with gonadal dysgenesis should be noted, if present: webbed neck, cubitus valgus, low-set ears and hairline, shield chest, and short metacarpal. Cranial nerve I should be evaluated with a "smell" test because congenital hypothalamic GnRH deficiency (Kallmann's syndrome) is associated with anosmia. The pelvic examination should be thorough but gentle. Outflow tract abnormalities can often be diagnosed by examination alone. Presence of vagina, cervix, and uterus can usually be determined easily with examination. Rectal examination may be preferable to vaginal examination to ascertain the presence and size of the uterus and is often sufficient to detect any adnexal masses.

The first step in the diagnosis of amenorrhea lies in characterizing the ovarian steroid production. Basal body temperature charts require daily charting of the temperature before the patient begins any activities. A sustained thermogenic rise of 0.5°F or greater implies ovulation. Although temperature charting requires a compliant patient, much information can be obtained in an easy, noninvasive manner. There is a limitation of the test, however, in that approximately 10% of ovulatory women have monophasic temperature charts. Excess androgen production is often reflected by clinical symptoms such as increasing hair growth in the androgen-sensitive areas of the face, breast, pubic, and perineal areas; acne; clitoral hypertrophy; and temporal hair regression. Hirsutism and acne are often the only symptoms present, however.

A vaginal smear for maturation index, evaluation of cervical mucus, and response to progestational challenge can be helpful in assessment of estrogen status. The sensitivity of these tissues to estrogens is considerably different; the vaginal mucosa is the most sensitive to estrogens, the cervical mucus is intermediate, and the endometrium is the least sensitive. Therefore, progestin withdrawal bleeding implies a level of estrogens sufficient to produce proliferation of the endometrium, ordinarily a relatively high level. Because the test is all-or-none, two patients having the same condition but with slightly different levels of estrogens may, therefore, respond in opposite ways to progestin. By relying too much on the progestin challenge test as the only discriminant, there is the danger of separating into different categories patients who are qualitatively identical and only quantitatively different.

Following a careful assessment of their ovarian steroid production, patients with amenorrhea can be put into one of three major diagnostic categories: (1) those with normal ovarian steroid production, (2) those with decreased ovarian steroid production, or (3) those with increased ovarian steroid production. The initial steps of the evaluation serve to differentiate between these three categories.[4]

A pregnancy test should be performed in all amenorrheic females of reproductive age. Girls can ovulate and conceive before initiation of menses. After a negative pregnancy test, the evaluation begins with the measurement of thyroid-stimulating hormone (TSH), a prolactin level, and a progestational challenge. If a patient also presents with galactorrhea, evaluation should also include a coned-down, lateral x-ray view of the sella turcica. Although only a few patients presenting with amenorrhea or galactorrhea have hypothyroidism that is not clinically apparent, the cost of measuring TSH is warranted because the treatment of hypothyroidism is simple and followed by a prompt return of ovulatory cycles.

HYPERPROLACTINEMIC AMENORRHEA

Increased prolactin level is measured in approximately one third of women with no obvious cause of amenorrhea. Only about 30% of women with high prolactin levels have galactorrhea, possibly secondary to structural modifications of the polypeptide that may result in a compound detectable by radioimmunoassay but that has decreased bioactivity. Another possible explanation for the lack of galactorrhea may be the hypoestrogenic state associated with the amenorrhea, which inhibits the lactogenic response to prolactin. About one third of women with galactorrhea experience normal menses. Up to one third of women with secondary amenorrhea have a pituitary adenoma, and if galactorrhea is also present, half have an abnormal sella turcica.[5] The sella turcica should be imaged in women with hyperprolactinemia. Although the coned-down view of the sella turcica cannot detect small pituitary adenomas, it usually can detect macroadenomas or invasive lesions. Because microadenomas (<1 cm) are slow growing and require therapy only to restore menstrual function or to treat galactorrhea, it is generally unnecessary to perform computed tomography (CT) scan or magnetic resonance imaging (MRI) of the pituitary region in women whose prolactin is less than 100 ng/mL. In the presence of an abnormal coned-down view or prolactin level greater than 100 ng/mL, a CT scan or MRI should be obtained. Both MRI and CT scan with intravenous contrast enhancement are capable of imaging the sella turcica and the suprasellar area. Although MRI is more expensive than the CT scan, it is not associated with radiation exposure and is better for evaluation of extension and the empty sella turcica. Because of the expense, however, MRI should be reserved for those patients requiring the added resolution. Patients with pituitary tumors should be referred for consultation.

Prolactin-secreting adenomas are the most common pituitary tumors, and they account for 50% of pituitary tumors at autopsy. Even small pituitary adenomas may be associated with ovulatory disturbances. The clinical symptoms do not always correlate with the prolactin level, and patients with normal prolactin measurement can have pituitary tumors.[6] The degree of menstrual irregularity, however, usually varies directly with prolactin level, and amenorrhea is more likely at higher prolactin concentrations, whereas less severe abnormalities such as luteal phase defect or oligomenorrhea typically occur at lower prolactin concentrations. For this reason, some women may be hypoestrogenic, whereas others are euestrogenic. High prolactin levels (>1000 ng/mL) are associated with invasive tumors and with amenorrhea, with or without galactorrhea.

The mechanism of action of prolactin-associated amenorrhea is secondary to prolactin inhibition of the pulsatile secretion of GnRH, mediated by increased opioid activity. The pituitary glands in these patients respond normally or in augmented fashion to GnRH administration (possibly owing to increased pituitary stores of gonadotropins), indicating that decreased GnRH results in the amenorrhea. Treatment that decreases the circulating prolactin concentration restores menstrual function, whether the treatment is surgical removal of a prolactin-secreting tumor or medical suppression of prolactin secretion.

Improved imaging techniques have increased ability to detect pituitary tumors and have also been accompanied by the development of microscopic surgical techniques, which are safer and less invasive. Patients with prolactin levels in the 150 to 500 ng/mL range have the best results; the higher the prolactin, the lower the cure rate. Unfortunately, surgical approaches are associated with significant risk of development of panhypopituitarism (up to 30%) and other complications, including cerebrospinal fluid leaks, meningitis, and postoperative diabetes insipidus. The diabetes insipidus is usually transient; however, it can be permanent. For this reason, medical therapy is usually the first treatment of choice for prolactin-secreting tumors, although surgical debulking for large tumors with or without invasion should be considered before long-term medical therapy.

Medical therapy employs dopamine agonists, which bind to dopamine receptors and inhibit pituitary prolactin secretion. Bromocriptine is the most commonly used dopamine agonist and is a lysergic acid derivative with a bromine substitute at position 2. Bromocriptine is available in short-acting or slow-release oral preparations or as a long-acting depot form for intramuscular injection. The standard oral preparation is rapidly but incompletely absorbed from the gastrointestinal tract. Decreases in prolactin concentrations can be detected within 2 hours of administration. The therapeutic dose that suppresses prolactin ranges from 2.5 to 7.5 mg daily, with an occasional patient requiring 10 mg/day to suppress adenoma secretion of prolactin. This dose is 10 times lower than that which improves the symptoms of Parkinson's disease. The oral slow-release formulation is administered in a dose of 5 to 15 mg daily; the dose of depot bromocriptine is 50 to 75 mg monthly. The response to the intramuscular form appears to be more rapid, which may be an advantage in cases with large tumors with visual field impairment.[7]

All forms of the medication are equally effective as the standard oral preparation and are associated with the same side effect severity and prevalence.[8] Nausea, headache, and faintness are common when the agonist is first initiated. Orthostatic hypotension occurs secondary to relaxation of smooth muscle in the splanchnic and renal beds as well as inhibition of transmitter release at noradrenergic nerve endings and central inhibition of sympathetic activity. Neuropsychiatric symptoms, occasionally with hallucinations, occurs in less than 1% of patients. This may be due to hydrolysis of the lysergic acid part of the molecule. Other side effects include dizziness, fatigue, nasal congestion, vomiting, and abdominal cramps. Side effects can be minimized by initiating the medication at reduced doses (1.25 mg/day) given at bedtime. Usually the dose can be increased to 2.5 mg/day within several days, and the second 2.5-mg dose can be added at breakfast or lunch approximately 1 week later. Vaginal administration can be attempted in an effort to avoid side effects. One 2.5-mg tablet is inserted high into the vagina at bedtime. This dose usually provides excellent clinical results with few side effects.[9] Vaginal absorption is rapid and nearly complete, compared to about 28% absorption of oral bromocriptine. Because vaginal absorption avoids the first-pass effect with its rapid liver metabolism, longer maintenance of systemic levels occurs, which allows achievement of therapeutic results at a lower dose.

For women who desire pregnancy, bromocriptine can be administered by either of two regimens. It can be given daily until the patient achieves pregnancy as documented by pregnancy test or by the basal body temperature chart. Alternatively, bromocriptine can be administered during the follicular phase and discontinued after ovulation, as documented by elevation of the basal body temperature, thus avoiding high drug levels early in pregnancy. The drug is resumed at menses when it is apparent that the patient is not pregnant. There are no comparative studies of the two methods to determine relative efficacy; however, there is no evidence that bromocriptine ingestion in early pregnancy is harmful to the fetus.[10]

The effect of bromocriptine has been extensively studied.[11] Eighty percent of women with amenorrhea/galactorrhea, associated with hyperprolactinemia but no demonstrable tumors, had menses restored. The average treatment time to the initiation of menses was 5.7 weeks. Response time for galactorrhea was slower and less certain than return of menstrual function. A 75% reduction of breast secretions was achieved in 6.4 weeks, whereas complete cessation of galactorrhea occurred in only 50% to 60% of patients in an average time of 12.7 weeks.

POSITIVE PROGESTATIONAL CHALLENGE

While awaiting the results of the thyroid test and the prolactin level, a progestational test should be administered. The purpose of the progestin challenge is to assess the level of endogenous estrogen and the competence of the outflow tract. It is important that a progestational agent devoid of estrogenic activity be used; oral contraceptives are not appropriate because they contain an estrogen formulation and do not exert a purely progestational effect. Progestational agents appropriate for this purpose include orally active medroxyprogesterone acetate 10 mg daily for 5 days or parenteral progesterone in oil 200 mg intramuscularly. Within 2 to 7 days after the conclusion of progestational medication, the patient demonstrates a response. If the patient bleeds, the presence of sufficient amounts of endogenous estrogen to prime the endometrium and a functional outflow tract is confirmed. Intact function of the ovary, pituitary, and hypothalamus has been demonstrated by the presence of estrogen. In the absence of galactorrhea, with a normal prolactin and a normal TSH, further evaluation is not necessary because the diagnosis of anovulation has been established.

All anovulatory patients require therapy because of the potential for rapid progression from normal endometrial tissue to precancerous and cancerous conditions.[12] Chronic anovulation can begin at menarche, and endometrial atypia and cancers have been demonstrated in young women. Therefore, women with a long history of anovulation should undergo endometrial evaluation regardless of age; an in-office endometrial biopsy with a suction pipelle is generally adequate. The choice of therapy is based on the woman's desire for pregnancy and sexual activity. For anovulatory women who are not sexually active, minimum therapy requires the monthly administration of a progestational agent such as 10 mg medroxyprogesterone acetate daily for the first 10 days of the month. At least 10 days of progestational exposure is necessary to provide adequate protection against the growth-promoting effects of continuous estrogen exposure. Low-dose oral contraceptives are an appropriate alternative for those women who require reliable contraception and are probably the therapy of choice for anovulatory teenagers. It is important to emphasize to anovulatory women that their irregular menses may recur after cessation of oral contraceptives but are not the result of the medication. Women desirous of pregnancy are candidates for ovulation induction after appropriate infertility evaluation.

If a previously anovulatory woman fails to have withdrawal bleeding on a monthly progestin program, pregnancy should be ruled out. If the pregnancy test is negative, this is a sign that she has moved to the negative withdrawal bleed category, and the remainder of the evaluation must be pursued. Occasionally the progestational challenge triggers an ovulation in an anovulatory patient, resulting in a later withdrawal bleed 14 days after the progestin.

Rarely, adequately estrogenized women fail to bleed in response to progestins. High androgen levels (e.g., associated with ovarian tumors or hyperthecosis) or high progesterone levels, secondary to an adrenal enzyme deficiency, may result in decidualization of the endometrium. In both states, the decidualized endometrium is not shed following the withdrawal of exogenous progestin.

MANAGEMENT OF THE NEGATIVE PROGESTATIONAL CHALLENGE

Failure to bleed to a progestational challenge implies either end-organ failure or inadequate endogenous estrogen to stimulate the endometrium. To differentiate these two conditions, exogenous estrogen is administered in dose and duration sufficient to produce endometrial proliferation and withdrawal bleeding, provided that a normal uterus and patent outflow tract exist. An appropriate regimen consists of conjugated estrogens 1.25 mg daily for 21 days with addition of medroxyprogesterone acetate 10 mg for the last 5 days of the regimen. In the absence of withdrawal flow, a validating second course of estrogen is suggested. If there is no withdrawal flow, the diagnosis of a defect in the endometrium or outflow tract can be made with confidence. Table 11–2 shows causes of end-organ failure. If withdrawal bleeding does occur, this implies normal functional abilities of the endometrium and outflow tract when properly stimulated by estrogen. Thus, a state of inadequate endogenous estrogen is documented consistent with hypothalamic pituitary dysfunction or ovarian failure.

Evaluation of End-Organ Failure

Müllerian Anomalies

A careful physical examination is usually adequate to diagnose müllerian anoma-

Table 11–2. Uterine and Outflow Tract Disorders

Asherman's syndrome
  Curettage
  Myomectomy
  Cesarean section
  Tuberculosis
  Schistosomiasis
Müllerian anomalies
  Imperforate hymen
  Transverse vaginal septum
  Absence of lower vagina
  Müllerian agenesis
Cervical stenosis
Testicular feminization

lies. It is unnecessary to perform an estrogen/progestin test if the physical examination reveals a müllerian anomaly. A spectrum of abnormalities has been described ranging from complete absence of müllerian structures (the Mayer-Rokitansky-Küster-Hauser syndrome) to segmental disruptions of the müllerian tube.[13] Imperforate hymen, obliteration of the vaginal orifice, and cervical agenesis are ruled out by direct observation. With the exception of uterine agenesis or congenital absence of the endometrium, the clinical problem of obstruction is compounded by the painful distention of hematocolpos, hematometra, or hematoperitoneum. Distal obstruction of the genital tract is a condition that requires prompt treatment. Delay in surgical treatment can lead to infertility secondary to inflammatory changes and endometriosis. Diagnostic needling should be avoided because of the potential for converting a sterile hematocolpos or hematometra into a pyocolpos or pyometra. MRI has proven useful in accurately delineating the anatomic abnormality, which facilitates the planning and execution of surgery. Effort must be made to incise and drain from below at the points of closure of the müllerian tube. Surgeries are often complex; however, an experienced surgeon can usually reestablish the continuity of the müllerian tract.

Müllerian agenesis is a relatively frequent cause of primary amenorrhea and is second only to gonadal dysgenesis in frequency. These patients have an absence or hypoplasia of the vagina. The uterus may be normal but lacking a conduit to the perineum, or there may be only rudimentary, bicornuate cords present. If a partial endometrial cavity is present, girls may present with cyclic abdominal pain. Because the clinical presentation is similar to some forms of male pseudohermaphroditism, it is necessary to document the normal female karyotype. Ovarian function is normal, and these patients can potentially undergo assisted reproductive techniques using a surrogate to produce a biologic child.

Approximately one third of patients have urinary tract abnormalities, and 12% or more have skeletal anomalies, most involving the spine. Urinary tract anomalies include renal agenesis, ectopic kidney, horseshoe kidney, and abnormal collecting ducts. Ultrasound can be used to visualize pelvic structures, and laparoscopic visualization is not necessary. Müllerian remnants need not be excised unless they are causing a problem, such as hematometra, endometriosis, leiomyoma uteri, or symptomatic herniation into the inguinal canal.

Progressive dilatation is preferable to surgical construction of an artificial vagina because it avoids many of the potential complications of surgery. Beginning first in a posterior direction and then after 2 weeks changing upward to the usual line of the vaginal axis, pressure is applied for 20 minutes daily with commercially available vaginal dilators. Using increasingly larger dilators, a functional vagina can be created in approximately 6 to 12 weeks. Operative treatment is reserved for those women in whom dilatation is unacceptable or fails or when a well-formed uterus is present and fertility might be preserved. Except when the cervical canal is intact, the uterus should probably be removed in cases of vaginal agenesis because surgical series have generally reported poor outcomes with attempted recanalization. It is suggested that the procedure be delayed until full growth has been attained and the patient is sufficiently mature to participate in the postoperative care of the neovagina. Reassurance and support are necessary to help a patient through these procedures and to encourage development of a normal body image and healthy sexual function.

Testicular Feminization

Müllerian anomalies must be differentiated from testicular feminization, in which a blind vaginal canal is encountered and the uterus is absent. The patient with testicular feminization is a male pseudohermaphrodite, having testes and an XY karyotype. Pseudohermaphrodite means that the genitalia are opposite of the gonads; thus, the individual is phenotypically female but with absent or meager pubic and axillary hair. Clinically, this syndrome should be considered in (1) a patient with primary amenorrhea and an absent uterus; (2) a female child with inguinal hernias, as the testes are frequently partially descended; and (3) a patient with absent body hair.[14]

These patients appear normal at birth except for the possible presence of an inguinal hernia. They experience normal growth and development, although overall height may be greater than average. The breasts are usually well developed but lack normal glandular tissue; nipples are small and areolae are pale. The labia minora are usually underdeveloped, and the vaginal pouch is shorter than normal. More than 50% have an inguinal hernia, which often contains the testes. Transmission of this disorder is by means of an X-linked recessive gene that is responsible for the androgen intracellular receptor. The plasma levels of testosterone are in the normal-to-high male range, and the plasma clearance and metabolism of testosterone are normal. These patients produce testosterone but are incapable of responding to it. Aromatization of testosterone to estrogen accounts for the development of secondary female sex characteristics.

The testes are not capable of spermatogenesis, and there is approximately 50% risk of neoplasia and 22% incidence of malignancy. Therefore, the gonads should be removed and the patient placed on hormonal replacement therapy once full pubertal development has been attained. Because gonadal tumors do not occur before puberty, the surgery may be delayed until after puberty in this condition. The development achieved with hormonal replacement does not seem to match the smooth pubertal changes caused by endogenous hormones. Incomplete testicular feminization represents an incomplete androgen receptor defect in which some androgen effect is present. These individuals often present with virilization at puberty, and gonadectomy should not be delayed in these cases.

Tact and sensitivity is necessary in dealing with these patients. Many endocrinologists have advocated a policy of nondisclosure regarding the gonadal and chromosomal sex to a patient with testicular feminization. Others, however, suggest that a straightforward, accurate discussion has less psychological impact. The female gender identity should be reinforced in either case.

Asherman's Syndrome

Outflow tract problems are most commonly iatrogenic and may occur after uterine surgery for myomectomy, cesarean section, or curettage. Partial or complete obliteration of the cavity results from destruction of the endometrium. The postpartum or postabortal uterus is especially susceptible to injury because the softness of the gravid uterus permits injury to the basalis layer of the endometrium, hindering endometrial regeneration and promoting adherence of the opposing walls. A typical pattern of multiple synechiae is seen on a hysterogram; however, hysteroscopy is more accurate and detects minimal adhesions that are not apparent on a hysterogram. The adhesions may partially or completely obliterate the endometrial cavity, the internal cervical os, the cervical canal, or a combination of these areas. Despite interruption of the outflow tract, hematometra does not frequently occur. The endometrium becomes refractory, perhaps in response to the increased intracavitary pressure, and simple cervical dilatation cures the problem in some cases. Because of the variable extent of cavity affected, the condition has several potential clinical presentations, including repetitive miscarriage, amenorrhea, dysmenorrhea, hypomenorrhea, or even otherwise unexplained infertility.

Although uncommon in the United States, amenorrheic women from Third World countries should be evaluated for the presence of tuberculosis or schistosomiasis, which may produce dense intrauterine adhesions. Diagnosis is made by examination and culture of the menstrual discharge or tissue obtained by endometrial biopsy. Schistosomiasis eggs additionally may be found in urine, feces, or rectal scrapings.

Intrauterine synechiae are best treated with hysteroscopic lysis of adhesions by scissors, cautery, or laser.[15] Blind dilatation and curettage has been shown to result in poorer outcome. It has been suggested that a pediatric Foley catheter be placed postoperatively into the uterine cavity to prevent the uterine walls from adhering. The Foley bulb is filled with 3 mL fluid, and the catheter is removed after 7 days. A prostaglandin synthetase inhibitor can be used if uterine cramping is bothersome. A broad-spectrum antibiotic is started preoperatively and maintained for 10 days. The patient is treated for 2 months with stimulatory doses of estrogen (e.g., conjugated estrogens 2.5 mg daily 3 weeks out of 4 with medroxyprogesterone acetate 10 mg daily added during the third week). It may be necessary to repeat the procedure to restore the normal cavity configuration; however, approximately 70% to 80% of patients with this condition have achieved a successful pregnancy. Pregnancy is frequently complicated by premature labor, placenta accreta, placenta previa, or postpartum hemorrhage.[14]

Evaluation of Decreased Endogenous Estrogen Production

In a patient with decreased ovarian steroid production and normal prolactin level, the next important step lies in determination of the level of gonadotropins. Because administration of exogenous estrogen may temporarily alter endogenous gonadotropin baseline levels, an interval of 2 weeks should ensue before gonadotropins are assayed.

The gonadotropin assay determines whether inadequate estrogen results from a defect in the ovary or in the hypothalamic-pituitary axis. The distinction between ovarian failure and hypogonadotropic states is critical, in terms both of cause and of prognosis and therapy. Primary ovarian failure is almost always irreversible, and there is little chance for successful therapy. Hypogonadotropic hypogonadism, however, is associated with a good prognosis for future pregnancy.

Elevated Gonadotropins

In many cases, a single determination of plasma gonadotropins allows diagnosis of ovarian failure. Although the midcycle surge of serum LH is greater than 40 IU/L, the level also associated with hypergonadotropic states such as menopause and ovarian failure, serum FSH levels greater than 40 IU/L are diagnostic of ovarian failure. Rarely, high gonadotropins can be accompanied by residual ovarian follicles. On rare occasions, tumors (particularly lung cancer) can produce gonadotropins. Single gonadotropin deficiency states have been reported in which high levels of one gonadotropin are associated with a normal baseline level of the other.

Amenorrhea associated with hypergonadotropism has been classified by Rebar and Cedars[16] (Table 11–3). About 1% of women experience premature menopause, defined as ovarian failure before the age of 40. All patients under the age of 30 who have been diagnosed with

Table 11–3. Classification of Hypergonadotropic Amenorrhea

Cytogenetic alterations
  Reduced germ cell number
  Accelerated atresia
  Structural alterations or absence of an X chromosome
  Trisomy X with or without mosaicism
  In association with myotonia dystrophica
Enzymatic defects
  17α-Hydroxylase deficiency
  Galactosemia
Physical insults
  Chemotherapeutic (especially alkylating) agents
  Ionizing radiation
  Viral infection
  Cigarette smoking
  Surgical extirpation
Immune disturbance
  In association with other autoimmune disorders
  Isolated
  Congenital thymic aplasia
Defective gonadotropin secretion or action
  Secretion of biologically inactive gonadotropin
  Gonadotropin receptor or postreceptor defects
Idiopathic

ovarian failure on the basis of elevated gonadotropins must have a karyotype determination. Although karyotypic abnormalities account for only 13% of cases of secondary amenorrhea, they are the most common cause of primary amenorrhea (56%). The presence of a Y chromosome requires excision of the gonadal tissue because the presence of any testicular component within the gonad is associated with malignant germ cell tumors: gonadoblastomas, dysgerminomas, yolk sac tumors, and choriocarcinoma. Genetic evaluation after age 30 is unnecessary because gonadal tumors usually appear before age 20 and are quite rare after age 30.[17] It is recommended that all patients with ovarian failure have an annual pelvic examination as an added precaution regardless of karyotype.

All patients with absent ovarian function and quantitative alterations in the sex chromosomes are categorized as having *gonadal dysgenesis*. Problems in gonadal development can present with either primary or secondary amenorrhea. Gonadal streaks secondary to abnormal development are present in 30% to 40% of women with primary amenorrhea. Turner's syndrome (45,X) is the most common karyotypic abnormality and accounts for approximately 50% of streak ovaries. A mosaic karyotype (multiple cell lines of varying sex chromosome composition) accounts for 25%, whereas the remainder have a normal (i.e., 46,XX) karyotype.[18]

Turner's syndrome (45,X) has been well characterized and is associated with several phenotypic anomalies, including short stature, webbed neck, shield chest, and increased carrying angle at the elbow. Several less common features may also be associated, including cardiovascular and renal abnormalities. Because other gonadal dysgenesis states may be confused with Turner's syndrome, a karyotype is necessary even in the presence of the classic phenotype. 45,X karyotype has been associated with the loss of the Y chromosome during meiosis, and 45,X/46,XY karyotypes have been reported. The presence of a Y chromosome in the karyotype requires laparotomy and excision of the gonadal areas because the presence of any testicular component within the gonad is a predisposing factor to tumor formation and to virilization. Only in the patient with the complete form of testicular feminization can laparotomy be deferred until after puberty. In all other patients with a Y chromosome, gonadectomy should be performed before puberty to avoid virilization and early tumor formation.

Mosaicism with an XX component (e.g., 46,XX/45,X) may be associated with some functional ovarian tissue within the gonad. The degree of ovarian function may be determined by the relative proportion of normal tissue; however, menopause is usually early, presumably because the functioning follicles undergo an accelerated rate of atresia.

Patients with gonadal dysgenesis may also present with secondary amenorrhea. The karyotypes associated with this presentation are, in order of decreasing frequency, 46,XX (most common), mosaics (e.g., 45,X/46,XX), deletions of varying segments of the X chromosome, 47,XXX, and 45,X.[18] The mechanism of ovarian failure in women with normal karyotype is not known; however, an autosomal recessive defect in meiosis has been proposed. Because of the association of 46,XX gonadal dysgenesis with neurosensory deafness, auditory evaluation should be considered.

Insensitive ovary syndrome is associated with elevated gonadotropins despite the presence of ovarian follicles. Ultrasound may yield evidence of follicular activity; however, response to treatment with exogenous gonadotropins is limited. Another situation in which ovarian follicles are associated with elevated serum FSH is the perimenopause. FSH levels begin to rise before cessation of menses, probably secondary to declining inhibin production by the less competent residual ovarian follicles. During this period, it is not uncommon for FSH levels to fluctuate significantly, and pregnancy can follow intervals of elevated FSH levels. Serial measurements of FSH, noting the differential increase of FSH levels greater than LH levels, aid to identify those women most likely to benefit from therapy.

Autoimmune disease may be associated with premature ovarian failure; although the ovaries contain normal appearing primordial follicles, lymphocytes and plasma cells have been demonstrated in the theca cell and granulosa cell layers.[16] Complete thyroid testing is necessary in all patients with premature ovarian failure because abnormal thyroid function is commonly associated with autoimmune syndromes. Some patients also have antibodies that react with steroid hormone–producing cells in all three layers of human adrenal cortices or with interstitial cells in testes and trophoblastic epithelium. Although the extensive polyglandular syndrome, including hypoparathyroidism, adrenal insufficiency, thyroiditis, and moniliasis, is rare, other diseases associated with autoimmune mechanisms have been associated with premature ovarian failure. These include myasthenia gravis, idiopathic thrombocytopenic purpura, rheumatoid arthritis, and autoimmune hemolytic anemia. For this reason, it has been suggested that selected blood tests for autoimmune disease be performed: complete blood count and sedimentation rate; antinuclear antibody; rheumatoid factor; TSH, thyroxine (T_4); antithyroglobulin antibody; antimicrosomal antibody; calcium; phosphorus; A.M. cortisol; and total protein, albumin, and globulin ratio. Testing for adrenocorticotropic hormone (ACTH) reserve does not seem necessary if clinical appearance and other laboratory tests are normal.

Rarely, 17α-hydroxylase deficiency has been associated with primary amenorrhea and failure to develop secondary sexual characteristics. Galactosemia also may be associated with early depletion of ovarian follicles; whether this represents a gonadal factor or inactivation of FSH and LH is not clear.

Low or Normal Gonadotropins

A low or normal level of gonadotropins in the presence of deficient ovarian hormone production and normal prolactin implies hypothalamic-pituitary dysfunction or failure. Intrinsic hypothalamic or pituitary conditions such as tumors or granulomatous disease should be considered, and the sella turcica should be imaged.

Patients with low ovarian hormone production without galactorrhea and with normal x-ray studies are classified as having hypothalamic amenorrhea. The mechanism of the amenorrhea is the suppression of pulsatile GnRH secretion below its critical range.[19] Frequently, there is an association with stress, such as school or business. Hypogonadotropic amenorrhea is also frequently associated with weight loss or with exercise. It is thought that increased central dopaminergic tone inhibits GnRH pulse secretion, resulting in decreased FSH and LH release in some women, whereas increased endogenous opioids may result in GnRH suppression in others.

Rarely, women may be diagnosed with the congenital syndrome known as Kallmann's syndrome, congenital hypogonadotropic hypogonadism associated with anosmia or hyposmia. In the female, this problem is characterized by primary amenorrhea, infantile sexual development, low gonadotropins, a normal female karyotype, and the inability to perceive odors (e.g., perfume or coffee). This defect is a consequence of the failure of GnRH neuronal and olfactory axonal migration from the olfactory placode in the nose and is demonstrated on MRI as hypoplastic or absent olfactory sulci in the rhinencephalon.[20] The mutations responsible for this syndrome involve a single gene on the short arm of the X chromosome.[21] The syndrome is more common in males than females because of the localization of the mutation to the X chromosome. Variable penetrance has been postulated with isolated GnRH deficiency representing one variant.

A good practice is to evaluate these patients annually using the coned-down view of the sella turcica and a prolactin assay because small tumors may be missed on the initial studies. After several years with no change, sellar films may be obtained at 2- to 3-year intervals. Although few long-term studies of secondary amenorrhea exist, Hirvonen[22] found that only 73% of women with amenorrhea associated with stress or weight loss experienced spontaneous recovery after 6 years. Thus, long-term follow-up is needed in about 30% of amenorrheic patients. Because the ovaries are normal and lack only stimulation to resume folliculogenesis, the potential for pregnancy is excellent.

AMENORRHEA ASSOCIATED WITH WEIGHT LOSS

Amenorrhea associated with weight loss is a well-characterized clinical syndrome. Amenorrhea in these cases is thought to result from abnormal patterns of GnRH release and subsequent disruption of gonadotropin secretion and regulation. The incidence of weight-related amenorrhea ranges from 15% to 34.5%, depending on the referral center seeing the patient.

Body weight and level of body fat are critical factors in the timing of the menarche. The minimum level of body fat necessary for initiating menarche is 17% or greater, corresponding to a body mass index of 19 kg/m². The 10th percentile at age 16 is equivalent to about 22% body fat, the minimal weight for height necessary for sustaining menstruation. A loss of body weight in the range of 10% to 15% of normal weight for height represents a loss of about one third of the body fat, which results in a drop below the 22% level and may result in abnormal menstruation.[23]

Anorexia was once thought to occur exclusively in young, white middle-class to upper-class women but is now known to occur at all socioeconomic levels. The syndrome is associated with varying psychiatric/psychosomatic dysfunction, the major components included variations on the themes of inappropriate body image perception and bizarre eating patterns. Excessive physical activity may be associated. The children are characteristically overachievers and often the family is dysfunctional. Bulimic behavior is frequently seen in patients with anorexia nervosa (about half) but not in all. Patients with bulimia have a high incidence of depressive symptoms.[25] Bulimic anorectics tend to be older, less isolated socially, and have a higher incidence of family problems.

Anorexia is associated with neuroendocrine dysfunctions that are orchestrated by the hypothalamus: appetite, thirst and water conservation, temperature, sleep, autonomic balance, and metabolic homeostasis. Relative hypercortisolemia and relative hypothyroidism have been noted, and many of the symptoms of anorexia can be explained by the relative hypothyroidism (constipation, cold intolerance, bradycardia, hypotension, dry skin, low metabolic rates, hypercarotenemia). FSH and LH levels are low, prolactin levels are normal, and TSH and T_4 levels are normal, but the reverse 3,5,3'-triiodothyronine (T_3) is high, and (T_3) level is low.[26] With weight gain, all of the metabolic changes revert to normal; however, approximately 30% of patients remain amenorrheic.

Neuroendocrine testing demonstrates persistently low gonadotropins similar to prepubertal children. As weight increases, the subsequent recovery of the hypothalamic-pituitary-ovarian axis resembles that seen in the neuroendocrine activation of the GnRH pulse generator at puberty.[27] Amplification of pulsatile LH activity associated with sleep is first noted, whereas full recovery is marked by pulsatile LH secretion throughout the day, similar to that of adults. Extensive testing is not necessary in these patients once other pathologic processes have been excluded. Often, it is necessary only to reveal gently the association between the amenorrhea and the low body weight to stimulate the patient to return to normal weight and normal menstrual function. Because of the association with dysfunctional families, it is recommended that psychological consultation be included in the therapy of these young women. Failure to change eating habits when faced with life changes such as going away to school or dating are predictive of a protracted illness.

EXERCISE AND AMENORRHEA

The rapid increase in popularity of physical exercise during the past decade has led to the recognition of deleterious effects of strenuous exercise on reproductive function. Menstrual abnormalities have been reported in connection with a wide variety of sports, including middle-distance and long-distance running, swimming, ballet dancing, and field events.[19] Varying degrees of menstrual disorders are related to the length and intensity of the activity. There is a positive correlation between weekly mileage and the incidence of amenorrhea. Even mild physical activity as seen in joggers, however, can result in fewer menstrual cycles per year or in decreased luteal phase length.

Significant variability between sports has been noted, with a much higher incidence of amenorrhea in long-distance runners and ballet dancers (40% to 50%) than in swimmers (approximately 12%). The difference may be attributable to the higher percent body fat among swimmers compared with runners and ballet dancers.[28] As in anorexia, menses often becomes progressively abnormal as body fat drops below the 22% line in the nomogram derived from Frisch, which is based on the calculation of the amount of total body water as a percentage of body weight. The competitive female athlete has about 50% less body fat than the noncompetitor, often much under the 10th percentile line associated with secondary amenorrhea. This change in body fat can occur with no discernible change in total body weight because fat is converted to lean muscle mass. There is, however, considerable variation in menstrual function at all levels of body fat content. In addition to the role of body fat, stress and energy expenditure also play important roles in initiation and maintenance of menstrual function. Ballet dancers often experience a return of menses during intervals of rest, despite no change in body weight or percent body fat.[29]

Abnormalities of GnRH secretion, as reflected by pulsatile LH frequency and amplitude, have been observed in patients with exercise amenorrhea. A spectrum similar to that seen in anorexia has been noted, including reduction of frequency or amplitude of LH pulses. The mechanism by which exercise affects the neuroendocrine axis is unclear. Hypercortisolism has been noted in women athletes.[30] The adrenal sensitivity to ACTH appears to be increased as judged by the ratio of cortisol/ACTH in response to exogenous corticotropin-releasing hormone (CRH). In view of the maintenance of normal ACTH secretion in the face of elevated cortisol levels, an increased endogenous CRH drive may be implicated. If proven, the inhibitory effect of CRH on GnRH pulse generator activity may be accountable, at least in part, for the alterations in LH pulses in these patients. Another unproven but plausible mechanism is suppression of GnRH pulsatility by the increased endorphins induced by exercise. Whatever the mechanism, LH pulse frequency and amplitude have been demonstrated even in athletes with regular menstrual periods. Progressive dysfunction in ovarian cyclicity can include delayed menarche in prepubertal girls, luteal phase defect, anovulatory cycles, and amenorrhea.

TREATMENT OF HYPOESTROGENIC STATES

The patient who is hypoestrogenic and who is not a candidate for induction of ovulation should receive hormone replacement therapy. This includes patients appropriately diagnosed with gonadal failure, patients with hypothalamic amenorrhea, and postgonadectomy patients. Data from menopausal women suggest increased risk for cardiovascular disease and osteoporosis in conjunction with hypoestrogenic states. Similar patterns of bone loss have been seen in both amenorrheic and postmenopausal women, with the most rapid loss in the first few years, emphasizing the need for early treatment.[31]

Therefore, treatment of hypoestrogenic amenorrhea with appropriate hormone replacement therapy is an important therapeutic option. A standard program for hormone replacement therapy should be used. One possible regimen is daily administration of 0.625 mg conjugated estrogens, adding 5 mg medroxyprogesterone acetate on the first 12 days of each month. In patients who have not developed secondary sexual characteristics, it is usually advisable to initiate treatment with 0.3 mg conjugated estrogens; creating a more physiologic environment encourages more natural breast development.

The importance of monthly menstruation to a young woman cannot be overemphasized. Regular and visible menstrual bleeding serves to reinforce her identification with the feminine gender role. Menstruation usually occurs within 3 days after the medroxyprogesterone acetate is stopped each month. Bleeding that occurs at any time other than the usual expected time may be a sign that endogenous function has returned. The hormone replacement program may be discontinued and the patient monitored for the resumption of ovulation. For those women who wish to avoid menstrual bleeding, utilization of a continuous regimen of 2.5 mg medroxyprogesterone acetate daily along with 0.625 mg conjugated estrogens usually prevents withdrawal bleeding.

Patients with hypothalamic amenorrhea must be cautioned that replacement therapy will not protect against a pregnancy should normal function resume. In those patients who must have reliable contraception, use of a low-dose oral contraceptive provides a reasonable option for hormone replacement as well as effective contraception.

Those women desiring pregnancy should be referred to an infertility specialist. Women with hypothalamic amenorrhea have an excellent prognosis for pregnancy, approximately 90% if there are no other factors that might have an adverse effect. Therapy, however, is somewhat complex and requires ovulation induction using either a pump injecting GnRH in a pulsatile fashion or administration of gonadotropins. Both therapies use rapid serum estradiol measurement and ultrasound to monitor folliculogenesis. Both therapies offer approximately the same success rate; however, the risk of multiple gestation is significantly higher with gonadotropin therapy.

Anorectics should not undergo attempts at pregnancy until weight is stabilized and disease is in full remission. Women with eating disorders have increased rates of preterm labor and delivery as well as problems with intrauterine growth retardation. Women in remission are more likely to gain sufficient weight, resulting in higher birth weights and 5-minute Apgar scores. Women with active disease often demonstrate worsening symptoms and psychological problems during pregnancy.[32] Because intrauterine growth retardation before the third trimester and preterm delivery are associated with significant long-term morbidity, physicians treating amenorrhea associated with weight loss should insist on solving the dietary problem before embarking on a program of ovulation induction. Patients with an eating disorder who are considering a pregnancy must be made aware of the potential adverse impact on fetal growth and development. The reward of pregnancy should be offered as an inducement to reach a normal prepregnancy weight.

Women with premature ovarian failure have a poor prognosis for a biologic pregnancy; however, there have been reports of occasional pregnancies in this group. Spontaneous pregnancies occurred most frequently in women receiving hormone replacement therapy. Assisted reproductive techniques offer a more promising therapy, with many centers reporting delivery rates of approximately 40% per attempt.

AMENORRHEA ASSOCIATED WITH INCREASED OVARIAN STEROID PRODUCTION

Amenorrhea may rarely result from ovarian tumors, either primary to the ovary or metastatic from a primary site in another organ. Dysfunction can also be caused by tumors that secrete gonadotropins ectopically.

Tumors Producing Estrogens

Estrogen-producing tumors are the most common functioning ovarian neoplasms and are referred to as granulosa-theca cell tumors. They account for 10% to 20% of all solid ovarian neoplasms and usually contain cells of both granulosa and theca type. Virilization can accompany signs of estrogen excess because androstenedione is the primary secretory product, with peripheral aromatization to estrone resulting in the estrogen effects. Eighty percent or more of feminizing tumors are palpable on pelvic examination.

Tumors Producing Androgens

Androgen-secreting tumors are of sex-cord, germ cell, or stromal origin. They include gonadoblastomas, Sertoli-Leydig cell tumors, lipoid cell tumors, and hilar cell tumors. Although hilar cell tumors are often quite small and can be easily missed even by transvaginal sonography, other androgen-producing tumors are usually palpable. Virilization usually accompanies these neoplasms, although in some cases they may produce estrogenic hormones or may be hormonally inactive. Dysgerminomas are sometimes discovered incidentally in patients evaluated for primary amenorrhea and in those cases are frequently associated with gonadal dysgenesis. Menstrual and endocrine abnormalities are more common in patients with dysgerminoma combined with other neoplastic germ cell elements, especially choriocarcinoma.

REFERENCES

1. Schachter M, Shoham Z: Amenorrhea during the reproductive years—is it safe? Fertil Steril 1994; 62:1–16.
2. Soules MR: Primary and secondary amenorrhea and hirsutism. *In* Stenchever MA, ed: Office Gynecology. St. Louis, Mosby-Year Book, 1992.
3. Marshall WA, Tanner JM: Variation in pattern of pubertal changes in girls. Arch Dis Child 1969; 44:291.
4. Ross GT: Disorders of the ovary and female reproductive tract. *In* Wilson JD, Foster DW, eds: Williams Textbook of Endocrinology. Philadelphia, WB Saunders, 1985, pp 233–250.
5. Schlechte J, Sherman B, Halmi N, et al: Prolactin-secreting pituitary tumors. Endocr Rev 1980; 1:295.
6. Speroff L, Levin RM, Haning RV Jr, Kase NG: A practical approach for the evaluation of women with abnormal polytomography or elevated prolactin levels. Am J Obstet Gynecol 1979; 135:896.
7. Brue T, Lancranjan I, Louvet J-P, et al: A long-acting repeatable form of bromocriptine as a long-term treatment of prolactin-secreting macroadenomas: A multicenter study. Fertil Steril 1992; 57:74.
8. Merola B, Colao A, Caruso E, et al: Oral and injectable long-lasting preparations in hyperprolactinemia: Comparison of their prolactin lowering activity, tolerability, and safety. Gynecol Endocrinol 1991; 5:267.
9. Ginsburg J, Hardiman P, Thomas M: Vaginal bromocriptine—clinical and biochemical effects. Gynecol Endocrinol 1992; 6:119.
10. Weil C: The safety of bromocriptine in long-term use: A review of the literature. Curr Med Res Opin 1986; 10:25.
11. Cuellar FG: Bromocriptine mesylate (Parlodel) in the management of amenorrhea/galactorrhea associated with hyperprolactinemia. Obstet Gynecol 1980; 55:278.
12. Coulam CB, Annegers JF, Kranz JS: Chronic anovulation syndrome and associated neoplasia. Obstet Gynecol 1983; 61:403.
13. Jones HW Jr: Mullerian duct anomalies. *In* Wallach EE, Zacur HA, eds: Reproductive Medicine and Surgery. St. Louis, Mosby, 1995, pp 1093–1114.
14. Speroff L, Glass RH, Kase NG: Amenorrhea. *In* Clinical Gynecologic Endocrinology and Infertility, 5th ed. Baltimore, Williams & Wilkins, 1994, pp 401–456.
15. Valle RF: Lysis of intrauterine adhesions (Asherman's syndrome). *In* Sutton C, Diamond MP, eds: Endoscopic Surgery for Gynecologists. Philadelphia, WB Saunders, 1993, pp 338–344.
16. Rebar RW, Cedars MI: Hypergonadotropic forms of amenorrhea in young women. Endocrinol Metab Clin North Am 1992; 21:173.
17. Manuel M, Katayama KP, Jones HW Jr: The age of occurrence of gonadal tumors in intersex patients with a Y chromosome. Am J Obstet Gynecol 1976; 124:293.
18. Portuondo JA, Barral A, Melchor JC, et al: Chromosomal complements in primary gonadal failure. Obstet Gynecol 1984; 64:757.
19. Yen SC: Female hypogonadotropic hypogonadism: Hypothalamic amenorrhea syndrome. Endocrinol Metab Clin North Am 1993; 22:29.
20. Knorr JR, Ragland RL, Brown RS, Gelber N: Kallmann's syndrome: MR findings. Am J Neuroradiol 1993; 14:845.
21. Hardelin JP, Levilliers J, Young J, et al: Xp22.3 deletions in isolated familial Kallmann's syndrome. J Clin Endocrinol Metab 1993; 76:827.
22. Hirvonen E: Etiology, clinical features and prognosis in secondary amenorrhea. Int J Fertil 1977; 22:69.
23. Warren MP, Jewelewicz R, Dyrenfurth I, et al: The significance of weight loss in the evaluation of pituitary response to LH-RH in women with secondary amenorrhea. J Clin Endocrinol Metab 1975; 40:601.
24. Frisch RE: Body fat, menarche, and reproductive ability. Semin Reprod Endocrinol 1985; 3:45.

25. Herzog DB, Coopeland PM: Eating disorders. N Engl J Med 1985; 313:295.
26. Garner DM: Pathogenesis of anorexia nervosa. Lancet 1993; 341:1631.
27. Berga SL, Mortola JF, Suh GB, et al: Neuroendocrine aberrations in women with functional hypothalamic amenorrhea. J Clin Endocrinol Metab 1989; 68:301.
28. Frisch RE, Snow RC, Johnson LA, et al: Magnetic resonance imaging of overall and regional body fat, estrogen metabolism, and ovulation of athletes compared to controls. J Clin Endocrinol Metab 1993; 77:471.
29. Warren MP: Effect of exercise and physical training on menarche. Semin Reprod Endocrinol 1985; 3:17.
30. Barbarino A, de Marinis L, Tofani A, et al: Corticotropin-releasing hormone inhibition of gonadotropin release and the effect of opioid blockade. J Clin Endocrinol Metab 1989; 68:523.
31. Drinkwater BL, Nilson K, Chestnut CH III, et al: Bone mineral content of amenorrheic and eumenorrheic athletes. N Engl J Med 1984; 311:277.
32. Stewart DE, Rasking J, Garfinkel PE, et al: Anorexia nervosa, bulimia, and pregnancy. Am J Obstet Gynecol 1987; 157:1194.

CHAPTER 12

Hirsutism

Michael A. Allon

Michael P. Diamond

Hirsutism has been defined as the excess of hair growth in women occurring in androgen-dependent areas, such as the upper lip, chin, sideburn area, neck, midchest, areolae, linea alba, and inner thighs. It is usually a benign condition caused by excess androgen production or increased androgen skin sensitivity. The quantity and distribution of hair vary with ethnicity and may take months or years to develop. Hirsutism may first appear after the time of menarche and increase through the late teen years and early 20s and subsequently decrease in later years. The typical patient seeks medical attention because of loss in menstrual cyclicity and infertility but rarely presents with signs of virilization, such as clitoral enlargement, voice deepening, temporal balding, or changes in body contour. The underlying cause for hirsutism most often is benign, but certain conditions may also be associated with hirsutism and should not be discounted.

PHYSIOLOGY OF HAIR GROWTH

Human hair begins as a condensation of basal cell nuclei in the epidermis around 8 to 10 weeks of gestation in the regions of eyebrow, upper lip, and chin.[1] The process of hair follicle development is completed by 22 weeks of gestation marking the complete hair complement because new hair follicles no longer form after birth. The hair follicle contains two swellings in its posterior edge. The upper swelling gives rise to the sebaceous gland, and the lower swelling forms the attachment of the arrector pili muscles. Next a multilayer of cells forms a solid column that elongates to the cluster of mesodermal cells, which then give rise to the dermal papilla. The inner cells of the hair column degenerate or keratinize, eventually hollowing out and forming a canal. This process marks the final formation of the pilosebaceous unit (Fig. 12–1). Postnatally the hair follicle grows in a cyclic fashion, beginning with the active phase termed the *anagen phase*. The duration of the anagen phase is the major determinant of hair length and varies with hair follicle location. Next the hair undergoes a shortening phase termed the *catagen phase*, and with time, the hair column shrinks and the hair bulb shrivels leading to the resting state termed the *telogen phase*. Scalp hair remains in the anagen phase for 3 years and has a short telogen phase. Because of its asynchronous growth, the scalp hair appears to be al-

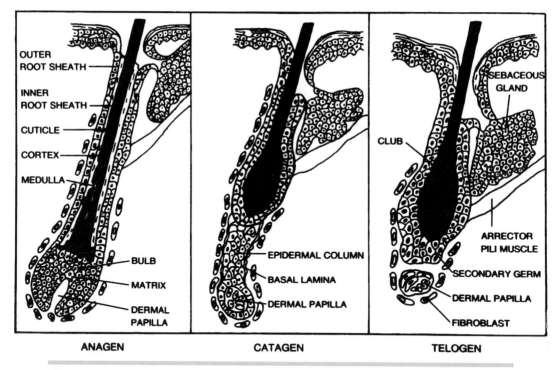

Figure 12–1. Physiology of pilosebaceous unit. (From McCarthy JA, Seibel MM: Physiologic hair growth. Clin Obstet Gynecol 1991; 34:799–804.)

ways growing. In the forearm, however, the anagen phase is short, and the telogen phase is long, leading to short hair of stable, nongrowing length. The evidence for continuous hair growth is determined by the degree of hair follicle's asynchronous growth when compared with its neighbors.

Certain hormones have an effect on hair growth and pigmentation. Androgens, specifically testosterone, increase hair growth as well as diameter and pigmentation. Androgens also increase the rate of matrix cell mitosis in most areas except the scalp. In the scalp, androgens and their metabolism have been found to play a major role in the balding of susceptible men. There is evidence that testosterone uptake, 5α reduction and metabolism is increased in the scalp hair follicles of balding men compared to nonbalding control men.[2] Furthermore the balding areas also have increased 5α reduction of testosterone when compared to the nonbalding areas of the same individual. Estrogen retards the hair growth causing finer, less pigmented, and slower-growing hair. The estrogen effect is seen well in pregnancy. In the second and

third trimester, there is an increase in the length of the anagen phase. This creates a heavier than normal growth of scalp hair in the latter part of pregnancy, followed by hair shedding in the first 3 months postpartum.

After birth, the fetus is covered by fine, soft, lightly pigmented hair called lanugo. This hair is replaced by the vellus downy hair found on bodies of children and adults. In some body areas, particularly the sexual hair areas, the vellus hairs are replaced by terminal hairs that are long, coarse, and darkly pigmented. Before puberty, the androgen-dependent pilosebaceous unit consists of the vellus follicle with fine hair and a small sebaceous gland. At puberty, the sensitivity of the pilosebaceous unit to androgens depends on their distribution. The sensitivity increases as their location changes from the mons pubis toward the head. There is a dose-response curve to testosterone as the mustache appears at plasma testosterone levels just above the upper limits of normal for women, and a beard requires 10-fold higher levels to grow (Fig. 12–2).

The dermal papilla is the major factor

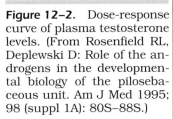

Figure 12–2. Dose-response curve of plasma testosterone levels. (From Rosenfield RL, Deplewski D: Role of the androgens in the developmental biology of the pilosebaceous unit. Am J Med 1995; 98 (suppl 1A): 80S–88S.)

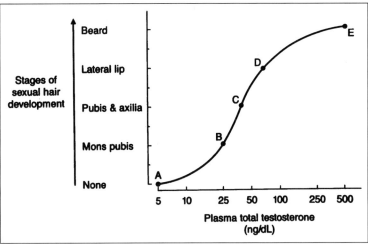

in controlling hair growth. In the event of injury to the hair follicle, if the dermal papilla survives, the hair follicle regenerates and regrows hair. In an experiment done by Oliver,[3] when the lower halves of rat hairs were removed, they no longer were able to regenerate, but hair growth can be reinduced with implantation of the dermal papillae into their base.

EVALUATION OF HIRSUTISM

Hirsutism results from the development of excessive terminal hair on the face or body and is a function of the local levels of androgen, the status of the androgen receptor, and the ability to form dihydrotestosterone by 5α-reductase activity.

Most common causes of hirsutism are idiopathic and secondary to chronic anovulation in women with a history of polycystic ovary syndrome (PCOS). The increase in androgens can occur from the adrenal gland or the ovary, and both must be evaluated (Figs. 12–3 through 12–5).

Sources of Androgens

The C19 steroids are formed from progestin precursors by 17α-hydroxylase/C-17, 20-lyase activity. Dehydroepiandrosterone (DHEA) (Table 12–1) is formed from the delta 5 steroid pathway, and androstenedione is formed from the delta 4 pathway. The delta 4 androgens can be converted from the delta 5 androgens by the enzyme 3β-hydroxysteroid dehydrogenase/delta 4-5 isomerase. The 17β-hydroxysteroids, such as testosterone or dihydrotestosterone (DHT), are the most potent androgens. The delta 4 saturation of testosterone can be reduced to either the nonandrogenic 5β-derivatives or the highly potent 5α derivatives (DHT) by 5α-reductase activity. DHT is the primary nuclear androgen in the pilosebaceous unit, and with its rapid cellular turnover and affinity for sex hormone–binding globulin, it has a limited use as a serum marker for peripheral androgen production. Its metabolite, 3α-androstenediol glucuronide, is produced exclusively in peripheral tissues and has been shown to correlate both with androgenicity and skin 5α-reductase activity.[4]

Causes of Androgen Excess

Ovarian Hyperandrogenism

The most frequently seen ovarian cause of hirsutism in women is PCOS.[5] This is a heterogeneous clinical syndrome that may be characterized as the syndrome of hyperandrogenism and chronic anovulation and usually with a perimenarcheal onset. Hirsutism is seen in about 70% of patients with this syndrome.[6] Laboratory

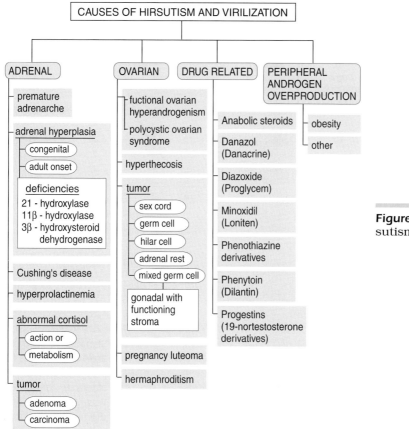

Figure 12–3. Causes of hirsutism and virilization.

findings in PCOS include high luteinizing hormone–to–follicle-stimulating hormone ratio (about 3:1) with elevated luteinizing hormone and normal or low levels of follicle-stimulating hormone. Other findings include mild elevation of testosterone, androstenedione, and dehydroepiandrosterone sulfate (DHEAS).[7] Usually the testosterone levels in PCOS are no more than twice the upper normal range (20 to 70 ng/dL) and rarely exceed 150 ng/dL. Hyperinsulinemia and insulin resistance have also been found in PCOS and are well documented in normal-weight PCOS patients.[8] A syndrome of hirsutism, hyperandrogenism (HA), insulin resistance (IR), and acanthosis nigricans (AN) has been termed the *HAIR-AN syndrome* and occurs in a small subset of PCOS patients. Acanthosis nigricans is characterized by a hyperpigmented, thickened verrucous skin change around the neck, axilla, or intertriginous areas. This skin lesion is thought to be a manifestation of hyperinsulinemia. The reason for insulin resistance was thought to be secondary to the hyperandrogenism or the obesity associated with PCOS; however, this has been disputed by the fact that in some reports, but not in others, a reduction in the concentration of androgens does not necessarily improve insulin sensitivity.[9]

Hyperinsulinemia has been implicated in the cause of ovarian hyperandrogenism through several observations.[46] Receptors for insulin have been found to be structurally related to insulin-like growth factor (IGF)-I in human ovarian tissue.[47] It is hypothesized that with hyperinsulinemia, the elevated levels of insulin bind to IGF-I receptors in a spillover phenomenon, leading to thecal stimulation and increased androgen production. Insulin has also been found to enhance androgen production in ovarian theca and stroma cell cultures from both hyperandrogenic and normal women.[48] Also, there is evidence to suggest that short-

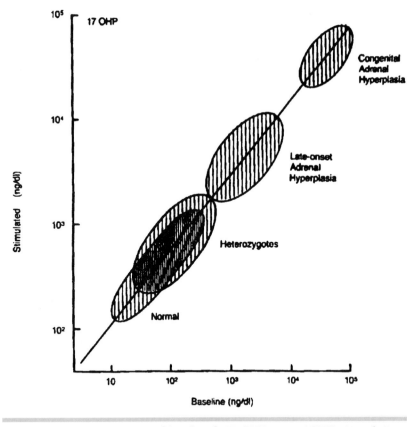

Figure 12-4.   Nomogram of levels of 17-OHP post ACTH stimulation.
(From Kessel B, Liu J: Clinical and laboratory evaluation of hirsutism.
Clin Obstet Gynecol 1991; 34:805–816.)

term suppression of serum insulin levels results in reduction of serum androgen levels in some individuals with PCOS.[49] Elevated levels of insulin in obese women with PCOS have been found to inhibit the hepatic synthesis of sex hormone–binding globulin,[50] thus leading to elevated levels of free testosterone. Finally, elevated levels of luteinizing hormone often found in patients with PCOS may increase IGF-I production by thecal cells within the polycystic ovary and enhance androgen production.[11]

Hyperthecosis

This benign histologic diagnosis is characterized by ovarian stromal hyperplasia and an excess of testosterone production from the luteinized theca cells. The histologic features of hyperthecosis are similar to those of PCOS,[43] yet unique

steroidal differences can be identified between hyperthecosis and PCOS. With hyperthecosis, luteinizing hormone levels tend to be lower secondary to the higher testosterone levels blocking the estrogen action at the hypothalamic-pituitary level.[44,45] A greater degree of insulin resistance can be correlated with the degree of hyperthecosis.[45] With hyperthecosis, signs of virilization are also more common, and testosterone levels may exceed 150 to 200 ng/dL.

Ovarian Neoplasms

Ovarian tumors, derived from sex cord stromal cells including Sertoli-Leydig cells, hilar cells, lipoid cells, and adrenal rest,[12,13] are a rare cause of hyperandrogenism. With tumors, there is typically a rapid progression of hirsutism and virilization along with higher levels of

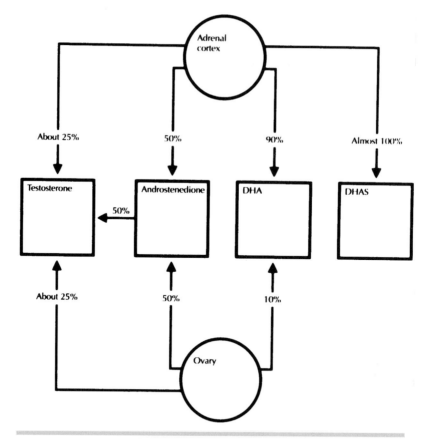

Figure 12–5. (From Hirsutism. *In* Speroff L, Glass RH, Kase NG (eds): Clinical Gynecologic Endocrinology and Infertility, 5th ed. Baltimore, Williams & Wilkins, 1994, pp 483–513.

Table 12–1. Sources of Androgens

Ovary
Production of testosterone is about 25%, the rest is from conversion from adrenal and ovarian precursors. Daily production of 0.2–0.3 mg/d
Production of androstenedione is about 50%
Production of DHEA is about 10%

Adrenal
Production of testosterone is about 25%
Production of androstenedione is about 50%. Androstenedione is a source for peripheral conversion of testosterone
Production of DHEAS, a weak androgen (20 mg/d) is almost exclusively formed in the adrenal gland

DHEA = Dehydroepiandrosterone; DHEAS = dehydroepiandrosterone sulfate.

serum testosterone (>200 ng/dL). Additionally, there is a unilateral adnexal mass palpable on pelvic examination in greater than 80% of the cases.[5]

Adrenal Androgen Excess

Cushing's Syndrome. A rare cause of hirsutism is a state of hypercortisolism (Fig. 12–6). About 60% of Cushing's Syndrome is due to Cushing's disease, which is caused by excess pituitary secretion of adrenocorticotropic hormone (ACTH). Primary adrenal disease, adenoma, or carcinoma accounts for about 25% of the cases, and the rest are accounted for by an ectopic secretion of ACTH or corticotropin-releasing hormone (CRH). Tumors

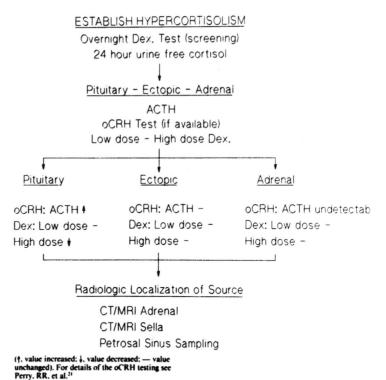

Figure 12-6. Workup of hypercortisolism. (From Kessel B, Liu J: Clinical and laboratory evaluation of hirsutism. Clin Obstet Gynecol 1991; 34:805-816.)

ESTABLISH HYPERCORTISOLISM
Overnight Dex. Test (screening)
24 hour urine free cortisol

Pituitary – Ectopic – Adrenal
ACTH
oCRH Test (if available)
Low dose – High dose Dex.

Pituitary	Ectopic	Adrenal
oCRH: ACTH ↑	oCRH: ACTH –	oCRH: ACTH undetectab
Dex: Low dose –	Dex: Low dose –	Dex: Low dose –
High dose ↓	High dose –	High dose –

Radiologic Localization of Source
CT/MRI Adrenal
CT/MRI Sella
Petrosal Sinus Sampling

(↑. value increased; ↓. value decreased; — value unchanged). For details of the oCRH testing see Perry. RR. et al.[21]

of the lung or pancreas are the most likely source of ectopic ACTH secretion.[14] Hirsutism occurs in about 75% of patients with Cushing's syndrome and Cushing's disease.

Adrenal Neoplasm. Excess production of adrenal androgen usually accompanies excessive production of cortisol. Some adrenal neoplasms secrete only androgen. Pure virilizing adrenal neoplasm is a rare disorder.

Hyperprolactinemia. Hyperprolactinemia is associated with increased adrenal androgens and hirsutism. Mild to moderate hirsutism is seen in 40% of hyperprolactinemic patients.[15] With hyperprolactinemia, there is an increase in DHEA, DHEAS, androstenedione, and free testosterone levels as well as a low DHT and low ratio of DHT to testosterone.[16,17] Prolactin affects adrenal androgens in at least two ways. It appears to stimulate the production of adrenal androgens by having a synergistic effect with ACTH because in hyperprolactinemic women, either dexamethasone or bromocriptine can reverse the androgen abnormalities.[15,17] Second, hyperprolactinemia depresses sex hormone–binding globulin, leading to an increase in free testosterone.

3β-Hydroxysteroid–Delta 5 Steroid Dehydrogenase (3β-HSD)

This enzyme converts the metabolically inactive delta 5 steroids to the active delta 4 steroids. Late-onset 3β-HSD deficiency may be a cause of adrenal and ovarian hyperandrogenism in perhaps 10% to 40% of hirsute women.[18] The diagnosis can be made after adrenal stimulation with ACTH with an altered 17-hydroxypregnenolone-to-17-OHP ratio usually greater than 6;[51] ovarian stimulation by a gonadotropin-releasing hormone (GnRH) agonist markedly increases the delta 5 steroids and delta 5-to-delta 4 steroids ratio.

17-Hydroxylase/17,20-Lyase

This cytochrome P-450 17 enzyme has both 17-hydroxylase and 17,20-lyase activity and is essential in the formation of 17-hydroxyprogesterone from progesterone and its subsequent conversion to androstenedione. In the delta 5 pathway, this enzyme converts pregnenolone to 17-hydroxypregnenolone and then to DHA. This enzyme is thought to have increased activity in the ovary and adrenal leading to dysregulation[19] of the enzyme products found in PCOS. It could then explain the increased response of 17-hydroxyprogesterone and androstenedione to GnRH agonist testing in PCOS women compared to normal. Also, abnormal activity of this enzyme may help explain the increased responses to ACTH with increases in both 17-hydroxysteroids and 17-ketosteroids that occur in PCOS women.

Congenital Adrenal Hyperplasia

Adrenal 21-hydroxylase deficiency accounts for 90% to 95% of the cases of classic congenital adrenal hyperplasia.[20] Infants with this diagnosis have ambiguous genitalia (simple virilizing), and they may also have adrenal crisis (salt-wasting congenital adrenal hyperplasia). An autosomal recessive disorder that is manifested around puberty has been described as late-onset or nonclassic 21-hydroxylase deficiency. Patients with this disorder develop acne, hirsutism, and menstrual irregularities. This phenomenon accounts for about 1% to 2% of the cases of hirsutism[21] and occurs in about 0.3% of the white population, although a higher propensity (3%) is found with Jews of European descent.

11β-Hydroxylase

This enzyme accounts for 5% to 8% of the cases of classic congenital adrenal hyperplasia.[22] A deficiency of this enzyme causes excessive production of androgenic precursors as well as 17-hydroxyprogesterone and the 11-deoxysteroids.

Other Causes of Hyperandrogenism

About 10% of women with hirsutism are characterized with idiopathic hyperandrogenism or hirsutism, which occurs when ACTH stimulation, GnRH agonist, and dexamethasone suppression tests do not reveal adrenal or ovarian basis for androgen excess.[23] The reason for the elevated androgens could be due to increased peripheral metabolism of inactive steroid precursors to active androgens. Here, both glucocorticoids and estrogen-progesterone combinations may be required to suppress the elevated plasma-free testosterone to normal.

Physical Examination

Hirsutism is clinically assessed using the semiquantitative scale by Ferriman and Gallwey[24,25] (Fig. 12–7). Nine body areas are graded on a scale of 0 (no hirsutism) to 4 (severe). Other investigators such as Bardin and Lipsett[26] use a simplified system that grades for the presence (1+) or absence (0) of facial hair in three regions: upper lip, chin, and sideburns. Those with a full beard received a 4+. In the evaluation of hirsutism, it is also important to consider the patient's ethnic background because the number of hair follicles per unit skin area varies (Mediterranean > Nordic > Asian), and hair patterns are similar within families. A pelvic examination is necessary as part of the evaluation of hirsutism. The pelvic examination may sometimes be inadequate or unsatisfactory in obese patients. If there is a high clinical suspicion, a further workup with a pelvic ultrasound may be justified. It is also imperative to look for galactorrhea, hypertension, central obesity, muscle weakness, suboccipital fat pad, and red striae as part of the signs and symptoms associated with Cushing's syndrome.

Diagnosis of Hyperandrogenic States

Initial laboratory evaluation of hirsutism should include total serum testosterone for ovarian hyperandrogenism, DHEAS, and 17-hydroxyprogesterone (17-OHP) for adrenal assessment. If late-onset CAH is suspected, 17-OHP (measured in the morning to avoid elevation from diurnal ACTH secretion) levels are greater than 200 ng/dL. If abnormal 17-OHP is found,

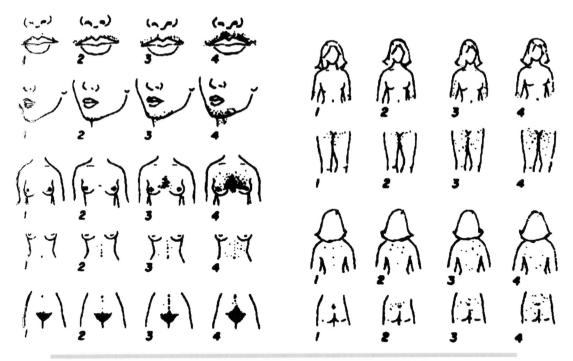

Figure 12–7. Assessment of hirsutism. (From Kessel B, Liu J: Clinical and laboratory evaluation of hirsutism. Clin Obstet Gynecol 1991; 34:805–816.)

an ACTH-stimulation test is performed by measuring basal 17-OHP followed by a repeat sample 60 minutes after an intravenous administration of 0.25 mg synthetic 1-24 ACTH (cosyntropin [Cortrosyn]) in the follicular phase of the menstrual cycle. The basal and stimulated values can then be plotted on a standard nomogram (see Fig. 12–4). When 17-OHP levels are greater than 800 ng/dL, the diagnosis of 21-hydroxylase deficiency can be assigned. If Cushing's syndrome is suspected, a screening test can be performed using 24-hour urine levels of free cortisol and an overnight dexamethasone suppression test. A cortisol level (drawn at 8 A.M.) less than 5 μg/dL after 1 mg of dexamethasone (given at 11 P.M. the night before the test) along with 24-hour urinary cortisol less than 100 μg excludes Cushing's syndrome. With established hypercortisolism, pituitary, ectopic, or adrenal sources of ACTH should be investigated (see Fig. 12–6). This is performed by the measurement of basal ACTH and post-CRH test as well as a low-dose and high-dose dexamethasone test (2 mg every 6 hours for

48 hours). With a pituitary source, ACTH increases in response to CRH and decreases in response to a high-dose dexamethasone test. With an ectopic source of ACTH, no change is seen in response to CRH or high-dose dexamethasone test. With an adrenal neoplasm as the source of ACTH, levels are undetectable after CRH stimulation and do not change with the high-dose dexamethasone test. In patients with pituitary Cushing's syndrome, computed tomography (CT) and magnetic resonance imaging (MRI) of the sella can be diagnostic of a pituitary microadenoma. More recently, the technique of bilateral inferior petrosal sinus sampling has been used for the measurement of ACTH before and after CRH administration. The values obtained are compared to peripheral blood measurement of ACTH, and a sinus to peripheral gradient of greater than 3 indicates a pituitary source of the ACTH.[51] In patients with a suspected adrenal tumor, CT and MRI scans almost always demonstrate one gland being larger and distorted, with the other small and atrophic. Elevated serum level of DHEAS (>700

μg/dL) is also suggestive of adrenal tumor, but it should be emphasized that normal DHEAS levels do not rule it out because only about half of the patients with virilizing adrenal carcinoma have elevated DHEAS levels.[27,28]

TREATMENT OF HIRSUTISM

Patient education is imperative for the success of the treatment program for the patient with hirsutism. Patients should be informed that mechanical means of hair removal are required for existing hair, and medical therapy is primarily used to decrease hair growth. Furthermore, medical therapy requires at least 6 months before success can be achieved, and it is effective only in regions where the hair is responsive to sex hormones. This includes hair on the face, chest, abdomen, and upper thighs. Hair around the nipples, on arms, on back, and on lower legs is often unresponsive to medical therapy. Patients should also be informed that most medications cannot be used during pregnancy and that discontinuation of treatment is usually associated with return of symptoms.

Hormonal Suppression

Oral Contraceptives

The progestin component of the oral contraceptive pill decreases leutinizing hormone secretion and decreases ovarian estrogen and androgen production. The estrogen component increases sex hormone–binding globulin by a direct effect on the liver, which leads to a decrease in free levels of testosterone. In addition to the decrease in androgens, oral contraceptives also has the added benefit of providing contraception, controlling dysfunctional uterine bleeding, and preventing endometrial hyperplasia often found in these patients. The ideal oral contraceptive should be estrogen dominant and with the least androgenic progestin, such as ethynodiol diacetate (Demulen), desogestrel, or gestodene (Ortho-Cyclen, Norgestimate).[29]

Gonadotropin-Releasing Hormone Agonist

GnRH agonists, given in a continuous fashion, result in decreased gonadotropin secretion and subsequent decrease in ovarian androgen production. GnRH analogues (leuprolide) can be given by subcutaneous injections two to three times a day, by daily nasal spray (nafarelin), by monthly intramuscular depot injection of leuprolide, or by monthly subcutaneous implant (goserelin). The hypoestrogenic side effect of bone loss that is seen after 6 months of therapy can be minimized by the concurrent administration of estrogen/progestin replacement.[30] GnRH analogues are most effective in reducing ovarian hyperandrogenism but have little or no apparent effect on adrenal androgens.

Adrenal Suppression

Glucocorticoids can be used with adrenal hyperandrogenism, although their optimal regimen remains a matter of debate.[31] Effective regimens include 10 to 20 mg hydrocortisone, 2.5 to 5 mg prednisone, and 0.25 to 0.5 mg dexamethasone given nightly. Glucocorticoids decrease the levels of DHEAS but do not have as great effect on testosterone, and effective hirsutism therapy requires other forms of medical treatment.

Ketoconazole

Ketoconazole has been found to have antiandrogenic effects by blocking both adrenal and gonadal steroid biosynthesis. Its effects are explained by the inhibition of several cytochrome P-450–dependent enzymes, including 17,20-desmolase, 17α-hydroxylase, and 11β-hydroxylase. Doses ranging from 400 to 1200 mg/day are used,[32–34] and its antiandrogen effects are dose dependent. Treatment is initiated with low doses because this drug has several side effects. Potential side effects include hepatotoxicity as well as scalp hair loss, dry skin, abdominal pain, and iatrogenic Addison's disease occurring with high doses.

Spironolactone

Spironolactone is a potassium-sparing diuretic acting via aldosterone antagonism. It has antiandrogenic actions by inhibiting testosterone production and competitively binding to the androgen receptor. It also acts peripherally by inhibiting 5α-reductase activity. Levels of serum cortisol, DHEA, and DHEAS do not change.[35] High levels of spironolactone decrease cytochrome P-450 activity and could explain its antiandrogenic effects.[36] Spironolactone was shown to have a greater decrease in hair shaft diameter using doses of 200 mg/day compared to women receiving 100 mg/day.[37] Side effects of this drug include menstrual irregularities, nausea, dyspepsia, fatigue as well as feminization of the male fetus. The menstrual irregularities and the risk of teratogenicity can be avoided by the addition of oral contraceptives.

Flutamide

Flutamide is a pure nonsteroidal antiandrogen and is used in higher doses (125 to 250 mg twice daily). In a study by Cusan and co-workers,[38] the use of the combination of flutamide (500 mg total) and Triphasil (Tri-Levelen) was more effective than a combination of spironolactone (100 mg total) and Triphasil. The major side effect of drug-induced hepatitis is found to occur in less than 0.5% of patients given this drug.[39] Flutamide has also been found to cause ambiguous genitalia in male offspring of rats given high doses, so a means of contraception (such as oral contraceptives) should also be prescribed when flutamide is used.

Cyproterone Acetate

Cyproterone acetate is not currently available in the United States but can be a potent antiandrogen with its competitive inhibition of testosterone and DHT receptor binding. It is a synthetic progestin and inhibits gonadotropin secretion and reduces ovarian androgen production. It also induces hepatic enzymes and increases testosterone clearance. Because cyproterone acetate is stored in the ad-ipose tissue and released slowly, it is administered on days 5 to 14 of the menstrual cycle (50 to 200 mg/day), with ethinyl estradiol given on days 5 to 25.[40] As with other antiandrogens, cyproterone acetate can cause feminization of the male fetus as well as rarely seen drug-induced hepatitis. It is prudent to monitor liver enzymes and use oral contraceptives when cyproterone acetate is considered.

Finasteride

Finasteride is the only available 5α-reductase inhibitor; it has been used for the treatment of benign prostatic hyperplasia. The recommended dose for benign prostatic hyperplasia is 5 mg/day. A study by Wong and colleagues[41] has found 5 mg of finasteride daily to be as effective as 100 mg spironolactone daily in reducing the hair shaft diameter by 14% after 6 months. Clinical effects of finasteride have been shown to be improved when used in conjunction with oral contraceptives according to Mogheti and associates.[42] No side effects have been noted in women, and this drug has a good safety profile when given to men for male pattern hair baldness.

Physical Methods

Medical therapy does not remove hair already present, and it does not completely prevent hair growth. The only method of permanent hair removal is electrolysis and temporary methods such as depilation or removal of only part of the hair (shaving and depilatory cremes) and epilation or removal of the entire hair shaft (plucking and waxing). In general, the best results are obtained when cosmesis is used in conjunction with appropriate medical treatment.

CONCLUSION

The patient who presents with hirsutism may often have serious concerns regarding her sexuality, her social acceptance, and her fertility. Frequently, hirsutism accompanies other manifestations of androgen excess, such as acne, anovulation, and menstrual dysfunction. With rare occasions, hirsutism is often a benign condition. The physician has the responsibility of identification of any underlying disorders and applying specific treatments. Because several medications are now available for the treatment of hirsutism, the patient's current reproductive plans should be considered, and cost-effective treatment should then be used.

REFERENCES

1. Pinkus H: Embryology of hair. *In* Montoya W, Elhs RA, eds: The Biology of Hair Growth. New York, Academic Press, 1958.
2. Price VH: Testosterone metabolism in the skin. Arch Dermatol 1975; 111:1496.
3. Oliver RF: The dermal papilla and the development and growth of hair. J Soc Cosmet Chem 1971; 22:741–755.
4. Lobo RA, Goebelsmann V, Itorton R: Evidence for the importance of peripheral tissue events in the development of hirsutism in polycystic ovarian syndrome. J Clin Endocrinol Metab 1983; 58:393.
5. Rebar RW: Hirsutism, hyperandrogenism, and polycystic ovarian syndrome. *In* DeGroot LJ, Besser GM, Cahil GF Jr, et al, eds: Endocrinology, 2nd ed. Philadelphia, WB Saunders, 1989, pp 1982–1993.
6. Goldzieher JW, Axelrod LR: Clinical and biochemical features of polycystic ovarian disease. Fertil Steril 1963; 14:631.
7. Kazer RR, Kessel B, Yen SSC: Circulating luteinizing hormone pulse frequency in women with polycystic ovary syndrome. J Clin Endocrinol Metab 1987; 65:233.
8. Chang RJ, Nakamura RM, Judd HJ, Kaplan SA: Insulin resistance in non-obese patients with polycystic ovarian disease. J Clin Endocrinol Metab 1983; 57:356.
9. Dunaif A, Green G, Futterweit W, et al: Suppression of hyperandrogenism does not improve peripheral or hepatic insulin resistance in the polycystic ovary syndrome. J Clin Endocrinol Metab 70:699, 1990.
10. Barbieri RL, Smith S, Ryan KJ: The role of hyperinsulinemia in the pathogenesis of ovarian hyperandrogenism. Fertil Steril 1988; 50:197–212.
11. Bergh C, Carlsson B, Olsson JH, et al: Regulation of androgen production in cultured human thecal cells by insulin-like growth factor I and insulin. Fertil Steril 1993; 52:323–331.
12. Morris M: Virilizing tumors of the ovary. Cancer Bull 1987; 39:300–303.
13. Scully RE: Ovarian tumors with endocrine manifestations. *In* Degroot LJ, Besser GM, Cahil GF Jr, et al, eds: Endocrinology, 2nd ed. Philadelphia, WB Saunders, 1989, pp 1994–2008.
14. Bondy PK: Disorders of adrenal cortex. *In* Wilson JD, Foster DW, eds: Textbook of Endocrinology. Philadelphia, WB Saunders, 1981, p 816.
15. Glickman SP, Rosenfield RL, Bergenstal RM, Helke J: Multiple androgenic abnormalities, including elevated free testosterone, in hyperprolactinemic women. J Clin Enocrinol Metab 1982; 55:251.
16. Adashi EY, Levin PA: Pathophysiology and evaluation of adrenal hyperandrogenism. Semin Reprod Endocrinol 1986; 4:155.
17. Lobo RA, Kletzky OA: Normalization of androgen and sex hormone-binding globulin levels after treatment of hyperprolactinemia. J Clin Endocrinol Metab 1983; 56:562.
18. Barnes RB: Polycystic ovary syndrome and ovarian steroidogenesis. Semin Reprod Endocrinol (in press).
19. Rosenfield RL, Barnes RB, Cara JF, Lucky AW: Dysregulation of cytochrome p 450-c17 as the cause of polycystic ovarian syndrome. Fertil Steril 1990; 55:785.
20. White PC, New MI, Dupont B: Congenital adrenal hyperplasia (first of two parts). N Engl J Med 1987; 316:1519.
21. New MI: Polycystic ovarian disease and congenital and late-onset adrenal hyperplasia. Endocrinol Metab Clin North Am 1988; 17:637.
22. White PC, New MI, Dupont B: Congenital adrenal hyperplasia (second of two parts). N Engl J Med 1987; 316:1580–1586.
23. Ehrmann DA, Rosenfield RL, Barnes RB, et al: Detection of functional ovarian hyperandrogenism in women with androgen excess. N Engl J Med 1992; 327:157.
24. Ferriman D, Gallwey JD: Clinical assessment of body hair growth in women. J Clin Endocrinol Metab 1961; 21:1440.
25. Hatch R, Rosenfield RL, Kim MH, Tredway D: Hirsutism: Implications, etiology and management. Am J Obstet Gynecol 1981; 43:74.

26. Bardin CW, Lipsett MB: Testosterone and androstenedione blood production rates in normal women with idiopathic hirsutism or polycystic ovaries. J Clin Invest 1967; 46:891.

27. Gagrilove JL, Seman AT, Sabet R, et al: Virilizing adrenal adenoma with studies on the steroid content of the adrenal venous effluent and a review of the literature. Endocrine Rev 1981; 2:462.

28. Derksen J, Haak HR, Moolenaar AJ, van seters AP: Endocrine evaluation of hirsute women to detect adrenal cancer [abstract]. J Steroid Biochem 1990; 36(suppl):78S.

29. Godsland IF, Crook D, Simpson R, et al: The effects of different formulations of oral contraceptive agents on lipid and carbohydrate metabolism. N Engl J Med 1990; 323:1375–1382.

30. Tiitinen A, Simberg N, Stenman U-H, Olavi Y: Estrogen replacement does not potentiate gonadotropin-releasing hormone agonist-induced androgen suppression in treatment of hirsutism. J Clin Endocrinol Metab 1994; 70:642–645.

31. Rittmaster RS, Givner ML: Effects of daily and alternate day low dose prednisone on serum cortisol and adrenal androgens in hirsute women. J Clin Endocrinol Metab 1988; 67:400–403.

32. Weber MM, Luppa P, Engelhardt D: Inhibition of human adrenal androgens secretion by ketoconazole. Klin Wochenschr 1989; 67:707.

33. Sonino N, Scaroni C, Biason A, et al: Low-dose ketoconazole treatment in hirsute women. J Endocrinol Invest 1990; 13:35.

34. Venturoli S, Fabbri R, Dal Prato L, et al: Ketoconazole therapy for women with acne and/or hirsutism. J Clin Endocrinol Metab 1990; 71:335.

35. Serafini P, Lobo RA: The effects of spironolactone on adrenal seroidogenesis on hirsute women. Fertil Steril 1985; 44:595.

36. Menard RH, Stripp B, Gillete JR: Spironolactone and testicular cytocrome p-450: Decreased testosterone formation in several species and changes in hepatic drug metabolism. Endocrinology 1974; 94:1628.

37. Lobo RA, Shoue D, Serafini P, et al: The effects of two doses spironolactone on serum androgens and anagen hair in hirsute women. Fertil Steril 1985; 43:200.

38. Cusan L, Tremblay RR, Dupont A, et al: Comparisons of flutamide and spironolactone in the treatment of hirsutism: A randomized controlled trial. Fertil Steril 1994; 61:281–287.

39. Wysowski DK, Fourcroy JL: Safety of flutamide? Fertil Steril 1994; 62:1089–1090.

40. Biffignandi P, Massuccheti C, Molinatti GM: Female hirsutism: Pathophysiological considerations and therapeutic implications. Endocrine Rev 1984; 5:498.

41. Wong IL, Morris RS, Chang L, et al: A prospective randomized trial comparing finasteride to spironolactone in the treatment of hirsutism. J Clin Endocrinol Metab 1995; 80:233–238.

42. Moghetti P, Castello R, Magnani CM, et al: Clinical and hormonal effects of the 5α-reductase inhibitor finasteride in idiopathic hirsutism. J Clin Endocrinol Metab 1994; 79:1115–1121.

43. Judd HL, Scully RE, Herbst AL, et al: Familial hyperthecosis: Comparison of endocrinologic and histologic findings with polycystic ovarian disease. Am J Obstet Gynecol 1973; 117:979.

44. Nagamani M, Lingold JC, Gomez LG, Barza JR: Clinical and hormonal studies in hyperthecosis of the ovaries. Fertil Steril 1981; 36:326.

45. Nagamani M, Dinn TV, Kelver ME: Hyperinsulinemia in hyperthcosis of the ovaries. Am J Obstet Gynecol 1986; 154:384.

46. Buyalos R: Insulin-like growth factors: Clinical experience in ovarian function.

47. Poretsky L, Grigorescu F, Seibel M, et al: Distribution and characterization of insulin and insulin-like growth factor I receptors in normal human ovary. J Clin Endocrinol Metab 1991; 72:582–587.

48. Barbieri RL, Makris A, Randall RW, et al: Insulin stimulates androgen accumulation in incubations of ovarian stroma obtained from women with hyperandrogenism. J Clin Endocrinol Metab 1986; 62:904–909.

49. Nestler JE, Barlascani CO, Matt DW, et al: Suppression of serum insulin by diozoxide reduces serum testosterone levels in obese women with polycystic ovary syndrome. J Clin Endocrinol Metab 1989; 66:1027–1032.

50. Nestler JE, Powers LP, Matt DW, et al: A direct effect of hyperinsulinemia on serum sex hormone-binding globulin levels in obese women with the polycystic ovary syndrome. J Clin Endocrinol Metab 1991; 72:83.

51. Pang S, Lerner AJ, Stoner E, et al: Late-onset adrenal steroid 3β-hydroxysteroid dehydrogenase deficiency:

I. A cause of hirsutism in pubertal and postpubertal women. J Clin Endocrinol Metab 1985; 60:428.

52. Oldfield EH, Doppman JL, Nieman LK, et al: Petrosal sinus sampling with and without corticotropin releasing hormone for the differential diagnosis of Cushing syndrome. N Engl J Med 1991; 325:897–905.

CHAPTER 13

Infertility

Kenneth A. Ginsburg

Dorcas C. Morgan

. . . Be fruitful and multiply . . .

Genesis 1:28

The early writings of all cultures speak of the importance of conception, birth, parenting, and family. The inability to accomplish this can be quite devastating to a couple. In modern times, infertility is one of the most common reasons for a couple of childbearing age to seek medical care.

For conception to occur, the female partner must have an intact hypothalamic-pituitary-ovarian axis, normal folliculogenesis and ovulation, an effective luteal phase, and normal anatomy. The male partner must have adequate spermatogenesis, normal anatomy, and normal sexual function to enable him to deposit semen in the vaginal vault. Once the ovum is released by the ovary and picked up by the fallopian tube, it travels to the ampullary portion with the assistance of ciliary motion and tubal peristalsis to meet the sperm. The sperm that had been deposited into the vagina traveled into and resided within the cervical mucus wherein the process of capacitation—the acquisition of fertilizing ability—is initiated,[1] then migrated through the internal os of the cervix, into the uterus, and through the tubal ostium to meet the ovum in the tubal ampulla. It is here that fertilization occurs. Once fertilized, the embryo is then propelled to the endometrial cavity, where the endometrium under the influence of the corpus luteum has developed adequately to receive the embryo for implantation. After a variable period, the embryo attaches to the endometrium and implants, and the pregnancy is thus established.

Any disruption along this complex pathway can lead to infertility. This chapter discusses the diagnostic evaluation of the infertile couple within the context of three major infertility mechanisms (Table 13–1): (1) disordered sperm production, function, or both; (2) abnormalities of the ovulatory process; and (3) female anatomic abnormalities. Immunologic infertility, the fourth mechanism of infertility, denotes the production of antisperm antibodies in either partner. These antibodies inhibit sperm migration through the female reproductive tract or interfere with sperm-oocyte interaction. Also included in this category is the antiphospholipid syndrome associated with early pregnancy loss. Because diagnosis and treatment of these conditions are less

Table 13–1. Mechanisms of Female Infertility

Mechanism	Examples or Potential Causes
Ovulatory failure	Turner's syndrome
	Premature ovarian failure
	Kallmann's syndrome
	Hyperprolactinemia
	Hypogonadotropic hypogonadism (anorexia nervosa, weight loss or weight gain, stress, athletic training)
Ovulatory dysfunction	Polycystic ovarian syndrome
	Oligo-ovulation due to stress or obesity
	Luteal phase defect
	Congenital adrenal hyperplasia
Cervix	Absolute dysmucorrhea (dry cervix) after treatment with laser, cold knife cone biopsy, or electrosurgical excision
	Stenosis
	Relative dysmucorrhea from ovulatory failure/dysfunction with hypoestrogenism or idiopathic
	Cervicitis
Uterus	Asherman's syndrome
	Leiomyoma uteri
	Müllerian defect (septum, bicornuate) with habitual abortion
Fallopian tubes	Obstruction due to infection, mechanical compression, endometriosis
Peritoneum	Endometriosis
	Peritoneal adhesions disturbing tubo-ovarian relationships and mobility
Immunologic	Secretion of antibodies into cervical mucus, follicular fluids, or other sites in the reproductive tract that compromise sperm transport or sperm-oocyte interaction

settled and more controversial than male, ovulatory, or anatomic abnormalities, however, immunologic mechanisms are not discussed. After a brief discussion of epidemiologic considerations, the appropriate tests to evaluate these mechanisms are reviewed. Specific diagnostic entities and treatment considerations are also mentioned. Because many of these therapeutic options are labor intensive and expensive, however, it is often in the patient's best interest to refer most treatment to a specialist.

EPIDEMIOLOGY

Infertility is defined as the inability to conceive after regular unprotected sexual intercourse for at least 1 year. This definition is not arbitrary but is based on apparent human fecundity (per cycle probability of pregnancy) of 20%. It is additionally supported by past studies, which confirm that with regular sexual intercourse[2] or insemination,[3] more than half of the women studied were pregnant within 3 months, and approximately 85% of them conceived within 12 months. This definition of 1 year's unsuccessful intercourse is not inviolate, however, because circumstances may be present that demand earlier intervention. For example, couples 35 years or older should be encouraged to seek infertility evaluations earlier because the incidence of infertility increases with the age of the female partner.[2,4] Women experience a gradual decrease in fertility after the age of 25 and more rapid decline after age 35.[5] Even with this recognition of declining female fertility, it must be emphasized that the couple's infertility could still be caused by either the male or female partner. Evaluation of both members of the infertile couple is always imperative.

The prevalence of infertility in the

United States is approximately 14% as reported by the National Survey of Family Growth in 1982 and has remained relatively stable over the past several decades. The perception that infertility has increased in the United States is the result of delays in childbearing in women born during the "baby boom," who have now come to the age when infertility is more prevalent.[6] The risk of infertility is 1.5 times higher in African-American than white couples.[7]

EVALUATION OF THE INFERTILE COUPLE

The initial evaluation of an infertile couple should begin with a complete history and physical examination. This history should be thorough and include detailed discussion of any past evaluation and the results of that testing and therapy, with review of supporting records, if possible. Pertinent issues include discussion of pubertal progression and normality in both partners; urologic or genital injury, infection, or surgery in men; and menstrual, gynecologic, and obstetric histories in women. A history of sexually transmitted disease or pelvic inflammatory disease, diethylstilbestrol (DES) exposure, menorrhagia, uterine enlargement, prior pelvic or abdominal surgery, or treatment for abnormal cervical cytology suggests possible female anatomic abnormalities. Menstrual disorders or evidence of hyperandrogenism (seborrhea, acne, hirsutism, decrease in breast size), hypothyroidism, or hyperprolactinemia (galactorrhea) suggests underlying ovulatory dysfunction. In addition to the infertility and reproductive history, past medical, surgical, and social histories are equally important. The physician should emphasize the importance of evaluating both the male and the female partner. It has been documented that in 30% to 40% of infertile couples, a male factor is the sole or contributing (along with a female factor) cause of infertility. Social factors that could influence fertility, such as tobacco, alcohol, or recreational drug use, should be addressed at the initial visit and behavior modification recommended. Even early in the discussion of infertility the physician should at-

tempt to analyze the couple's goals (to have a biologic child or to have a family) so that other parenting options such as surrogacy, gamete donation, or adoption can be offered when appropriate. In addition, the physician should be aware of religious and social limitations set by the couple. Finally, a reasonable time should be set for completion of the diagnostic evaluation.

Social Factors Influencing Fertility

Numerous social factors influence a couple's ability to conceive. Not infrequently, identification and correction of these factors alone may allow conception to occur without the need for medical intervention. In the young couple without obvious risk factors by history and physical examination, some period of time might be allowed for spontaneous conception after behaviors are modified before further testing or referral.

Many drugs have been associated with alteration of fertility. Tobacco use has been associated with impaired fertility. The Oxford Family Planning Association Study demonstrated that the incidence of infertility in women increased with the number of cigarettes smoked.[8] Nicotine in tobacco is reported to affect fallopian tube peristalsis and motility.[9] Also, tobacco use has been associated with the finding of chlamydia in cervical cultures, therefore increasing the risk for fallopian tube disease and hence ectopic pregnancy.[10] Additionally, although no studies to date have been conducted in humans, exposure of rodents *in utero* to polycyclic aromatic hydrocarbons (a class of compounds found in cigarette smoke) destroyed oocytes in fetal ovaries,[11,12] leading to early reproductive failure in these animals.[10] Therefore, it is possible that maternal smoking could lead not only to tubal infertility, but also reduced fertility in female offspring. In the male, some studies have found impairment of sperm density, motility, and morphology in smokers, although these findings are inconsistent.

Excessive alcohol intake and marijuana use have been associated with reduction in serum testosterone, sperm density, motility, and number of normal appearing sperm.[13–16] Anabolic steroid use may result in hypogonadotropic hypogonadism in men as well. The effects of excessive alcohol intake on female fertility are not well documented, although the consequences of alcohol intake during pregnancy (i.e., the fetal alcohol syndrome) are known to be profound.

In some couples, lubricants are necessary to facilitate coitus. Lubricants such as K-Y jelly, Keri lotion, Lubrifax, and saliva, however, are reported to affect sperm motility *in vitro* and hence could possibly diminish sperm function. Couples should be advised that vegetable oil, petroleum jelly, raw egg white, and peanut oil do not appear to have this effect *in vitro* and hence may be safer for use.

Coital frequency and timing are important in couples trying to conceive. Macleod and Gold[17] found that couples who engaged in sexual intercourse more than three times a week were more likely to conceive within 6 months than couples who had a lower coital frequency. Additionally, when coital frequency is optimal, sperm should be present in the fallopian tubes at the time of ovulation, enhancing the chances of conception. Therefore, knowledge of the approximate time of ovulation and optimal coital timing improve a couple's chance for conception.

DIAGNOSTIC EVALUATION

The initial infertility evaluation should consist of evaluation for male factors, documentation of ovulation, and evaluation for female anatomic factors. In most cases, when a problem in any of these areas is identified, referral to a specialist is necessary to initiate treatment. As well, couples with unexplained infertility based on this diagnostic algorithm should be referred for advanced testing or empiric infertility therapy.

Male Factor Evaluation

The male evaluation should start with a complete history and physical examination. The historical survey should include a search for congenital anomalies such as cryptorchidism and hypospadias, which could effect sperm quality or delivery. In addition, a history of abnormal pubertal development could suggest the diagnosis of central endocrine disorders causing hypogonadotropic hypogonadism, adrenogenital syndrome, or Klinefelter's syndrome. A history of prepubertal or adult genital trauma should alert the practitioner to the possibility of defective sperm production or the presence of autoantibodies to sperm.

The physical examination should be complete and include a thorough examination of the body habitus, degree of masculinization, and genitalia. The length of the penis should be 5 cm with minimal stretch, and the position of the meatus is noted. The testicles should be palpated for consistency and size. Normal adult testes are somewhat firm, 4.6 cm in length and 2.6 cm in width, with a mean volume of 18.6 ± 4.8 ml.[18] Because the seminiferous tubules constitute most of the testicular volume, diminished volume is associated with loss of seminiferous tubules and germinal epithelium. Hence, shrinkage and softening of the testicles are often associated with abnormal exocrine (spermatogenic) function. The spermatic cords are palpated for thickening or enlargement possibly indicative of a varicocele. The Valsalva maneuver should be a part of this evaluation to determine the presence of a varicocele. Ninety percent of varicoceles occur on the left side. If suspected from the examination, an ultrasound examination of the scrotum can be obtained to confirm the findings. The significance of this finding is controversial because a varicocele is present in approximately 8% to 23% of all men and 17% of men with proven fertility. Although not yet settled, some investigators advocate surgical correction of the varicocele in infertile men with grossly abnormal sperm density or sperm motility.

Central to the laboratory evaluation of male reproductive potential is the semen analysis, which should be obtained at a reputable laboratory after a 48- to 72-hour period of abstinence. At least two, and preferably three, semen analyses over 2 to 3 months are necessary to characterize semen quality adequately because some variability is inherent. Furthermore, because spermatogenesis is a continuous process occurring in cycles of approximately 74 days, between 2 and 3 months should elapse between analyses to sample different cycles of spermatogenesis. This is especially important when abnormalities are found on the initial semen analysis or when transitory insults such as febrile illness or medications occur.

The basic semen analysis assesses the physical characteristics of semen (volume, pH, liquefaction, color) and sperm density, morphology, and motility. Table 13–2 defines the 1992 World Health Organization criteria for normal semen.[19] There is no threshold value, however, below which pregnancy will not occur because fertility has been associated even with multiple severe abnormalities in semen parameters. Further, normal sperm concentration, morphology, and motility do not guarantee optimal or even normal sperm function, and they cannot be used to define male fertility; the semen analysis is viewed, therefore, as a screening test to determine who should be evaluated further. In addition, these normal

criteria must now be reassessed in light of emerging assisted reproductive technologies such as in vitro fertilization with gamete micromanipulation, which have allowed conception when literally only several sperm have been recovered.

Based on the results of several semen analyses, the male partner is provisionally classified as having normal or abnormal reproductive potential. When semen abnormalities are demonstrated, further testing by a specialist attempts to describe the nature of sperm dysfunction, its possible cause, and best treatment available. Some other tests to evaluate male reproductive function include serum endocrine testing, testicular biopsy, radiographic evaluation of the exocrine ducts (vas deferens, ejaculatory ducts), assays of sperm penetration into zona free hamster oocytes or attachment to human hemizonae, and tests of semen and serum for the presence of autoantibodies to sperm antigens.

Ovulation Assessment

The only definitive proof that ovulation has occurred is pregnancy. There are known physiologic changes, however, that occur at or around the time of ovulation that can be measured and used as indirect evidence of ovulation. These include measurement of basal body temperature (BBT), detection in blood or urine of a luteinizing hormone (LH) surge, measurement of serum progesterone levels in the luteal phase, or a luteal phase endometrial biopsy. Transvaginal ultrasound to assess ovarian follicular growth serially is an excellent means of monitoring the ovulatory process, especially when used in conjunction with serum estradiol determination. The combination of follicular ultrasound determination with estrogen measurement is more involved than the other methods mentioned, and is probably best relegated to the specialist.

The measurement of BBT is the least expensive and simplest test to assess ovulation. The disadvantages in using this method are that it is not accurate and it provides only a retrospective evaluation of ovulation. Therefore, one cannot use BBT charting to determine

Table 13–2. Normal Values of Semen Variables

Variables	Normal Values
Volume	>2.0 mL
pH	7.2–7.8
Sperm concentration	20×10^6/mL or greater
Total sperm count	40×10^6 or greater
Motility	≥50% with forward progression or ≥25% with rapid linear progression within 60 min after collection
Morphology	≥30% normal morphology
Viability	≥50% live
White blood cells	$<1 \times 10^6$/mL
Mixed antiglobulin test	<10% spermatozoa with adherent particles
Immunobead test	<10% spermatozoa with adherent beads

Data from the World Health Organization: Laboratory Manual for the Examination of Human Semen and Sperm-Cervical Mucus Interaction. Cambridge, Cambridge University Press, 1992.

whether coitus occurred at the appropriate time in the cycle until after ovulation has occurred. With that caveat in mind, the BBT chart does provide useful information about ovulation and the length of the luteal phase. In taking the BBT, the patient is instructed to record her temperature immediately on awakening after at least 4 hours of uninterrupted sleep. Just before ovulation, there is a reported dip in the curve thought to represent impending ovulation, although this nadir is not consistently found. With ovulation, there is the production of progesterone by the corpus luteum, which has a thermogenic effect on the hypothalamus causing a 0.4 to 0.6°F rise in temperature.[20] It should be recognized that although BBTs are used frequently to determine if ovulation has occurred, numerous factors may affect the accuracy of the results. These include an illness, interrupted sleep, medication, reader's error, and cycle variability.

Another indirect predictor of ovulation is measurement of relative urinary LH concentration using commercially available test kits. The ovum is released from the mature graafian follicle 32 to 34 hours after the onset of the ovulatory surge of LH in blood. As serum LH levels rise, the hormone spills into the urine, where its increased level can be detected with monoclonal qualitative colorimetric assays. Using prior cycle length as a guide (BBT chart from previous cycles or menstrual history), the woman begins daily urinary LH testing several days before anticipated ovulation. The day of the LH surge is defined as the first day when the test switches from negative to positive, reflecting the appearance of LH in the urine above some basal amount. Ovulation can be predicted to occur within 1 to 2 days. With the detection of an LH surge, one can time coitus or schedule inseminations to facilitate conception.

With ovulation, there is the formation of a corpus luteum from the mature follicle, which now secretes progesterone in addition to estrogen. These steroids prepare the proliferative endometrium to accept the fertilized ovum and support the resulting early pregnancy. Serum progesterone normally rises to peak levels 6 to 8 days after the LH surge. Therefore, measuring serum progesterone at this time of the cycle provides additional evidence that ovulation has occurred. A serum progesterone level of 10 ng/mL or greater is usually taken to be suggestive of ovulation. A value between 3 and 10 ng/mL may suggest luteal phase deficiency, and a value less than 3 ng/mL suggests anovulation.[21] Owing to the pulsatile release of progesterone from the corpus luteum, there is as yet no agreement on a single serum progesterone value that is indicative of normal luteal function. Consequently the clinical use of these assays to determine luteal adequacy is neither sensitive nor specific.

An endometrial biopsy during the late luteal phase of the menstrual cycle can provide not only evidence of probable ovulation, but also allows evaluation of endometrial maturation in response to the progesterone and estrogen secreted by the corpus luteum.[22] For evaluation of ovulation and luteal adequacy, it is recommended that the biopsy be done 10 to 12 days after ovulation (determined by BBT, urinary LH surge). To be considered abnormal, the endometrium must be out of phase more than 2 days with the retrospectively determined ovarian cycle day. This luteal phase defect should be confirmed in at least one additional cycle because in approximately 15% of random cycles, individuals with normal ovulation and fertility have out of phase endometrial biopsy specimens by these criteria.[23] The disadvantages of this method include (1) the pain associated with the procedure, which may be overcome by administering an analgesic before performing the procedure; (2) the possibility of disrupting an established pregnancy with the introduction of the biopsy instrument during the late luteal phase, even before serum human chorionic gonadotropin is detectable; and (3) the inherent cost. Those concerns aside, the authors recommend endometrial biopsy to confirm luteal adequacy in the routine infertility evaluation; the biopsy is performed in a cycle in which the patient does not attempt conception, using a nonsteroidal anti-inflammatory agent as an analgesic administered 0.5 hour before the procedure for patient comfort.

Numerous causes of anovulation exist, such as polycystic ovarian disease, androgen excess of adrenal or ovarian origin, hypogonadotropic hypogonadism (pituitary or hypothalamic dysfunction or failure, resulting in inadequate or inappropriate gonadotropin production), hyperprolactinemia, and ovarian failure. Once ovulatory dysfunction has been documented by the aforementioned tests, further evaluation is warranted. Various endocrine axes can be probed for normality under baseline conditions (e.g., serum gonadotropins, androgens, thyroid-stimulating hormone, prolactin) and after provocative or suppressive challenges. Again the complexity and cost of these additional tests suggest that they be done by practitioners experienced in their performance and interpretation.

Mechanical Factors

Cervical Factors

In addition to facilitating sperm transport and acting both as a reservoir for and as a filter of sperm, cervical mucus plays an important role in sperm capacitation, a poorly understood process by which sperm acquire the ability to bind to and penetrate the oocyte, resulting in fertilization. The process includes alterations in sperm motility and energy state and modifications in the apical sperm plasma membrane (the outer acrosomal membrane) rendering it capable of undergoing the acrosome reaction when in the vicinity of the oocyte. The acrosome contains enzymes necessary for dispersion of the cumulus cells and digestion of the zona pellucida surrounding the oocyte. With the acrosome reaction, these enzymes are released into the extracellular milieu surrounding the oocyte and its cumulus complex. This dispersion of cumulus cells and digestion of the zona pellucida facilitates penetration of the oocyte by sperm.

The cervical mucus is produced by nonciliated cells of the cervical epithelium under hormonal control. The amount of mucus produced varies directly with the estrogenic effect on the cervix, from as little as 60 mg/day in the early follicular phase to 700 mg/day at midcycle. Preovulatory (estrogenic) mucus is abundant in amount, is highly elastic (spinnbarkeit), watery and thin, clear,

and supportive of sperm transport. Early in the follicular phase, or once ovulation occurs and progesterone is produced by the corpus luteum, the cervical mucus becomes thick, scant, and impenetrable by sperm.[24] Sperm survive approximately 48 hours in favorable cervical mucus.[25]

The evaluation of the cervical factor in infertility is initiated with the postcoital test (PCT). Period of abstinence since last ejaculation, elapsed time between coitus and the examination, and the timing of the PCT relative to ovulation are critical variables to control relative to proper interpretation. The PCT should be done after an abstinence period (usually 2 to 3 days) so as to allow adequate restoration of motile sperm concentration in the man[26] and in the midcycle periovulatory interval when cervical mucus is at its peak quality (high volume, lowest viscosity, highest elasticity, and lowest cellularity). The patient is instructed to have sexual intercourse, and the mucus is recovered from the exocervix and endocervix 6 to 24 hours thereafter.[19,27,28] The mucus quality is determined according to established criteria evaluating such physical factors as amount, spinnbarkeit, ferning pattern, viscosity, cellularity, and pH, using an established scoring system (Table 13–3) such as the one developed by Moghissi.[27] In addition to the mucus quality described, one evaluates the number and motility of sperm present in the cervical mucus. Although controversy exists as to the number and type of sperm motility necessary in the PCT for pregnancy to occur, it is generally accepted that the presence of any progressively motile sperm is acceptable.

If the PCT is abnormal, further specialized testing is sometimes warranted. For example, a semen-mucus crossed penetration test may be performed in a four-way comparison with semen and cervical mucus from fertile donors. Briefly, mucus penetration by the sperm in question is tested with the partner's mucus and donor mucus, and a similar test is carried out with the mucus in question using the partner's and donor sperm. This allows one to determine if the abnormality on the PCT is the result of an abnormality in the male or female partner. Another test to measure cervical mucus–

Table 13-3. Cervical Mucus Evaluation

Score	Volume
0	0 mL
1	0.1 mL
2	0.2 mL
3	≥0.3 mL
	Consistency
0	Thick, highly viscous, premenstrual mucus
1	Mucus of intermediate viscosity
2	Mildly viscous mucus
3	Watery, minimally viscous, midcycle (preovulatory) mucus
	Ferning
0	No crystallization
1	Atypical fern formation
2	Primary and secondary stem ferning
3	Tertiary and quaternary stem ferning
	Spinnbarkeit
0	<1 cm
1	1-4 cm
2	5-8 cm
3	≥9 cm
	Cellularity
0	20 cells/hpf
1	11-20 cells/hpf
2	1-10 cells/hpf
3	0 cells

sperm interaction is the sperm–cervical mucus contact test.[29] This test involves examining sperm at an *in vitro* interface with mucus by placing drops of semen and mucus in contact under a glass coverslip. The test is positive if progressive sperm motility is reduced or penetration into the mucus does not occur, and the investigation should then search for antisperm antibodies in both partners.

Uterine Factors

Abnormalities of the uterus that could adversely affect reproductive potential include those that distort the uterine cavity or its muscular wall (or both), and endometrial abnormalities. The former category includes uterine fibroids, polyps, adhesions, and müllerian anomalies such as uterine septum or bicornuate uterus. Endometrial abnormalities include chronic or acute endometritis and luteal phase deficiency (LPD). In LPD, the endometrium is insufficiently stimulated by luteal progesterone and estrogen or, less commonly, is unable to respond normally to these steroids. In either case, endometrial maturation is delayed relative to the ovarian cycle such that the embryo is attempting to implant into an endometrium that is not prepared to receive it.

The routine evaluation of endometrial maturation for LPD involves either luteal phase serum progesterone determinations or endometrial biopsy (discussed previously). Serum progesterone levels are measured during the midluteal or late luteal phases of the menstrual cycle for determination of luteal adequacy. Unfortunately, no progesterone level is significantly associated with endometrial adequacy or LPD; hence, serum progesterone determination is not a sensitive determinant of ovarian function or endometrial maturation. At present, the best way to diagnose LPD is via a timed endometrial biopsy. Two consecutive biopsies greater than 2 days out of phase is diagnostic of LPD.

Evaluation of the uterine cavity can be accomplished using either hysterosalpingography or hysteroscopy. The hysterosalpingogram (HSG) allows delineation of the uterine (and tubal) internal architecture. Areas of dye exclusion within the uterine cavity could be submucous myomas, polyps, adhesions (Fig. 13–1), or evidence of müllerian anomaly. Details on performing the HSG are given later. Hysteroscopy involves transcervical placement of an endoscopic instrument into the uterine cavity, with distending media (carbon dioxide or various aqueous media such as dextran or 10% dextrose in water) used to separate the uterine walls so that the cavity can be inspected. The complete hysteroscopic examination allows inspection of the internal tubal ostia; the configuration of the cavity and the presence of adhesions, myomas, and müllerian defects; and the normality of the endometrial surfaces. The procedure can be performed within the office setting with suitable analgesia or in the operating room under anesthesia. In the latter case, hysteroscopy is often done in conjunction with laparoscopy for complete evaluation of the pelvis.

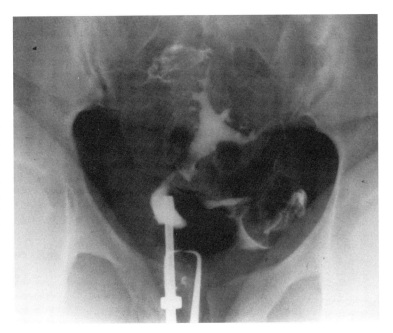

Figure 13–1. Hysterosalpingogram demonstrating marginal filling defects in both uterine horns associated with intrauterine synechiae or adhesions (Asherman's syndrome). Although not well delineated on this film, both tubes filled with dye, and patency was demonstrated bilaterally.

Tubal and Peritoneal Factors

Determining tubal patency is a crucial part of an infertility evaluation. It should be performed early in the evaluation of all patients, especially those with a history of pelvic inflammatory disease, gonococcal or chlamydial infection, previous pelvic surgery, prior intrauterine device use,[30] postpartum curettage, or in utero exposure to DES. Determining tubal patency can be accomplished either with an HSG or by direct visualization at laparoscopy with transcervical instillation of dye (endoscopic tubal dye perfusion).

The HSG is an invaluable nonsurgical examination in a patient with infertility because it provides information about the internal anatomy of the uterus and the fallopian tubes.[31] In the case of the fallopian tubes, visualization of the internal architecture cannot be accomplished even at laparoscopy or hysteroscopy. It is less invasive and less expensive than laparoscopy and should be performed, in most cases, before laparoscopy is considered. The HSG provides information about intrauterine contour and the presence or absence of intrauterine pathology such as synechiae or myomas. In addition, it provides information about the presence of tubal disease such as salpingitis isthmica nodosa, obstruction,

or hydrosalpinx (Fig. 13–2) and the state of the tubal architecture (the presence or absence of rugal folds). An increased pregnancy rate has been associated with the cycles immediately following the HSG procedure. Therefore, if a patient has an otherwise normal evaluation including a normal HSG, an interval of time could be allowed between the HSG and other intervention for spontaneous conception to occur.

The HSG should be performed in the early follicular to midfollicular phase of the menstrual cycle after completion of menstrual bleeding because during menstruation there is the theoretical risk of refluxing dislodged endometrium through the tubes, which could lead to the development of endometriosis. Also, in the early proliferative to midproliferative phase, there is still a thin endometrial lining, which would decrease the possibility of false occlusion of the tubal ostia by late proliferative or secretory endometrium. The HSG is never performed during the luteal phase because there is the possibility of disruption of an established pregnancy at that time.

Performance of the HSG entails injecting a radiopaque medium into the uterus via a cannula placed into the endocervix or uterine cavity. Several different cannulas are commercially available, each

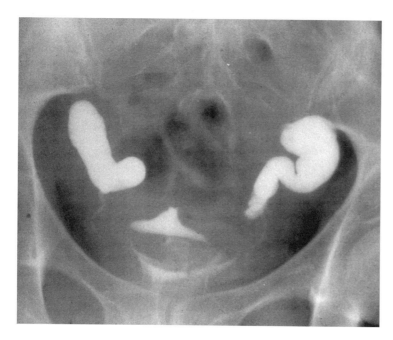

Figure 13-2. Hysterosalpingogram demonstrating bilateral distal tubal occlusion or hydrosalpinx. The uterine cavity in this delayed film appears unremarkable. Both tubes, however, remain dilated with dye that has failed to escape from the fimbriated end.

with advantages and disadvantages. Single-use disposable and reusable instruments can also be found. The authors prefer an instrument that attaches to the exocervix and hence allows examination of the cervical canal and internal cervical os; balloon-tipped cannulas that wedge inside the uterine cavity necessarily obscure the lower uterine segment such that the contour there cannot be evaluated. Image intensification fluoroscopy allows the examiner to follow the retrograde progress of radiopaque dye through the reproductive tract. Several spot films are sequentially taken when the uterus fills, when the tubes fill, when spillage of dye from the tubes is seen, and then later to demonstrate emptying of the tubes and normal dye dispersion through the pelvis. With good technique and timing, the HSG can be completed with three to four spot films, thus limiting radiation exposure to considerably less than 1 rad.[21]

Both water-based and oil-based radiopaque media can be used for the HSG. Each has inherent advantages and disadvantages associated with its use. Both preparations contain iodine and therefore should not be used in patients with iodine sensitivity. Both have been associated with exacerbation or reactivation of acute pelvic inflammatory disease in patients with prior history or possibly causing *de novo* pelvic inflammatory disease as a result of bacteria ascending to the uterus during the procedure itself. Many practitioners recommend that patients with suspected or known prior tubal disease receive prophylactic antibiotics before or immediately after HSG to decrease the incidence of this complication.[32] The authors prefer to treat all women prophylactically with a broad-spectrum antibiotic (e.g., doxycycline) beginning 24 hours before the HSG. The water-based preparations are absorbed more quickly; however, their use is associated with more pain than the oil-based media. The oil-based media better delineate the rugal folds of the fallopian tubes; however, they have been associated with a greater inflammatory response and a higher risk for granuloma formation possibly because of their slow absorption and resulting risk of a foreign body reaction. The most dramatic complication associated with the HSG is lymphatic or venous intravasation of contrast media with embolization. The results of embolization can be more serious with the oil-based media. Symptoms may vary from minor complaints to chest pain, cough, dyspnea, light-headedness, cardiopulmonary compromise, and death.[33,34] Although these complications are reported rarely, their potential should be kept in mind. With fluoroscopy, when the intravasation of contrast media is noted, it is imperative to terminate the procedure before a large quantity of contrast media is injected.

Evaluation of the pelvis by direct visualization to examine the pelvic anatomy, especially the relationship of the ovarian surfaces to the fallopian tube, and to document the presence of any other pathology such as endometriosis or adhesions, is accomplished via laparoscopy. Diagnostic laparoscopy is an invasive surgical procedure that requires the use of either regional or general anesthesia. Briefly the technique is as follows: With the patient anesthetized, pneumoperitoneum is first established by instilling gas into the peritoneal cavity via a needle inserted transcutaneously, usually at the umbilicus. The patient is placed in deep Trendelenburg position, in which the bubble of gas pushes the intestinal contents downward, away from the pelvic organs. The laparoscope, inserted at the umbilicus, is then used to inspect the pelvic organs. Transcervically instilled colored dye can be used to document or confirm tubal patency.

At the time of laparoscopic examination, the surgeon should be prepared to perform operative laparoscopy to treat any endometriosis found or lyse any adhesions that may improve the tubo-ovarian relationship. The timing of this examination in an infertility evaluation is individualized and depends on the patient's past history, physical examination, and duration of infertility. Before initiating most infertility treatment, however, endoscopic examination of the pelvis is warranted to exclude otherwise undetected pathology that could compromise further treatment efficacy. In the future, the development of smaller endoscopes will allow routine performance of laparoscopy under local anesthesia in an office setting. The decreased cost and increased availability of this procedure will undoubtedly alter current recommendations regarding the sequence of tests in the routine evaluation of the infertile couple. Moreover, falloposcopy will one day allow direct examination of the internal tubal architecture, of particular significance when deciding between surgical repair of obstructed fallopian tubes or *in vitro* fertilization.

Hysteroscopy is a technique for evaluation of the internal anatomy of the uterus that can be performed at the time of laparoscopy. It requires the use of an analgesic or anesthetic and a distending medium to separate the uterine walls to allow adequate visualization. If intrauterine adhesions, myomas, polyps, or an intrauterine septum is identified, operative hysteroscopy for incision, excision, or resection can be performed. Often, this operative hysteroscopy is best performed with concomitant laparoscopy. Hence a thorough preoperative evaluation before endoscopic examination and possible treatment allows the physician and patient to plan the most efficient and cost-effective therapy.

TREATMENT CONSIDERATIONS

Once the evaluation is completed, all appropriate treatment options should be discussed with the couple. From this discussion, therapeutic plans can be initiated. Moreover, it must be emphasized that treatment should, with few exceptions, be deferred until the evaluation as outlined previously is completed. In this way, treatment is individualized and specific and is aimed at correcting *all* known fertility factors in the particular couple. Empiric therapy is, in general, less successful than specific therapy and can also result in significant frustration and expense.

Treatment of Male Factors

In male factor infertility, one of the most common diagnostic entities is a varicocele. If physical examination and appropriate diagnostic tests support the presence of a varicocele and semen analysis shows low motility (asthenospermia), low sperm concentration (oligozoospermia), or abnormal morphology (teratospermia), a varicolectomy can be recommended to the patient to improve semen quality. Alternatively a course of clomiphene citrate can be employed to stimulate sperm production with the hope of increasing the number of motile sperm in the ejaculate. Published results with this approach have, in general, been disappointing. As an alternative or if semen quality does not improve after surgery, in vitro fertilization with or without intracytoplasmic sperm injection can be offered. Another option for a couple with male factor infertility because of a varicocele is insemination with anonymous donor sperm.

Endocrinopathies are a rare cause of male infertility. When found, however, they offer the opportunity for endocrine therapy, which may be highly efficacious in selected patients. The treatment strategy is analogous to the anovulatory woman, wherein confounding endocrinopathies are treated, the hypothalamic-pituitary-gonadal axis is up-regulated, or replacement therapy with gonadotropins is used, depending on the exact diagnosis. Thus, patients with elevated prolactin levels should be evaluated for the presence of an adenoma and treated according to findings; as in the woman, bromocriptine lowers elevated prolactin levels in these men and helps restore normal spermatogenesis. In couples with male hypogonadotropic hypogonadism (e.g., Kallmann's syndrome), therapy using either human chorionic gonadotropin or menopausal gonadotropins can stimulate the germinal epithelium. These patients should be aware, however, that it may take several months to years before there is evidence of sperm production after beginning this replacement therapy. Clomiphene is also used in men to stimulate endogenous gonadotropin production, with the hope of stimulating sperm production. In carefully selected men with hypothalamic-pituitary dysfunction who can respond to clomiphene, improvement in semen quality can be seen; however, when used in other circumstances (especially as empiric therapy for idiopathic oligozoospermia), success rates have been disappointing.

In men with primary testicular diseases, such as Sertoli-cell only syndrome, Klinefelter's syndrome, or destruction of germ cells by chemotherapy or trauma, therapeutic donor insemination or adoption is the only alternative available. Today, therapeutic donor insemination is universally performed in the United States using cryopreserved semen that has been quarantined to allow adequate donor testing and retesting for sexually transmitted diseases. Hence the practice is safe, with little chance of communicating disease. Success rates remain quite high when donor insemination is properly timed with ovulation.

In general, the physiology, pathophysiology, and treatment of male fertility problems have not received the attention afforded various female diagnoses. As a result, less is known about male infertility, and fewer specific treatments are available. Intrauterine insemination with borderline or minor semen defects is at times recommended, often with concomitant superovulation protocols. The value of this approach, however, is as yet unproven. The ability to inject sperm successfully directly into the oocyte cytoplasm (intracytoplasmic sperm injection) with resulting fertilization, pregnancy, and live birth has opened innumerable opportunities for treatment of severely oligozoospermic men who would have been untreatable in the past. In addition, the use of testicular or epididymal sperm recovery allows clinicians to offer intracytoplasmic sperm injection to men who have *any* germinal epithelial function, regardless of whether or not mature spermatozoa are present within their semen. Finally, for some couples (with intractable male infertility problems when various religious, ethical, or moral beliefs preclude acceptance of donor insemination), adoption remains the only option for establishing a family. It is equally important for the physician to recognize these couples, so that help and guidance in the appropriate direction can be offered early in the therapeutic discussion.

Treatment of Female Factors

If infertility is the result of anovulation, the underlying cause should again first be investigated before treatment is initiated. Examples of treatment options include the following. In anovulation secondary to polycystic ovarian syndrome (in which the LH-to-follicle-stimulating hormone ratio is inverted and greater than 2:1), ovulation may be induced using either clomiphene citrate or gonadotropin therapy. Patients with ovulatory dysfunction of adrenal origin, such as in late-onset congenital adrenal hyperplasia (in which 17-hydroxyprogesterone response to an ACTH challenge is exaggerated), respond to supplementation of the deficient steroid with the return of regular ovulation and menses; after dexamethasone or prednisone replacement in these women, continued anovulation or ovulatory dysfunction is then treated using clomiphene or gonadotropin therapy. Anovulation secondary to hyperprolactinemia is treated with bromocriptine to lower endogenous prolactin levels. If hypogonadotropic hypogonadism is found, treatment either with pulsatile gonadotropin-releasing hormone or exogenous gonadotropin therapy is recommended, depending on measured pituitary responsiveness, experience of the physician, and the patient's wishes. Luteal phase deficiency represents a type of ovulatory dysfunction in which follicular development is in some way abnormal; despite this, ovulation occurs, but corpus luteum function is abnormal. When luteal phase defect is detected, treatment with clomiphene citrate during the follicular phase of the cycle is the preferred option. With this medication, improved folliculogenesis, enhanced follicular estrogen production, and enhanced luteal steroid production better prepare the endometrium for luteal transition and development. Alternatively, support of the luteal phase with additional progesterone has been used with variable success. The diagnosis of ovarian failure is based on the repeated demonstration of markedly elevated gonadotropins in a hypoestrogenic woman. In these patients, ovulation induction is not indicated because ovarian function cannot be recovered. Ovum donation or adoption should be offered at the same time that climacteric hormone replacement for prevention of osteoporosis and cardiovascular disease is discussed.

These two ovulation induction agents, clomiphene and gonadotropin preparations, have different mechanisms of action. Clomiphene citrate is a weak estrogen, which binds to estrogen receptors but results in a minimal estrogenic effect. In essence, therefore, clomiphene is an antiestrogen that acts at the hypothalamic-pituitary level via negative feedback to stimulate gonadotropin secretion. Given early in the follicular phase only for several days, the induced hypoestrogenic signal results in enhanced pituitary follicle-stimulating hormone secretion that stimulates follicular growth. Normally occurring estrogen feedback from the growing follicle then triggers the midcycle gonadotropin surge that results in oocyte release. Parenterally administered gonadotropin preparations act to stimulate the ovarian follicles directly; neither hypothalamic-pituitary function nor feedback is necessary for gonadotropin actions. Preparations available include human chorionic gonadotropin (seen as LH by the follicle) and human (urinary) menopausal gonadotropins with various ratios of follicle-stimulating hormone and LH. Formulations of recombinant follicle-stimulating hormone and recombinant LH are currently under review for eventual use in the United States.

Two strategies are employed in treating cervical factor infertility: attempting to improve mucus or bypassing the mucus barrier. The absence of good quality mucus may be due to inadequate stimulation of the cervical glands in an anovulatory or oligo-ovulatory woman. In this setting, successful ovulation induction or the use of exogenous preovulatory estrogen may improve cervical mucus quality. Alternatively, both for the problem of inadequate or hostile mucus and when antibodies are present, intrauterine insemination with the partner's sperm may be offered. If pregnancy is not obtained after several treatment cycles in cervical factor patients, in vitro fertilization and embryo transfer may be offered.

Intrauterine pathology is treated via the hysteroscope or laparotomy, depending on the exact abnormality found. If intrauterine adhesions, submucous myomas, polyps, or a septum is found, these can be surgically corrected by way of the hysteroscope. Intramural or subserosal fibroids can often be treated only by laparotomy. Metroplasty to correct some congenital uterine defects (including some uterine septa) may be performed by laparotomy as well.

The fallopian tubes are essentially a

site for gamete interaction and early embryo development and transport to the uterus. Options for the patient with tubal disease basically involve treatment to repair the tubes or treatment to bypass them; the situation is analogous to the cervical factor patient. If proximal tubal occlusion is detected and the remainder of the fallopian tube appears normal by direct visualization at the time of laparoscopy, selective proximal tubal canalization to attempt transcervical tuboplasty may be offered. Failed transcervical tuboplasty requires either laparotomy with segmental tubal resection and re-anastamosis, laparotomy with tubal reimplantation, or in vitro fertilization.

If distal tubal occlusion (a hydrosalpinx; see Fig. 13–2) is found, the internal architecture of the fallopian tubes at the time of HSG is important in predicting the success of reparative surgery. If the fallopian tubes are dilated with no rugal folds, the likelihood of that tube being able to pick up an oocyte and transport it to the uterus is poor. In this situation, a distal neosalpingostomy is not ideal, and in vitro fertilization should be offered to the patient. If the internal anatomy of the fallopian tubes is intact with just distal occlusion, however, the patient may be a candidate for neosalpingostomy. Unfortunately, even in experienced hands under the best of circumstances, the probability of intrauterine pregnancy after neosalpingostomy is never high. Assisted reproduction using in vitro fertilization is frequently the treatment of choice whenever intrinsic tubal disease is found. When the tubes themselves are normal and occlusion or malposition results from pelvic adhesive disease, lysis of adhesions by laparoscopy or laparotomy is a viable and appropriate treatment option.

Optimal treatment of the infertile patient with endometriosis is not settled. Early stages of disease (e.g., minimal or mild endometriosis based on the revised American Fertility Society Classification) do not appear to impair fertility. Hence, additional surgery (beyond the laparoscopy used to diagnose the condition) or medical therapy in the infertile patient with minimal or mild endometriosis fails to enhance fertility and therefore cannot be recommended in most circumstances.

Moderate or severe endometriosis should be treated surgically if found. Either a laparoscopic approach or laparotomy is appropriate, depending on the amount of disease, its location relative to other viscera, and the skill and experience of the physician. Laser vaporization, electrocauterization, and resection appear to be equally efficacious. Neither the role of preoperative or postoperative medical suppressive therapy for endometriosis nor the use of isolated 6- to 9-month treatment courses to enhance fertility potential is clear based on controlled clinical trials. In general, gonadotropin-releasing hormone analogues, danazol, and progestins appear to be approximately equally beneficial, and choices between them involve the patient's ability to tolerate different side effects along with physician preference.

CONCLUSION

An infertility evaluation begins with a complete history and physical examination. The major causes of infertility—male factors, ovulatory disturbances, and female anatomic abnormalities—should be investigated (Table 13–4) in every couple presenting for evaluation. It should be emphasized that all factors should be evaluated and excluded before therapy is begun because frequently more than one problem causes the couple's infertility. It should also be noted, however, that in approximately 15% of couples no cause for their infertility is identified. Once the diagnostic evaluation is completed, treatment directed toward correcting the underlying

---

Table 13–4. Routine Infertility Evaluation

History and physical examination of both
  partners
At least two (preferably three) semen analyses
Documentation of ovulation
Hysterosalpingogram
Postcoital test
Timed endometrial biopsy to document luteal
  adequacy
Endoscopic evaluation of the female pelvis

cause or causes is initiated. Empiric therapy involving insemination, super-ovulation, in vitro fertilization, or other such modalities is used when no cause is identified or when specific therapy is un-available or unsuccessful.

RECOMMENDED READINGS

Insler V, Lunenfeld B, eds: Infertility: Male and Female, 2nd ed. Edinburgh, Churchill Livingstone, 1993.

Keye WR, Chang RJ, Rebar RW, Soules MR, eds: Infertility Evaluation and Treatment. Philadelphia, WB Saunders, 1995.

Seibel MM: Infertility: A Comprehensive Text. Norwalk, CT, Appleton & Lange, 1990.

Sigman M, Lipshultz LJ, Howards SS. Evaluation of the subfertile male. In Lipshultz LJ, Howards SS, eds: Infertility in the Male. St. Louis, Mosby-Yearbook, 1991, 179.

Speroff L, Glass RH, Kase NG: Clinical Gynecologic Endocrinology and Infertility, 5th ed. Baltimore, Williams & Wilkins, 1994.

REFERENCES

1. Lambert H, Overstreet JW, Morales P, et al: Sperm capacitation in human fe-male reproductive tract. Fertil Steril 1985; 43:325.
2. Guttmacher AF: Factors affecting nor-mal expectancy of conception. JAMA 1956; 161:855.
3. Strickler RC, Keller DW, Warren JC: Ar-tificial insemination with donor semen. N Engl J Med 1975; 283:848.
4. Tietze C: Reproductive span and rate of reproduction among Hutterite women. Fertil Steril 1957; 8:89.
5. Hendershot GE, Mosher WD, Pratt WF: Infertility and age: An unresolved issue. Fam Plann Perspect 1982; 14:287.
6. Mosher WD, Pratt WE: Fecundity and infertility in the United States: Inci-dence and trends. Fertil Steril 1991; 56:192.
7. United States Congress, Office of Tech-nology Assessment: Infertility: Medical and Social Choices [OTA-BA-358]. Washington, DC, U.S. Government Printing Office, 1988.
8. Howe G, Westoff C, Vessey M, Yeate D: Effects of age, cigarette smoking, and other factors on fertility: Finding in a large prospective study. Br Med J 1985; 290:1697.
9. Weatherbee PS: Nicotine and its influ-ence on the female reproductive sys-tem. J Reprod Med 1980; 25:243.
10. Stillman RJ, ed: Smoking and repro-ductive health. Semin Reprod Endo-crinol 1989; 7:291–348.
11. Felton JS, Kwan TC, Wuebbles BJ, Dobson RL: Genetic differences in poly-cyclic-aromatic-hydrocarbon metabo-lism and their effect on oocyte killing in mice. In Mahlum DD, Sikov MR, Hack-ett PL, Andrew FD, eds: Developmental Toxicology of Energy-Related Pollu-tants. DOE Symposium Series 47, 1978.
12. Mackenzie KM, Angevine DM: Infertility in mice exposed in utero to ben-zo(a)pyrene. Biol Reprod 1981; 24:13.
13. Kolodny RC, Masters WH, Kolodner RM, et al: Depression of plasma tes-tosterone levels after chronic intensive marihuana use. N Engl J Med 1974; 290:872.
14. Mendelson JH, Kuehnle J, Ellinghoe J, et al: Plasma testosterone levels before, during and after chronic marihuana smoking. N Engl J Med 1974; 291:1051.
15. Smith CG, Asch RH: Drug abuse and reproduction. Fertil Steril 1987; 48:355.
16. Van Thiel DH, Lester R, Sherins RJ: Hypogonadism in alcoholic liver dis-ease: Evidence for a double defect. Gastroenterology 1974; 67:1188.
17. Macleod JM, Gold RZ: The male factor in fertility and infertility: VI. Semen quality and certain other factors in re-lation to ease of conception. Fertil Steril 1953; 4:10.
18. Griffin JE, Wilson JD. Disorders of the testes and the male reproductive tract. In Wilson JD, Forester DW, eds: Textbook of Endocrinology, 8th ed. Philadelphia, WB Saunders, 1992; p 818.
19. World Health Organization: WHO Labo-ratory Manual for the Examination of Human Semen and Sperm-Cervical Mucus Interaction, 3rd ed. Cambridge, Cambridge University Press, 1992.
20. McCarthy JJ, Rockette HE: Prediction of ovulation with basal body tempera-ture. J Reprod Med 1986; 31:412.
21. Glass RH: Female infertility. In Keye WR, Chang RJ, Rebar RW, Soules MR, eds: Infertility Evaluation and Treat-ment. Philadelphia, WB Saunders, 1995; p 57.
22. Rebar RW: Evaluation of the menstrual cycle: The normal menstrual cycle. In Keye WR, Chang RJ, Rebar RW, Soules

MR, eds; Infertility Evaluation and Treatment. Philadelphia, WB Saunders, 1995; p 85.

23. Davis OK, Berkeley AS, Naus GJ, et al: The evidence of luteal phase defect in normal, fertile women, determined by serial endometrial biopsies. Fertil Steril 1989; 51:582.

24. Hafez ESE: Histology and microstructure of the cervical epithelium secretory system. *In* Elstein M, Moghissi KS, Borth R, eds: Cervical Mucus in Human Reproduction. Copenhagen, Scriptor, 1973; p 23.

25. Hanson FW, Overstreet JW, Katz DF: A study of the relationship of motile sperm numbers in cervical mucus 48 hours after artificial insemination with subsequent fertility. Am J Obstet Gynecol 1982; 12:47.

26. Freund M: Effect of frequency of emission on semen output an estimate of daily sperm production in man. J Reprod Fertil 1963; 6:269.

27. Moghissi KS: Postcoital test: Physiologic basis, technique, and interpretation. Fertil Steril 1976; 27: 2:117.

28. Moghissi KS: Significance and prognostic value of postcoital test. *In* Insler V, Bettendirf G, eds: The Uterine Cervix in Reproduction. Stuttgart, Georg Thieme, 1977; p 231.

29. Kremer J, Jager S: The sperm-cervical mucus contact test: A preliminary report. Fertil Steril 1976; 27:335.

30. Daling JR, Weiss NS, Metch BJ, Chow WH: Primary tubal infertility in relation to the use of an intrauterine device. N Engl J Med 1985; 312:937.

31. Soules MR, Mack LA: Imaging of the reproductive tract in infertile women: Hysterosalpingography, ultrasonography, and magnetic resonance imaging. *In* Keye WR, Chang RJ, Rebar RW, Soules MR, eds: Infertility Evaluation and Treatment. Philadelphia, WB Saunders, 1995; p 85.

32. Pittaway DE, Winfield AC, Maxson W, et al: Prevention of acute pelvic inflammatory disease after hysterosalpingogram: Efficacy of doxycycline prophylaxis. Am J Obstet Gynecol 1983; 147:623.

33. Siegler AM: Dangers of hysterosalpingography. Obstet Gynecol Surv 1967; 22:284.

34. Zachariae F: Venous and lymphatic intravasation in hysterosalpingography. Acta Obstet Gynaecol Scand 1954; 34:131.

CHAPTER 14

Menopause

Susan L. Hendrix

Menopause is often approached as a condition to be tolerated, not understood or treated. The significant reduction in estrogen after menopause, however, contributes to a variety of symptoms and adverse long-term health effects. Although by definition, menopause is cessation of menstruation, this event is only one point in the continuum of declining ovarian function. It signals the time in a woman's life of change and loss of reproductive function. The process of transition has been termed the *climacteric* or *perimenopause;* however, it may more appropriately be termed the *transmenopause.* This chapter reviews the epidemiology, physiologic effects, and health impact of the menopause as well as indications and complications of hormone replacement therapy (HRT). It also describes a rational approach to patient selection and therapy.

EPIDEMIOLOGY

The U.S. Bureau of the Census has estimated that by 1990 there were 36 million women in the United States over age 50.[1] Given that the median age of menopause in the United States is 50[2] and the life expectancy for women is 83 years, the Census Bureau estimate means that nearly 15% of the population will live a third of their lives in an estrogen-deficient state. This population will increase, both in the United States and worldwide, so addressing healthier living after ovarian failure is a priority.

Frequency of ovulation begins to decrease at about age 40. This is often signaled by irregular menstrual function and intermittent symptoms of menopause. During this time, estrogen deficiency is not present; however, the follicular phase can shorten, and serum estradiol levels are lower than in younger women.[3] This era is commonly termed the *perimenopause.* Premature menopause, more appropriately termed *premature ovarian failure*, is the cessation of menses before age 40.

The age of menopause is genetically determined and is not related to the number of prior ovulations (i.e., pregnancy, lactation, use of metabolic contraceptives, or anovulatory cycles). Although the age of menopause has previously been described, the reports have been of white women of European descent in confined geographic areas.[4–7] Future studies need to determine if women of differing ethnic groups and geographic locations traverse the menopause at a similar biologic age. These studies also suggest age of menopause is unrelated to race, socioeconomic status, level of education, height, weight, age of menarche, or age at last pregnancy. Age at menopause does appear to be earlier with cigarette smoking,[8,9] living at high altitude, and poor nutritional status.

PHYSIOLOGY

Ovarian follicles are oldest as a woman reaches her 40s. These follicles remain in the ovary because of their inherent refractoriness to gonadotropin stimulation. When these follicles are finally activated, their degree of hormone production varies. This process begins well before menstrual cessation and can be surmised when a patient complains of hot flushes, night sweats, or menstrual dysfunction. The diagnosis of perimenopause can be made when the follicle-stimulating hormone (FSH) level rises to 30 mIU/mL.

Ovarian follicle depletion, accompanied by degeneration of the granulosa and theca cells, is the physiologic root of menopause. Theca cells become unable to respond to gonadotropin stimulation (FSH) and therefore produce less estrogen. As the pituitary attempts to correct the deficiency, the rise in FSH is the initial evidence of impending menopause. Typically, FSH levels rise above 40 mIU/mL, and estradiol levels fall below 15 pg/mL. Although the World Health Organization defines menopause as requiring 12 months of amenorrhea, gonadotropin levels are more accurate in diagnosing menopause.

PHYSIOLOGIC CHANGES

Hot Flushes

The neuroendocrine mechanisms responsible for the hot flush are not well understood. It is believed that during the transmenopause, falling estrogen results in lowering of the set-point of the thermoregulatory centers in the hypothalamus. The higher brain centers above the pituitary are responsible for the peripheral manifestation of the hot flush.[10] Although skin temperature rises with the flush, the core temperature actually falls.[11]

Regardless of cause, the vasomotor hot flush is experienced by nearly 75% of menopausal women with varying frequency, duration, and intensity. A hot flush is commonly described as a sudden sensation of intense upper body warmth, which usually begins in the chest region and rises to the neck and face. The flushes are often followed by intense sweating in this region.[12] They are particularly disturbing at night, causing night sweats, insomnia, and fatigue. Hot flushes can occur every 20 minutes to once or twice per month.[13] Furthermore, greater than 80% of menopausal women continue to experience hot flushes after 1 year and 25% after 5 years.[14] The hot flush is often preceded by subjective prodromal symptoms, including "increasing head pressure."[15]

Estrogen replacement therapy (ERT) has been documented to be up to 95% successful in the treatment of hot flushes.[6,16] Conjugated estrogen, 0.625 mg daily or its equivalent, generally controls hot flush episodes, but higher doses may be necessary. Schiff and colleagues[16] documented that conjugated estrogen, 0.625 mg/day, in addition to decreasing hot flushes, increased rapid-eye-movement sleep, improving sleep.[17] Medroxyprogesterone acetate (MPA), 10 mg daily, can also be effective and is a reasonable alternative therapy in women for whom estrogen therapy is contraindicated.[18] Megestrol acetate 10 to 40 mg/day has also been shown to be effective the treatment of hot flushes. There are no long-term data, however, on the effect of these drugs on bone mass. They should not be used as substitutes for proven methods unless contraindicated or not tolerated. Abnormal bleeding can occur in 25% to 50% of women, so this treatment is primarily of benefit in women who have previously had a hysterectomy.[19]

Other agents have been used with varying success. Bellergal-S, a mixture of ergotamine tartrate, levarotatory alkaloids of belladonna, and phenobarbital, has been used in the treatment of hot flushes. Lebherz and French[20] found significant reduction in the intensity of hot flushes with Bellergal-S. Bergmans and associates,[21] however, showed relief of symptoms only in the first 4 weeks of therapy. After 4 weeks, relief of hot flushes was no better than with placebo. Therapy is twice daily, and each tablet of Bellergal-S contains 40 mg phenobarbital. The patient should be warned about the drug's sedative effects as well as the addictive potential of the drug.

Clonidine, an α-adrenergic agonist commonly used as an antihypertensive agent, has been shown to be effective in reducing the frequency and severity of hot flushes.[22] Initiation of therapy begins with Catapres-TTS-1 0.1 mg/day patch to be worn for 1 week. The dose can be increased as needed for control of hot flushes; however, one must be careful to monitor the blood pressure when increasing the dosage. Side effects are mild and tend to decrease with continued therapy. Common complaints include dizziness, drowsiness, localized skin irritation, and dry mouth.

The use of propranolol to treat hot flushes has been associated with conflicting outcomes. Alocoff and associates[24] found significant benefit; however, the study was not controlled with placebo. Coope and associates[23] showed reductions in hot flushes were equal to placebo. It must be recognized that neither clonidine nor propranolol are approved by the Food and Drug Administration for treatment of hot flushes.

Changes in Menstrual Bleeding Patterns

Decreased frequency in menstrual bleeding, followed by complete amenorrhea, is the usual change in bleeding pattern as the transmenopause progresses. Many women, however, experience more frequent, heavier, or prolonged bleeding before the onset of oligomenorrhea. The diagnosis of the last menstrual period is made retrospectively and requires 6 to 12 months of amenorrhea to confirm. Once the menopause is confirmed by elevated gonadotropin levels, subsequent bleeding must be evaluated to rule out endometrial pathology.

Vaginal Atrophy

Normal vaginal moisture is influenced by both estrogens and progestins. Estrogens increase blood flow to the vagina, increasing the normal vaginal transudate and sensation of vaginal moisture. The absence of estrogen heralds profound morphologic changes in the lower genital tract. These are manifested as thinning of the vaginal mucosa, decreased rugae and vascularity, and changes in the normal bacterial flora. Typically the vaginal pH increases above 4.5. Altered vaginal pH allows recolonization of the vagina with enteric bacteria and may result in pruritus and discharge. Inflammation of the vaginal mucosa secondary to progressive estrogen loss, known as atrophic vaginitis, can cause the mucosa to have a *strawberry* appearance.

Atrophic changes are responsible for the common complaints of urinary frequency and urgency, vaginal dryness, and dyspareunia.[25] Urinary frequency can occur in both the daytime and nighttime. It is commonly accompanied by urinary urgency. Stress urinary incontinence and urge incontinence, which are common in this age group, can be exacerbated by estrogen deficiency.

The maturation index is a measure of the relative abundance of superficial cells, intermediate cells, and parabasal cells swabbed from the vaginal fornix. With estrogen depletion, there is diminution of the superficial cells and prevalence of the parabasal cells, or a *shift to the left*. This cellular distribution is reversed by the addition of estrogen.[26]

Other Changes

Psychological symptoms of the menopause have been one of the most contentious issues in menopause research. These symptoms include, but are not limited to, inability to concentrate, mood lability, irritability, anxiety, insomnia, mood depression, memory loss, lack of energy, aggressiveness, nervousness, and headache. Accompanying these symptoms can be complaints of myalgia, joint aches, lack of libido, and palpitations. These symptoms are often ill defined and nonspecific. It is important to recognize that although the relationship between the biologic and psychosocial nature of these complaints is not well understood, the complaints are nonetheless real and need attention.

Estrogen therapy is often accompanied by decreases in insomnia, anxiety, and irritability and improvement of memory compared with placebo.[27] The authors suggest that in decreasing hot flushes during sleep, the quality of sleep is improved, preventing chronic sleep disturbance. Campbell and co-workers[28] showed in a double-blind crossover study that estrogen was significantly more effective in relieving not only hot flushes, but also insomnia, irritability, headaches, and urinary frequency. Thus, estrogen improves many psychological symptoms in addition to relieving hot flushes.

HEALTH HAZARDS

Cardiovascular Disease

Among women over age 50, heart disease and stroke are responsible for more than 50% of deaths each year.[29] Coronary heart disease in women occurs 10 to 12 years later in life than men. Because their rates approach those of men in the older ages and there are more older women than men, overall about half of all coronary deaths occur in women. Almost all these deaths occur in postmenopausal women.

There is concern that women may develop more serious consequences after a coronary heart disease event than men. They also appear to have a higher incidence of certain types of cardiovascular disease, such as angina pectoris. Although the Women's Health Initiative (a longitudinal clinical trial examining causes and prevention of cardiovascular disease, breast and colorectal cancer, and osteoporosis in menopausal women) is still in its infancy, many of these issues will be better defined with results from this study.

Observational studies have suggested that women using menopausal estrogens have a 50% decrease in heart disease risk.[30–32] Although the addition of pro-

gestins was previously thought to attenuate the positive effects of estrogen, studies have confirmed a cardioprotective effect in combined regimens.[33–36]

Multiple mechanisms have been suggested to be estrogen-mediated factors in the prevention of cardiovascular disease. These include physiologic effects on lipid metabolism, blood pressure, coagulation factors, endothelial cells, and carbohydrate metabolism. The development of atherosclerosis is probably one of the main mechanisms for subsequent cardiovascular events and is related to increases in low-density lipoprotein cholesterol (LDL-C) and decreases in high-density lipoprotein cholesterol (HDL-C). Increases in total cholesterol and LDL-C and less dramatic decreases in HDL-C have been documented in postmenopausal women not undergoing estrogen therapy.[37] Furthermore, the addition of conjugated estrogen 0.625 mg has been shown to decrease LDL-C from 10% to 15%.[38–41] This translates to a 14% decrease in cardiovascular risk.[38]

HDL-C is the best risk predictor of coronary heart disease risk in women[42–44] and appears to be protective against coronary heart disease.[17,45] It has been documented that estrogen increases HDL-C from 10% to 14%.[46] It has been suggested that the first-pass hepatic effect may cause oral estrogen preparations to be more potent in causing the lipoprotein changes than nonoral preparations. There are no objective data, however, to confirm that hypothesis.

Multiple studies have suggested that the addition of progestin to ERT attenuates the beneficial effects of estrogen on lipoprotein profile, causing a decrease in HDL.[47–50] Two conflicting studies showed that women treated with combined estrogen and progestin had equivalent or improved levels of HDL-C.[51,52] The Postmenopausal Estrogen/Progestin Intervention Trial (PEPI) provides the best evidence to date and confirms previous studies that found estrogen alone or estrogen combined with progestin increases HDL-C and decreases LDL-C, improving cardioprotection.[36]

Another mechanism of improved cardiovascular risk for the postmenopausal woman taking estrogen is the evidence suggesting that natural estrogens may significantly decrease blood pressure.

This contrasts the evidence in oral contraceptive users, in which an increase in blood pressure can be seen in a small number of women. Three of six studies on the effect of natural estrogens on blood pressure show improvement with the addition of estrogen,[53-55] and three show no change in blood pressure.[33,56-58]

Concern has been raised over the issue of whether menopausal estrogen use increases a woman's risk for thromboembolism or thrombophlebitis. Epidemiologic studies have shown no increase in the incidence of thromboembolism or thrombophlebitis in women on menopausal replacement as compared with controls. Aylwood and colleagues[59] showed that natural estrogens do not increase clotting factors, as opposed to ethinyl estradiol. PEPI found no change in fibrinogen levels in women in the active treatment group, suggesting no increase in risk from thrombotic abnormalities.[36]

Osteoporosis

Osteoporosis remains a significant cause of morbidity and mortality in menopausal women. More than 1 million fractures are reported each year in menopausal women, and nearly 15% of women with hip fractures die within 3 months. The cause of osteoporosis has many contributing factors. Age, calcium metabolism, and estrogen status all play an integral role in maintaining bone integrity. Calcium supplementation alone does not prevent loss of bone mineral content.

Estrogen replacement therapy, if given, should start as soon as possible after natural menopause or opphorectomy because estrogen slows the rate of bone loss. Menopausal estrogen replacement, however, cannot restore bone mass to pretreatment levels. Riis and colleagues[60] studied three groups of menopausal women who received 17β-estradiol (1 mg) daily, calcium (2 g) daily, or placebo. Of the three groups, only the women receiving estrogen showed stable bone mass after 2 years.[60] Conjugated estrogen (0.625 mg), ethinyl estradiol (20 μg), and micronized estradiol (1 mg) have proven efficacy in the prevention of osteoporosis.[61-64] According to one study, bone loss can also be slowed when lower doses of estrogen (0.3 mg conjugated estrogen) and higher doses of calcium (1.5 g/day) are used.[63] Transdermal administration of 17β-estradiol has been equally effective in arresting bone loss.[65]

Other antiresportive agents such as calcitonin and bisphosphonates (etidronate, alendronate) have similar effects on bone density and appear to protect somewhat against fractures. Calcitonin prevents bone-resorbing cells from causing more bone breakdown. Bisphosphonates are incorporated into the bone matrix. It becomes part of the bone and has a long life in bone. There is a question, however, of whether this bone is of good quality and whether it is properly mineralized. Much less clinical information is available on these products, and risks are not known.

There is real risk in overdoing antiresorption therapy. In trying to prevent osteoporosis, clinicians are slowing the process of bone breakdown and production, which is critical for bone repair. If the antiresorptive effect is too strong, bone repair stops. If microfractures and other small areas of bone damage are not repaired, the bone becomes older and less healthy. The bone's resistance is less, and fatigue fractures can develop.

POSSIBLE ADVERSE EFFECTS OF ESTROGEN

Endometrial Hyperplasia and Cancer

Estrogen is a known cellular mitogen in the endometrium, and endometrial hyperplasia and cancer have been associated with unopposed estrogen use.[66] This effect is both dose and duration dependent, with an increase of 1.8-fold and 12.7-fold with conjugated estrogen dosages of 0.625 mg and 1.25 mg. Furthermore, when unopposed estrogen was given for 5 to 10 years or longer, the relative risk for endometrial cancer rose from 4.1 to 11.6.[67] The development of endometrial cancer while using unopposed estrogen is associated with a better prognosis. Women diagnosed with stage I, grade 1 adenocarcinoma demonstrated a 96.7% 5-year survival rate.[68,69] The PEPI Trial showed women on 0.625 mg of conjugated estrogens alone had a significantly higher chance of developing endometrial hyperplasia and recommended the addition of a progestin for women without a uterus.[70]

The addition of progestin to estrogen therapy has been shown to decrease the occurrence of endometrial hyperplasia and cancer.[71-73] This effect also appears to be dose and duration dependent. The addition of norethindrone for 7 and 10 days each month decreased the incidence of endometrial hyperplasia from 32% in the estrogen-alone group to 4% and 2%.[57] It appears that therapy for greater than 12 days each cycle is required to reduce endometrial hyperplasia to zero.[74] This makes intuitive sense because in ovulating women progesterone secretion affects the endometrium for 13 to 14 days. The most efficacious dose of progestin for endometrial stabilization with minimal metabolic impact on lipoprotein profiles remains to be determined.

Breast Cancer

Epidemiology literature over the past 20 years has attempted to determine if there is an association between postmenopausal estrogen use and breast cancer. The determination of this relationship is difficult because of the confounding variables of estrogen type, dosage, and duration of exposure.[75] There is the suggestion, however, of a 50% increase if estrogen use is greater than 20 years.[76] The type of estrogen appears to be of importance: One European study reported an 80% increase in the breast cancer rate among women using estradiol for longer than 9 years.[77] Using meta-analytic techniques, data from separate investigations can be analyzed to generalize conclusions.[78,79] One report using meta-analysis to review 556 articles found no significant increase in the risk of breast cancer with conjugated estrogen use.[78] Another report that used this technique to analyze specific types of estrogen reported a 30% increase in the risk of breast cancer among women taking estradiol.[79]

Most recently, there have been two conflicting articles in the literature on this issue. The latest report from the Nurse's Health Study found an increased risk of breast cancer 30% to 40% in women currently using estrogen or estrogen plus progestin for more than 5 years, as compared with menopausal women who had never used hormones.[80] As well, the risk of breast cancer with 5 or more years of menopausal hormone use was greater among older women. When looking at the study, however, the user and nonuser groups were different. The current users had a 14% higher prevalence of mammography, more benign breast disease, fewer childbirths, and earlier menarche. Differences in breast cancer risk may be related to these differences as opposed to an increased risk from using hormones.

In contrast, a large case-control study from Washington state published a short time later showed that estrogen plus progestin was not associated with an increase in breast cancer risk in middle-aged women.[81] In fact, long-term users (8 or more years) had a 60% reduction in risk.

Taken together, there is inconclusive evidence relating the causal effects of estrogen use and breast cancer, especially when considering conjugated equine estrogens. This current understanding should be discussed with each patient before estrogen therapy is instituted. There will be no definitive answer until data from the large randomized, controlled clinical trial, the Women's Health Initiative, become available.

THERAPY

Because exogenous estrogen therapy in estrogen-deficient women lessens and possibly prevents undesirable, potentially life-threatening sequelae, therapy should be seriously considered for all menopausal women.[10,46,82,83] Large-scale, cross-sectional, prospective studies confirm that the benefits of replacement therapy outweigh the risks.[84-87] Epidemiologic studies have estimated the number of preventable deaths to be hundreds per 100,000 estrogen users aged 65 to 75 and the cumulative preventable deaths to be in the thousands.[17] Patients with symptoms of menopause or at risk for osteoporosis or cardiovascular disease should be encouraged to join the Women's Health Initiative or offered therapy, even if there is concern about patient noncompliance. Therapy should be at the lowest dosage possible that maximizes relief from symptoms but minimizes bone resorption and slows the progression of atherosclerosis.

Defining Estrogen Deficiency

The primary premenopausal estrogen is 17β-estradiol, which is produced in the preovulatory follicle and corpus luteum each month.[88] With ovulatory cycles, the ovarian production of 17β-estradiol ranges from 60 to 600 µg/day, with circulating serum levels of 40 to 400 pg/mL.[89] After the cessation of menses, ovarian production of 17β-estradiol is less than 20 µg/day, and circulating serum levels are less than 30 pg/mL. In response, FSH levels rise, then fluctuate during the perimenopausal period until menopause is established, wherein levels remain elevated greater than 40 mIU/mL.

Estrone, the other major circulating estrogen, is produced primarily by either the metabolism of 17β-estradiol or the aromatization of androstenedione in adipose tissue. Little estrone is produced by the adrenal gland and the ovary.[90] Before menopause, the circulating serum estrone levels parallel the somewhat higher estradiol levels. In other words, the estradiol-to-estrone ratio is greater than 1.0.[26] After menopause, the adrenal gland continues to produce androstenedione, which is converted to estrone in peripheral fat. The ovarian production of estradiol is markedly decreased, and the estradiol-to-estrone ratio is reversed to less than 1.0. Thus, estrone is the primary postmenopausal estrogen.

Estrogens are present in blood in three forms: free, conjugated, and bound. The protein-bound estrogens are biologically inactive, whereas the free forms readily cross the cell membrane to bind with receptors. The conjugated forms are water-soluble and do not cross cell membranes as easily as the unbound species. The relative potency of an estrogen depends on its ability to cross the cell membrane, bind to its specific receptor, and initiate nuclear activation.

Estrogens are metabolized by the gastrointestinal mucosa and the liver.[91] The liver is the primary site for conjugation of estrogen before urinary excretion. The liver also excretes estrogen in the bile and is intimately involved in the enterohepatic circulation of estrogen metabolites. Sex hormone–binding globulin (SHBG) is produced in the liver and is the principal estrogen-binding hormone. Estradiol has the highest affinity for SHBG. Estrone, whose primary binding protein is albumin, binds poorly to SHBG. Estrogen therapy, hyperthyroidism, and pregnancy increase SHBG, and hypothyroidism, obesity, and androgen excess lower it. Specific clinical problems related to variable levels of SHBG are well documented. Phenytoin therapy enhances liver glucuronidation, and a higher dose of oral estrogen replacement is needed to obtain adequate serum levels of estrone and estradiol.

Contraindications

The medical history is used to determine if absolute contraindications are present (Table 14–1). Relative contraindications are listed in Table 14–2. Progestin-only therapy may be beneficial in patients who cannot undergo estrogen therapy. There is no evidence to deny use of HRT in women with controlled hypertension, diabetes mellitus, or biliary stones. Further prospective studies need to be performed to determine whether ERT can be used without harm in patients with previously removed breast or endometrial cancer or with acute myocardial infarction. There are studies that confirm stage I endometrial cancers do not have increased recurrence rates on HRT.[92] Stages II, III, and IV are still relative contraindications.

Table 14–1. Absolute Contraindications to Hormone Replacement Therapy

Suspected or previously diagnosed estrogen-dependent neoplasia (breast or advanced stage uterine cancer)
Active thrombosis or embolic disease
Undiagnosed uterine bleeding
Active liver disease or severely impaired hepatic function

Table 14–2. Estrogen Use
in Preexisting Conditions

Chronic liver dysfunction (may use smaller
and less frequent doses of estrogen)
Preexisting symptomatic uterine leiomyomas
or active endometriosis
Acute intermittent porphyria (estrogens pre-
cipitate attacks)

Commercially Available Estrogens

Estrogen preparations commonly used
for menopausal ERT are natural estrogens, whereas estrogens used in oral
contraceptive preparations are synthetic
(Table 14–3). Synthetic estrogens differ
from natural estrogens in their increased
target tissue potency.[93] Synthetic estrogens are known to increase circulatory
blood clotting factors, but no such association has been observed with natural
estrogens.[69] In contrast to oral contraceptives, postmenopausal estrogen replacement is not associated with an increased risk of thrombosis.

The rationale for any medical therapy
is to prescribe the lowest possible dose to
achieve the desired clinical effect. Studies have shown that 1 µg of ethinyl estradiol is comparable in biologic potency
to 0.625 mg of conjugated equine estrogens. The practice of prescribing low-
dose oral contraceptives for hormone replacement would provide four to seven
times the desired estrogen dosage and
cannot currently be endorsed. The administration of natural estrogens can
cause mild increases in hepatic
globulins. Although not thought to have

clinical significance, this effect can be
prevented by nonoral administration.[94]

Unopposed estrogen therapy is an option as long as proper precautions are
taken. Therapy is often reserved for the
patient who suffers intolerable adverse
side effects from progestin component. If
estrogen-alone therapy is ultimately desired in a woman with a uterus refusing
progestin, discussion regarding the increased risk of endometrial hyperplasia
and cancer should be undertaken. Pretreatment and annual endometrial biopsies are warranted. If abnormal endometrial histology is identified, estrogen
therapy should be stopped and the patient appropriately treated with observation or high-dose progestin therapy.

Conjugated equine estrogens (Premarin, PMB; Tables 14–4 through 14–6)
are derived from pregnant mares' urine,
which contains estrone, equilin, and a
mixture of other estrogen metabolites.
Equilin is a potent estrogen and, because
it is stored in fat, is also long-lasting. Premarin is available in 0.3-, 0.625-, 0.9-,
1.25-, and 2.5-mg tablets; the recommended starting dose is 0.625 mg. When
applied vaginally or transdermally, estrogens bypass the liver and act directly on
the target tissue. After prolonged treatment with conjugated equine estrogens,
serum equilin levels can remain elevated
for 13 weeks or more posttreatment because of storage and slow release from
adipose tissue.[95]

Estradiol (Estrace, Estraderm, Climara, and Vivelle) is a synthetically produced natural 17β-estradiol. Estrace is
the micronized form of estradiol, available in 0.05, 1, and 2-mg tablets for oral
use. The recommended starting dose is
1 mg. Estraderm, Climara, and Vivelle
are transdermal systems, available for in
vivo delivery of 0.0375, 0.05, 0.075, and
0.1 mg by patch twice weekly (Table 14–
5). The recommended starting dose is
0.05 mg, and the patch is applied to the
skin of the lower trunk and changed once
every 3.5 days. Serum levels remain constant for 84 hours, then fall rapidly.
Although Climara contains the same estrogen as Estraderm, the patch is manu-
factured differently, and it is applied once
weekly.

Estropipate (Ogen, Ortho Est) is a naturally produced estrogen prepared from

Table 14–3. Natural and
Synthetic Estrogens

Natural Estrogens	Synthetic Estrogens
Estrones	17β-ethinyl es-
Conjugated equine	tradiol
estrogens	Mestranol
Estropipate	Diethylstilbestrol
Estradiols	
Micronized estradiol	
Estradiol valerate	

Table 14–4. Available Oral Estrogens

Generic Name	Trade Name	Usual Dose	Manufacturer
Conjugated equine estrogen	Premarin	0.625–1.25 mg	Wyeth-Ayerst
17β-estradiol	Estrace	0.05–2 mg	Bristol-Myers Squibb
Estropipate	Ogen, Ortho-Est	0.625–5.0 mg	Upjohn, Ortho
Esterified estrogens	Estratab, Menest	0.3, 0.625, 1.25, 2.5 mg	Solvey, Smith-Kline Beecham
Estrogen/progestin combinations	Prempro, Premphase	0.625 mg premarin, 2.5 mg medroxypro-gesterone acetate	Wyeth-Ayerst
Estinyl estradiol	Estinyl	0.02, 0.05, or 0.5 mg	Schering-Plough
Estrone	Estrone (no longer available)	2 mg (no longer avail-able)	Legere
Estradiol cypionate	Ecypionate (no long-er available)	5 mg (no longer avail-able)	Legere
Quinestrol	Estrovis	100 μg/wk	Warner Lambert, Parke-Davis

Table 14–5. Transdermal Estrogen Replacement Therapy

Generic Name	Trade Name	Estrogen/g	Usual Dose	Site	Manufacturer
17β-Estradiol	Estraderm, Vivelle	0.037, 0.05, 0.075, 0.1 mg/d	0.05–0.1 mg every 3.5 d	Skin	Ciba
17β-Estradiol	Climara	0.05, 0.1 mg/d	0.05–0.1 mg once weekly	Skin	Berlex
Conjugated equine estrogens	Premarin vaginal cream	0.625 mg	1–4 g daily	Vagina	Wyeth-Ayerst
Estropipate	Ogen vaginal cream	1.5 mg	1–4 g daily	Vagina	Upjohn
17β-Estradiol	Estrace vaginal cream	1 mg	3–18 g weekly	Vagina	Bristol-Myers Squibb
Dienestrol	Ortho Dienestrol cream	0.1 mg	3–18 g weekly	Vagina	Ortho

Table 14–6. Injectable Estrogens

Generic Name	Trade Name	Usual Dose	Manufacturer
Conjugated equine estrogens	Premarin Injection	25 mg/mL	Wyeth-Ayerst
Estradiol cypionate	Estro V Injection	0.5 mg/mL	Legere
Polyestradiol phosphate	Estradurin (no longer available)	40 mg/mL IM every 2–4 wk	Wyeth-Ayerst

Table 14–7. Oral Estrogen/Testosterone Preparations

Generic Name	Trade Name	Usual Dose	Manufacturer
Conjugated equine estrogens and methyltestosterone	Premarin and Testosterone (no longer available)	0.625 mg/5 mg 1.25 mg/10 mg	Wyeth-Ayerst
Esterified estrogen and methyltestosterone	Estratest, H.S. Estratest	0.625 mg/1.25 mg 1.25 mg/2.5 mg	Solvay

purified crystalline estrone. It is available in tablets for oral use: 0.625 mg (0.75-mg estropipate), 1.25 mg (1.2-mg estropipate), 2.5 mg (3-mg estropipate), and 5 mg (6-mg estropipate). The recommended starting dose for estropipate is 0.625 mg.

Estradiol esters (Estratest; Tables 14–7 and 14–8) are available only in combination tablets. Menrium, which is no longer available, contained esterified estrogens and chlordiazepoxide (Librium) in three strengths. Estratest contains esterified estrogens and methyltestosterone available in two strengths.

Vaginal creams are also available. Estrogen is readily absorbed through the vaginal epithelium; however, circulating levels of estrogen are only one fourth the levels of an equivalent oral dose.[95] Disadvantages include messy application and variable absorption patterns resulting in widely different bioavailability.

Estrogen Side Effects

Studies by Sherwin at McGill University suggest that estrogen replacement in postmenopausal women may improve cognitive function.[83] Sherwin prospectively studied women who underwent bilateral oophorectomy and found that women who were started on estrogen in the immediate postoperative period performed better on tests of cognitive func-

tion than did women in the placebo group. In a similar study, Sherwin also found that women with Alzheimer's disease on estrogen were able to maintain their scores on a test of short-term memory, whereas those in the placebo group were not.[96]

Known side effects of estrogen include nausea, breast tenderness, and edema. These usually decrease in intensity and resolve with continued therapy.

Regimens

Before initiating therapy, a thorough discussion should include the indications for therapy, dosing schedule, possible side effects and alternative therapy, and the possible change in recommendations as new information becomes available. If the information is presented as an issue of prophylaxis against osteoporosis and cardiovascular disease, the patient will understand therapy as preventive health care. The concern about possible increased risk for breast cancer, however, must also be presented during informed consent. The informed patient is more likely to remain compliant with the recommended therapy.

Patients who have previously undergone hysterectomy for benign tumors can be placed on estrogen therapy alone. The addition of progestin in these patients remains controversial but cannot be en-

Table 14–8. Oral Estrogen/Tranquilizer Therapy

Generic Name	Trade Name	Usual Dose	Manufacturer
Esterified estrogen and chlordiazepoxide	Menrium (no longer available)	0.2 mg/5 mg 0.4 mg/10 mg	Roche

dorsed. Common oral therapeutic regimens include conjugated equine estrogens 0.625 to 1.25 mg or estradiol 1 mg all days. Transdermal application of estrogen 0.05 or 0.1 mg maintains a relatively constant circulatory drug level. It has added advantages of lower overall dose of estradiol with precise control, reduced frequency of dosing, and convenient administration and termination.[97] Although transdermal nitroglycerin is differentially absorbed by patients with differences in skin type, transdermal estradiol does not appear to have comparable problems.[98] Transdermal delivery systems avoid first-pass metabolism in the liver, thereby leaving more available to target tissues.

For patients with an intact uterus, progestin is added to the regimen for endometrial protection against atypical changes. A routine pretreatment endometrial biopsy is not necessary. Estrogen/progestin regimens can be sequential or continuous. The success of the therapy depends largely on the history of the patient. If the patient is bleeding monthly on a regular or semiregular schedule, sequential therapy offers a window for withdrawal bleeding and lessens the chance of intermittent abnormal uterine bleeding. Cyclic bleeding continues, however, as long as therapy does. Combined continuous therapy, although having the initial disadvantage of up to a year of irregular bleeding, offers the patient eventual relief from monthly bleeding episodes. If, however, she has been amenorrheic for 6 months or more, combined continuous therapy offers her the benefits of replacement without the added worry of monthly withdrawal bleeding and is the only logical choice.

Sequential Combined Therapy

Sequential therapy is defined by a hormone-free period when withdrawal bleeding is allowed to occur. Estrogen therapy can be administered for either 25 or 31 days (continuously) with the addition of a progestin for 10, 12, 14, or 25 days of the patient's cycle. Traditionally in the United States, estrogen has been given days 1 to 25 each month but is associated with postmenopausal symptoms

during the estrogen-free days. Continuous daily estrogen therapy provides for patient convenience and avoids annoying cyclic postmenopausal symptoms. There is no evidence that continuous combined estrogen therapy is associated with an increase in endometrial hyperplasia when compared with a cyclic combined regimen.[99]

Common regimens include conjugated equine estrogens 0.625 to 1.25 mg or estradiol 1 mg each day with 10 to 14 days of medroxyprogesterone acetate 5-10 mg or 25 days of medroxyprogesterone acetate 2.5 mg. Menses usually ensue within 5 to 6 days following the progestin withdrawal.[100] If withdrawal bleeding occurs during progestin therapy before the 11th day, an endometrial biopsy is warranted to investigate for abnormal endometrial histology.[101]

Medroxyprogesterone acetate 10 mg/day is a commonly used progestin that can be associated with the side effects of depression, fluid retention, and bloating in nearly 25% of women. Reducing the dosage to 5 mg/day often eliminates these complaints.[102] Alternative progestin therapies may also be substituted to ameliorate these untoward effects (Table 14–9). Norethindrone 0.7 mg has been shown to be endometrial protective when added to estrogen therapy and is less commonly associated with the side effects found with medroxyprogesterone acetate.[79,80] Megestrol acetate 10 mg/day also appears to have less unwanted side effects, although there are no data on benefits or risks.

Continuous Combined Therapy

Continuous combined therapy administers estrogen and progestin on a continuous, daily basis. The major benefit of this therapy is possible avoidance of cyclic bleeding and therefore better compliance as well as a lower progestin dose.[103] Daily progestin causes endometrial atrophy and protection from atypical changes.[104] The endometrial atrophy is probably protective from pregnancy implantation in much the same way as long-term progestin use and therefore offers a contraceptive side effect. Because the progestin is administered at a lower

Table 14–9. Progesterone and Progestins

Generic Name	Trade Name	Usual Dose	Manufacturer
Medroxyprogesterone acetate	Provera, Cycrin	2.5, 5, or 10 mg	Upjohn, ESI, Lederle
Norethindrone acetate	Norlutate (no longer available)	5 mg	Parke-Davis
Norethindrone tablets	Norlutin (no longer available)	5 mg	Parke-Davis
Norethindrone acetate	Aygestin	5 mg	ESI, Lederle
Norethindrone tablets	Micronor	0.35 mg	Ortho

total dose (medroxyprogesterone acetate 75 mg continuous versus 100 to 140 mg sequential dosing), its adverse effects on lipoproteins and side effects such as breast tenderness, bloating, headache, and emotional lability are minimized.[105–107]

Minimal spotting may occur during the first 6 months of therapy; however, 33% of patients do not experience bleeding at all, and 80% of patients who bleed stop within the first year.[100] Continuous dosing may decrease the incidence of additional problems associated with premenstrual symptoms and uterine fibroids. This approach, first described by Staland,[108] has received great attention.[109–112] In a prospective, randomized study of more than 300 postmenopausal women, the endometrial histologic response was compared between women treated with combined continuous therapy with conjugated estrogen (0.625 mg/day) and medroxyprogesterone acetate (2.5 or 5.0 mg/day) versus sequential therapy with conjugated estrogen (0.625 mg calendar days 1 to 25) and medroxyprogesterone acetate (5.0 mg days 14 to 25).[107] After 12 months of treatment, endometrial biopsy specimens from the group receiving continuous combined therapy showed an endometrium that was atrophic or proliferative-inactive. Five percent of the combined biopsy specimens from the group receiving sequential therapy, however, showed cystic or adenomatous hyperplasia. Varying doses of progestin (medroxyprogesterone acetate 2.5 to 5 mg or norethindrone 0.35 to 1.45 mg) have been examined using the continuous combined regimen.[108–112] In one study, 44 women received 2 mg of micronized

estradiol and 1 mg of norethindrone continuously for 12 months and a beneficial, persistent decrease in LDL was found over the study period.[110]

Early evidence suggests that combined continuous therapy may also protect bone as well as combined sequential therapy does.[111,113] Single tablet estrogen-progestin formations have been available in Europe for years. Wyeth-Ayerst recently released a combination of conjugated equine estrogens 0.625 mg with medroxyprogesterone acetate 2.5 mg for combined continuous use called Prempro. The potential advantages from continuous, daily administration of estrogen and progestin are summarized in Table 14–10.

CONCLUSION

With an ever-increasing number of women seeking health care during the menopause, it is important to provide these women with a rational plan for HRT. Before any therapeutic modality can be recommended, sound medical practice demands that inherent benefits of such therapy outweigh the identifiable associated risks for each patient. This chapter

Table 14–10. Potential Advantages of Continuous Dosing

Amenorrhea
Endometrial atrophy (protection from atypical changes and pregnancy)
Uterine atrophy (asymptomatic fibroids)
Less adverse effect on blood lipoproteins
Convenience, therefore better compliance

has reviewed the inherent health risks associated with estrogen deficiency and the associated benefits with HRT. The risks and side effects of this therapy known in advance to the patient, with a verbalized plan to address them, fosters an understanding that promotes patient compliance.

REFERENCES

1. U.S. Bureau of the Census: Population Estimates and Projections, Series P-25, no. 937, 12. Bethesda, MD, Government Printing Office, 1983.
2. Crailo MD, Pike MC: Estimation of the distribution of age at natural menopause from prevalence data. Am J Epidemiol 1983; 117:356.
3. Sherman B, West JH, Korenman S: The menopausal transition: Analysis of LH, FSH, estradiol and progesterone concentrations during menstrual cycles of older women. J Clin Endocrinol Metab 1976; 42:629.
4. Brambilla DJ, McKinlay SM: A prospective study of factors affecting the age of menopause. J Clin Epidemiol 1989; 42:1031–1039.
5. Krailo MD, Pike MC: Estimation of the distribution of age at natural menopause from prevalence data. Am J Epidemiol 1983; 117:356–361.
6. Frommer DJ: Changing age of the menopause. Br Med J 1964; 2:349–351.
7. McKinlay SM, Jefferys M, Thompson B: An investigation of the age of menopause. J Biosoc Sci 1972; 4:161–173.
8. Jick H, Porter J, Morrison AS: Relation between smoking and age of natural menopause. Lancet 1977; 1:1354.
9. Linquist O, Bengtsson C: The effect of smoking on menopausal age. Maturitas 1979; 1:171.
10. Haas S, Schiff I: Symptoms of oestrogen deficiency. In Studd J, Whitehead M, eds: The Menopause. Oxford, Blackwell Scientific, 1988.
11. Freedman RR, Norton D, Woodward S, Cornelissen G: Core body temperature and circadian rhythm of hot flashes in menopausal women. J Clin Endocrinol Metab 1995; 80:2354–2358.
12. Voda AM: Climacteric hot flash. Maturitas 1981; 3:73–90.
13. Tataryn IV, Lomax P, Meldrum, et al: Objective techniques for the assessment of postmenopausal hot flashes. Obstet Gynecol 1981; 57:340–344.
14. Thompson B, Hart SA, Durno D,et al: Menopausal age and symptomatology in general practice. J Biosoc Sci 1973; 5:71–82.
15. Tataryn IV, Lomax P, Bajorek JG, et al: Postmenopausal hot flushes: A disorder of thermoregulation. Maturitas 1980; 2:101–107.
16. Schiff I, Regestein Q, Tulchinsky D, et al: Effects of estrogens on sleep and the psychologic state of hypogonadal women. JAMA 1979; 242:2405–2407.
17. Campbell S, Whitehead M: Estrogen therapy and the postmenopausal syndrome. Clin Obstet Gynecol 1977; 4:31–47.
18. Albrecht BH, Schiff I, Tulchinsky D, et al: Objective evidence that placebo and oral medroxyprogesterone acetate therapy diminish menopausal vasomotor flushes. Am J Obstet Gynecol 1981; 139:631.
19. Schiff I, Tulchinsky D, Cramer D, Ryan K: Oral medroxyprogesterone in the treatment of postmenopausal symptoms. JAMA 1979; 242:2405–2407.
20. Lebherz TB, French LT: Nonhormonal treatment of the menopausal syndrome: A double blind evaluation of an autonomic system stabilizer. Obstet Gynecol 1969; 33:795.
21. Bergmans MGM, Merkus JMWM, Corby RS, et al: Effect of Bellergal retard on climacteric complaints: A double-blind, placebo controlled study. Maturitas 1987; 9:227.
22. Clayden JR, Bell JW, Pollard P: Menopausal flushing: Double blind trial of a nonhormonal preparation. Br Med J 1974; 1:409–412.
23. Coope J, Williams S, Parrerson JS: A study of the effectiveness of propanolol in the menopausal hot flash. Fr J Obstet Gynecol 1978; 85:472–475.
24. Alcoff JM, Campbell D, Tribble D, et al: Double blind placebo controlled cross-over trial of propanolol as treatment for menopausal vasomotor symptoms. Clin Ther 1981; 3:356–364.
25. Dewhurst J: Postmenopausal bleeding from benign causes. Clin Obstet Gynecol 1983; 26:769.
26. Hammond DO: Cytological assessment of climacteric patients. Clin Obstet Gynecol 1977; 4:49–69.
27. Campbell S, Whitehead M: Oestrogen therapy and the menopausal syndrome. Clin Obstet Gynecol 1977; 4:31–47.

28. Campbell S, Beard RJ, McQueen J, et al: Double blind psychometric studies on the effects of natural estrogens on post-menopausal women. *In* Campbell S, ed: Management of the Menopause and Post-Menopausal Years. Lancaster, England, MTP Press Ltd, 1976, p 33.

29. Bush TL, Barrett-Connor E, Cowan L, et al: Cardiovascular mortality and noncontraceptive use of estrogen in women: Results from the Lipid Research Clinics Program Follow-up Study. Circulation 1987; 75:1102–1107.

30. Bush TL: Noncontraceptive estrogen use and risk of cardiovascular disease: An overview and critique of the literature. *In* Korenman SG, ed: The Menopause: Biological and Clinical Consequences of Ovarian Failure; Evaluation and Management. Norwell, MA, Serono Symposia, 1990; pp 221–224.

31. Stampfer MJ, Colditz GA: Estrogen replacement and coronary heart disease: A quantitative assessment of the epidemiologic evidence. Prev Med 1991; 20:47–63.

32. Grady D, Rubin SM, Petitti DB, et al: Hormone therapy to prevent disease and prolong life in postmenopausal women. Ann Intern Med 1992; 117:1016–1037.

33. Hunt K, Vessey M, McPherson K, Coleman M: Long-term surveillance of mortality and cancer incidence in women receiving hormone replacement therapy. Br J Obstet Gynaecol 1987; 94:620–635.

34. Falkeborn M, Persson I, Adami HO, et al: The risk of acute myocardial infarction after oestrogen and oestrogen-progestogen replacement. Br J Obstet Gynaecol 1992; 99:821–828.

35. Psaty BM, Heckbert SR, Atkins D, et al: The risk of myocardial infarction associated with the combined use of estrogens and progestins in postmenopausal women. Arch Intern Med 1994; 154:1333–1339.

36. The Writing Group for the PEPI Trial: Effects of estrogen or estrogen/progestin regimens on heart disease risk factors in postmenopausal women. JAMA 1995; 273:199–208.

37. Gordon T, Kannel W, Hjortland M: Menopause and coronary heart disease. Ann Intern Med 1978; 89:157–161.

38. Walsh BW, Schiff I, Rosner B, et al: Effects of postmenopausal estrogen replacement on the concentrations and metabolism of plasma lipoproteins. N Engl J Med 1991; 325:1196–1204.

39. Miller VT: Dyslipoproteinemia in women: Special considerations. Endocrinol Metab Clin North Am 1990; 19:381–398.

40. Lobo RA: Effects of hormonal replacement on lipids and lipoproteins in postmenopausal women. J Clin Endocrinol Metab 1991; 73:925–930.

41. Rijpkema AH, van der Sanden AA, Ruijis AH: Effects of postmenopausal oestrogen-progestogen replacement therapy on serum lipids and lipoproteins: A review. Maturitas 1990; 12:259–285.

42. Goldbourt U, Medalie JH: High density lipoprotein cholesterol and incidence of coronary heart disease: The Israeli Ischemic Heart Disease Study. Am J Epidemiol 1979; 109:296–308.

43. Castelli WP: Cardiovascular disease in women. Am J Obstet Gynecol 1988; 158:1553–1560.

44. Bass KM, Newschaffer CJ, Klag MJ, Bush TL: Plasma lipoprotein levels as predictors of cardiovascular death in women. Arch Intern Med 1993; 153:2209–2216.

45. Gruchow HW, Anderson AJ, Barboriak JJ, Sobocinski VA: Postmenopausal use of estrogen and occlusion of coronary arteries. Am Heart J 1988; 115:954–963.

46. Silferstolpe G, Gustafsson A, Samsioe G, Syanborg A: Lipid metabolic studies in oopherectomized women: Effects on serum lipids and lipoproteins of three synthetic progestogens. Maturitas 1982; 4:103–111.

47. Wren B, Garrett D: The effects of low-dose piperazine oestrogen sulphate and low-dose levonorgestrel on blood lipid levels in postmenopausal women. Maturitas 1985; 7:141–146.

48. Tikkanen MJ, Kuusi T, Nikklia EA, Sipinen S: Postmenopausal hormone replacement therapy: Effects of progestogens on serum lipids and lipoproteins: A review. Maturitas 1986; 8:7–17.

49. Newnham HH: Oestrogens and artherosclerotic vascular disease: Lipid factors. Baillieres Clin Endocrinol Metab 1993; 7:61–93.

50. Lobo RA, Pickar JH, Wild RA, et al: Metabolic impact of adding medroxyprogesterone acetate to conjugated estrogen therapy in postmenopausal women. Obstet Gynecol 1994; 84:987–995.

51. Nabulsi AA, Folsom AR, White A, et al: Association of hormone-replacement therapy with various cardiovascular risk factors in postmenopausal women. N Engl J Med 1993; 328:1069–1075.

52. Barrett-Connor E, Laakso M: Ischemic heart disease risk in postmenopausal women: Effects of estrogen use on glucose and insulin levels. Arteriosclerosis 1990; 10:531–534.

53. Wren BG, Routledge AD: The effect of type and dose of oestrogen on the blood pressure of post-menopausal women. Maturitas 1983; 5:135.

54. Lind T, Cameron EC, Hunter WM et al: A prospective trial of six forms of hormone replacement therapy given to postmenopausal women. Br J Obstet Gynaecol 1979; 86 Suppl 3:1–29.

55. Regensteiner JG, Hiatt WR, Byyny RL et al: Short-term effects of estrogen and progestin on blood pressure of normotensive postmenopausal women. J Clin Pharmacol 1991; 31:543–548.

56. Barrett-Connor E, Brown WV, Turner J, et al: Heart disease risk factors and hormone use in postmenopausal women. JAMA 1979; 241:2167.

57. Pfeffer RI, Kurosaki TT, Charlton SK: Estrogen use and blood pressure in later life. Am J Epidemiol 1979; 110:469–478.

58. Kaplan NM: Hypertension induced by pregnancy, oral contraceptives, and postmenopausal replacement therapy. Cardiol Clin 1988; 6:475–482.

59. Aylwood M, Maddock J, Lewis PA, et al: Oestrogen replacement therapy and blood clotting. Curr Med Res Opin 1971; 4(suppl 3):83.

60. Riis B, Thomsen K, Christiansen C: Does calcium supplementation prevent postmenopausal bone loss? A double-blind controlled clinical study. N Engl J Med 1987; 316:173–177.

61. Christiansen C, Christiansen GS, McNair P, et al: Prevention of early postmenopausal bone loss: Controlled 2 year study in 315 females. Eur J Clin Invest 1980; 10:273–279.

62. Ettinger B, Genant HK, Cann CE: Postmenopausal bone loss is prevented by treatment with low-dosage estrogen with calcium. Ann Intern Med 1987; 106:40–45.

63. Lindsay RL, Hart DM: The minimum effective dose of oestrogen for prevention of postmenopausal bone loss. Obstet Gynecol 1984; 63:759–763.

64. Quigley MET, Martin PL, Burnier AM, Brooks P: Estrogen therapy arrests bone loss in elderly women. Am J Obstet Gynecol 1987; 156:1516–1523.

65. Chetkowski RJ, Meldrum DR, Steingold KA, et al: Biologic effects of transdermal estradiol. N Engl J Med 1986; 314:1615–1620.

66. Ziel HK, Finkle WD: Increased risk of endometrial carcinoma among users of conjugated estrogen. N Engl J Med 1975; 293:1167–1170.

67. Gray LS, Christopherson WM, Hoover RN: Estrogens and endometrial carcinoma. Obstet Gynecol 1988; 49:385–389.

68. Creaseman WT, Henderson D, Hinshaw W, et al: Estrogen replacement therapy in patients treated for endometrial cancer. Obstet Gynecol 1986; 67:326.

69. Gambrell RD: Estrogen Replacement Therapy. Dallas, Essential Medical Information Systems, 1989.

70. The Writing Group for the PEPI Trial: Effects of hormone replacement therapy on endometrial histology in postmenopausal women. JAMA 1996; 275:370–375.

71. Whitehead MI, King RB, McQueen J, et al: Endometrial histology and biochemistry in the climacteric woman during estrogen and estrogen/progestogen therapy. J R Soc Med 1979; 72:322–327.

72. Gambrell RD: Use of progestogen therapy. Am J Obstet Gynecol 1987; 156:1304–1313.

73. Persson I, Adami HO, Bergkvist L, et al: Risk of endometrial cancer after treatment with oestrogens alone or in conjunction with progestogens: Results of a prospective study. Br Med J 1989; 298:147–151.

74. Luciano A: Hormone replacement therapy in postmenopausal women. Infertil Reprod Med Clin North Am 1992; 3:109–128.

75. Kempers R: Hormone replacement therapy: The breast-cancer controversy. Postgrad Obstet Gynecol 1992; 12:1–5.

76. Hulka BS: Hormone replacement therapy and the risk of breast cancer. CA 1990; 40:289.

77. Bergkvist L, Adami H, Persson IM, et al: The risk of breast cancer after estrogen and estrogen-progestin replacement. N Engl J Med 1989; 321:293.

78. Dupont WD, Page DL: Menopausal estrogen replacement therapy and breast cancer. Arch Intern Med 1991; 151:67.

79. Steinberg KK, Thacker SB, Smith SJ, et al: A meta-analysis of the effect of estrogen replacement therapy on the risk of breast cancer. JAMA 1991; 265:1985.

80. Colditz GA, Hankinson SE, Hunter DJ, et al: The use of estrogens and progestins and the risk of breast cancer in postmenopausal women. N Engl J Med 1995; 332:1589–1593.

81. Stanford JL, Weiss NS, Voigt LF, et al: Combined estrogen and progestin hormone replacement therapy in relation to risk of breast cancer in middle-aged women. JAMA 1995; 274:137–142.

82. Dennerstein I, Burrows GD, Hyman GJ, et al: Hormone therapy and affect. Maturitas 1979; 1:247–259.

83. Sherwin BB: Affective changes with estrogen and androgen replacement therapy in surgically menopausal women. J Affect Dis 1988; 14:177–187.

84. Henderson BE, Ross RK, Paganini-Hill A, et al: Estrogen use and cardiovascular disease. Am J Obstet Gynecol 1986; 154:1181–1186.

85. Henderson BE, Ross RK, Lobo RA, et al: Re-evaluating the role of progestogen therapy after the menopause. Fertil Steril 1988; 49(suppl):9S–15S.

86. Cruqui MH, Suarez L, Barrett-Connor E, et al: Postmenopausal estrogen use and mortality: Results from a prospective study in a defined homogenous community. Am J Epidemiol 1988; 128:606–614.

87. Hammond CB, Maxon WS: Current status of estrogen therapy for the menopause. Fertil Steril 1982; 37:5.

88. Baird DT, Frazer IS: Blood production and ovarian secretion rates of estradiol-17β and estrone in women throughout the menstrual cycle. J Clin Endocrinol Metab 1984; 38:1009–1017.

89. Powers MS, Schenkel L, Darley PE, et al: Pharmacokinetics and pharmacodynamics of transdermal dosage forms of 17 β-estradiol: Comparison with conventional oral estrogens used for hormone replacement. Am J Obstet Gynecol 1985; 152:1099–1106.

90. Barnes RB, Lobo RA: Pharmacology of estrogens. In Mishell DR, ed: Menopause: Physiology and Pharmacology. Chicago, Year Book Medical Publishers, 1987, p 301.

91. Quirk JG, Wendel GD: Biologic effects of natural and synthetic estrogens. In Buchsbaum HJ, ed: The Menopause. New York, Springer-Verlag, 1983, pp 55–75.

92. Creasman W: Estrogen replacement therapy: Is previously treated cancer a contraindication? Obstet Gynecol 1991; 77:308.

93. Mashchack CA, Lobo RA, Dozono-Takano R, et al: Comparison of pharmacodynamic properties to various estrogen formulations. Am J Obstet Gynecol 1982; 144:511.

94. Chetowski R, Medrum D, Steingold K, et al: Biological effects of estradiol (E$_2$) administration by a transdermal therapeutic system (TTS) [abstract]. Presented at the 32nd Annual Meeting of the Society for Gynecologic Investigation, Phoenix, 1985, p 67.

95. Mandel FP, Geola FI, Meldrum DR, et al: Biologic effects of various doses of vaginally administered conjugated equine estrogens in post-postmenopausal women. J Clin Endocrinol Metab 1983; 57:133.

96. Skolnick AA: At third meeting, menopause experts make the most of insufficient data [Medical News and Perspectives]. JAMA 1992; 268:2483–2485.

97. Guy RH, Hadgraft J, Bucks DAW: Transdermal drug delivery and cutaneous metabolism. Xenobiotica 1987; 17:325.

98. Zwicke DL, Niazi I, Reeves WC, Wagel SS: Reduced transcutaneous nitroglycerin absorption in blacks. Circulation 1986; 74(suppl 2):543.

99. Schiff I, Sela HK, Cramer D, et al: Endometrial hyperplasia in women on cyclic or continuous estrogen regimens. Fertil Steril 1982; 37:79–82.

100. Birkenfeld A, Kase NG: Menopause medicine: Current treatment options and trends. Comp Ther 1991; 17:36–45.

101. Whitehead MI, Siddle N, Lane G, et al: The pharmacology of progestogens. In Mishell DR Jr, ed: Menopause: Physiology and Pharmacology. Chicago, Year Book Medical Publishers, 1987, pp 317–334.

102. Rebar RW, Thomas MA, Gass M, Liu J: Problems of hormone therapy: Evaluations, follow-up, complications. In Korenman SG, ed: Menopause. Boston, Serona Symposia, 1989.

103. Mugglestone CJ, Swinhoe JR, Craft IL: Combined estrogen and progesterone for the menopause. Acta Obstet Gynaecol Scand 1980; 59:327.

104. Gambrell RD: Prevention of endo-

metrial cancer with progestogens. Maturitas 1986; 8:159–168.

105. Weinstein L, Bewtra C, Gallagher CJ: Evaluation of continuous combined low dose regimen of estrogen-progestin for treatment of the menopause patient. Am J Obstet Gynecol 1990; 162:1534–1542.

106. Magos AL, Brincat M, Studd JWW, et al: Amenorrheas and endometrial atrophy with continuous oral estrogen and progesterone therapy in post-postmenopausal women. Obstet Gynecol 1985; 65:496–499.

107. Luciano AA, Turksoy RN, Carleo J, et al: Clinical and metabolic responses of postmenopausal women to sequential versus continuous estrogen and progestin replacement therapy. Obstet Gynecol 1988; 71:39–43.

108. Staland B: Continuous treatment with natural oestrogens and progestogens: A method to avoid endometrial stimulation. Maturitas 1981; 3:145–151.

109. Mattson LA, Samoie G: Estrogen-progestogen replacement therapy in climacteric women particularly as it regards a new type of continuous regimen. Acta Obstet Gynaecol Scand 1985; 130:53–58.

110. Jensoen J, Riis BJ, Strom V, et al: Continuous oestrogen-progestogen treatment and serum lipoproteins in postpostmenopausal women. Br J Obstet Gynaecol 1987; 94:130.

111. Riis BJ, Johansen J, Christiansen C: Continuous oestrogen-progestogen treatment and bone metabolism in postpostmenopausal women. Maturitas 1988; 10:51.

112. Williams SR, Frenchek B, Speroff T, Speroff L: A study of combined continuous ethinyl estradiol and norethindrone acetate for postpostmenopausal hormone replacement. Am J Obstet Gynecol 1990; 162:438.

113. Munk-Jensen N, Nielsen SP, Obel EB, et al: Reversal of postmenopausal vertebral bone loss by oestrogen and progestogen: a double blind placebo controlled study. Br Med J. 1988; 296–1150.

CHAPTER 15

Premenstrual Syndrome

Lisa B. Bazzett

Scott B. Ransom

EPIDEMIOLOGY

Approximately 30% of menstruating women are affected by premenstrual syndrome (PMS). Two to 10% of these women (about 3 to 7 million women) are disabled severely enough by their symptoms that work or social life is impaired.[1-4] All age groups are affected, with women in their 20s to 30s most frequently reporting symptoms.

DIAGNOSIS

PMS is "the cyclic recurrence, in the luteal phase of the menstrual cycle, of a combination of distressing physical, psychological, and behavioral changes of sufficient severity to result in deterioration of interpersonal relationships, and/or interference with normal activities."[5] It is the repeated occurrence of either irritability or depression and fatigue during the luteal phase of the menstrual cycle, accompanied by abdominal bloating and edema of the extremities, breast tenderness, or headache. At least one of the symptoms presents as behavioral, and one presents as a physical symptom.[6] The most common behavioral symptoms include irritability or depression, fatigue, labile mood, concentration difficulties, and forgetfulness. The core physical symptoms include bloating, headache, and breast tenderness and, less commonly, appetite changes, gastrointestinal upset, vasomotor flushing, heart palpitations, and dizziness. More than 150 behavioral, physical, and psychological symptoms are associated with PMS.[7] Because no symptoms are unique to PMS, widely accepted diagnostic criteria have been developed to aid further in the diagnosis (Table 15–1).

PHYSIOLOGY OF THE MENSTRUAL CYCLE

The menstrual cycle is divided into three main phases: follicular, ovulatory, and luteal. The menstrual cycle begins, by definition, on the first day of menstrual bleeding, which initiates the follicular phase. In the standard 28-day menstrual cycle, days 1 to 14 represent the follicular phase, and days 15 to 28 represent the luteal phase. The ovulatory phase is contained within the follicular phase at its terminal portion, consisting of a 36-hour period starting with onset of the luteinizing hormone (LH) surge and ending with ovulation. The extreme physiologic im-

Table 15–1. Diagnostic Criteria
for Premenstrual Syndrome

Cyclic recurrent physical and/or behavioral
symptoms are present in the luteal phase of
the menstrual cycle, specifically the 5 days
before menses

Luteal phase symptoms, which are relieved
within 4 days of the onset of menses and do
not recur until at least cycle day 12, are present in the majority of cycles

Cyclic, recurrent nature of the symptoms is
documented through prospective recording
by the patient for at least two menstrual cycles

Luteal phase symptoms do not represent a
worsening of a chronic physical or emotional disorder

Symptoms occur in the absence of hormone
or pharmacologic therapy, alcohol use, or
drug use

Symptoms are severe enough to cause physi-
cal or emotional distress leading to deterio-
ration in social or economical performance,
including:
   Marital relationship difficulties confirmed
      by partner
   Disruption of parenting skills
   Poor work or school performance such as
      poor attendance or tardiness
   Increased social isolation or withdrawal
   Legal problems
   Seeking medical attention for somatic
      complaints
   Suicidal ideations

portance of these 36 hours designates
the ovulatory phase as a separate entity.
Any deviation of the menstrual cycle
length is usually seen in the follicular
phase, which can be variable. Conversely
the luteal phase length is determined by
the life span of the corpus luteum, which
is consistently 14 days except in women
with a luteal phase defect.

During the follicular phase, follicles
mature within the ovary, and a dominant
follicle is selected. Follicle-stimulating
hormone (FSH) within the follicles induces estrogen production with the two
acting in concert to increase FSH receptor count. While estrogen exerts positive
feedback within the maturing follicle, its
negative feedback at the hypothalamic-
pituitary level withdraws support to less
developed follicles, supporting only the
selected dominant follicle. Throughout
the follicular phase, estrogen, being at

low levels, exerts a negative feedback on
LH. Estrogen rises throughout this phase
with a peak approximately 24 to 36 hours
before ovulation, resulting in the LH surge. The transition from estrogen suppression to stimulation of LH depends on the
concentration of estradiol being greater
than 200 pg/mL for a time of approximately 50 hours. Ovulation occurs around
10 to 12 hours after the LH surge. LH then
promotes luteinization of the dominant
follicle, forming the corpus luteum, which
leads to production of progesterone.

During the luteal phase, progesterone
levels rise sharply after ovulation, with
a peak approximately 8 days after the
LH surge, inhibiting any new follicular
growth. The corpus luteum has a pro-
grammed life span of approximately 12 to
14 days, which limits the luteal phase,
through an unknown mechanism of degeneration. Survival of the corpus luteum is prolonged with the production of
human chorionic gonadotropin (hCG).
hCG production begins 9 to 13 days after
ovulation. To assist in preparation for
possible implantation, estrogen stimulates the synthesis of endometrial progesterone receptors. Inhibin, originating
in the granulosa cells of the dominant follicle, also plays an important role
throughout the luteal phase. Its concentration rises with estradiol before the LH
surge and continues to increase to its
peak in the midluteal phase, acting together with estrogen and progesterone
negative feedback to inhibit follicular
growth. The decrease in inhibin seen with
luteolysis in the late luteal phase allows
for a rise in FSH approximately 2 days
before menses.

ETIOLOGY

It is often confusing separating the diagnosis of dysmenorrhea and PMS. The
cause of dysmenorrhea, however, is fairly
well defined as increased prostaglandin
$F_{2\alpha}$ stimulating uterine and other smooth
muscle contractions, with relatively successful treatment with prostaglandin synthetase inhibitors. This treatment is not
as successful with PMS.[14] Prostaglandins
appear to be responsible for some of the
symptoms of PMS, and multiple studies
have shown some relief of premenstrual

cramps, backache, headache, and gastrointestinal symptoms with prostaglandin synthetase inhibitors used in the luteal phase. Oral contraceptive pills (OCPs) relieve dysmenorrhea by ovulation suppression. This treatment leads to improvement of symptoms in approximately one third of women with PMS, worsening in one third, and no change in the remaining third. Also, patients often begin experiencing PMS-like symptoms after initiation of OCPs, which confuses the diagnosis if adequate prospective symptom recording in the absence of OCPs had not been performed.[15,16]

Progesterone, being the primary hormone produced in the luteal phase, has been evaluated in multiple studies with the majority finding no difference in peripheral blood levels in PMS sufferers and controls.[17] Estrogen appears to have almost an opposite effect, with many PMS patients feeling their best in the midfollicular phase as estrogen levels rise. Some women, however, complain of symptoms in the periovulatory period when estrogen is highest or during the midcycle nadir.[18] Also, in the early follicular phase when estrogen levels are low, some patients report severe symptoms.[19] In rat studies, progesterone has been shown to have a central sedative effect and estrogen a stimulatory effect. Because peripheral hormone levels may not reflect those within the central nervous system, ovarian hormones may still have an unproven direct effect on PMS. An interesting study was performed leading to further questions in the role these hormones actually play in the symptoms of PMS. Mifepristone (RU486) is an antiprogestational agent that when given in the midluteal phase of the menstrual cycle causes luteolysis with a rapid fall in progesterone and estrogen leading to the onset of menses. The patients received RU486, as well as a midluteal injection of placebo or hCG, which *rescued* the corpus luteum and maintained normal luteal phase serum progesterone levels but did not prevent menses. The PMS symptoms of both groups of patients continued in their normal pretreatment pattern, regardless of hormone alterations or the onset of menses.[20] Further studies have shown that severity of PMS symptoms rises before the rapid premenstrual fall in hormone levels, showing that symptoms cannot be brought on solely by a withdrawal of these sex steroids.[21] The conclusions made here can only suggest that endocrine events in the late luteal phase do not have a direct cause-and-effect relationship on the symptoms of PMS. There may, however, be endocrine events triggered earlier in the cycle that are unaffected by these late hormonal manipulations, with this indirectly supported by the fact that medical or surgical castration does relieve symptoms.[22,23]

Normal ovarian endocrine function triggers biochemical events within the central nervous system and other target tissues, with serotonin questionably being involved in these events, leading to serotonin deficiency as a suggested cause. Other theories have been developed to explain the cause of PMS, including endogenous opiate abnormalities, abnormal melatonin secretion and sleep patterns, stress, nutritional deficiencies (i.e., vitamin B_6 [pyridoxine] and magnesium), and the possibility of this disorder being a learned event. Still a direct cause-and-effect relationship in any of the theories has not been demonstrated, and, therefore, the theories remain under further investigation.

DIFFERENTIAL DIAGNOSIS

Considering the wide range of symptoms, PMS may be confused with many other disorders. The diagnosis of PMS relies on a relatively symptom-free interval during the follicular phase, recorded prospectively. A majority of patients that present complaining of PMS have another condition that can account for their symptoms or an additional complaint requiring correction before an accurate assessment may be made. Many of these patients on prospective recording are found to have no symptom-free interval or non–menstrually related exacerbation of symptoms. PMS is frequently equated with late luteal phase dysphoric disorder (LLPDD). The practitioner should be aware, however, that LLPDD is a subset of PMS in which mood disturbances are the primary complaint. Symptoms in women with LLPDD tend to be more severe with more significant impact on work or social life.

Hormonal contraceptive side effects, dysmenorrhea, eating disorders, substance abuse, and previously diagnosed medical conditions are commonly confused with PMS.[8] Up to 40% to 60% of women seeking treatment for or referred for PMS have a psychiatric disorder diagnosed, with the most common being depression and adjustment disorder. Only 20% to 25% actually suffer from PMS.[9–12] Worsening of psychiatric symptoms during the premenstrual period can make the diagnosis confusing; however, the prospective documentation of symptoms that includes the absence of an asymptomatic week during the follicular phase is required for the diagnosis of PMS.

MANAGEMENT

A standardized approach must be used in the patients presenting with PMS symptoms, and then treatment is individualized to the specific symptoms the patient is experiencing. During the first visit, the history should be the focus, with the development of a differential diagnosis. The clinician should keep in mind the wide range of symptoms that can present with PMS when considering the differential diagnosis. Fifty percent of women who ovulate have one or more mild menstrually related symptoms that are not perceived as distressing.[5] Medical disorders such as migraines, convulsive disorders, irritable bowel syndrome, and hypothyroidism often worsen symptoms in the luteal phase.[24] The patient should be instructed on how to chart symptoms throughout the next two full menstrual cycles (Fig. 15–1). This usually consists of assessing the three to five most severe symptoms and on a daily basis recording their absence or presence; their severity as mild, moderate, or severe; and when the menses occurs. Any further testing to aid in the evaluation of other conditions should also be ordered at this time, and the patient should return after two complete cycles of charting.

When the woman returns with her charts, it is best to divide them into three phases: premenstrual, menstrual and postmenstrual. This assists in developing a temporal relationship of the symptoms to the menses. Charting consistent with

PMS demonstrates symptoms at or after ovulation, resolving with the menses or within 4 days after its onset, and no symptoms in the postmenstrual phase. Other symptom patterns may present that the clinician should recognize.[24] The first is that of a cyclic recurrence of a medical disorder, such as migraines, herpes, or a convulsive disorder, in which symptoms most often recur in the late luteal or early menstrual phase. A more complex pattern is that of PMS with an additional disorder, showing symptoms throughout the cycle with different (PMS) symptoms in the late luteal phase. If non-PMS symptoms present in all three phases but with the same symptom throughout, increasing in severity in a particular phase, this represents a cyclic exacerbation of a chronic disorder. Finally the noncyclic pattern occurs when symptoms are present in all three phases either daily or sporadically without any consistency in severity. Systematic charting and evaluation helps determine if the symptoms are consistent with PMS.

The first step to consider in the management of PMS is usually self-help techniques (Fig. 15–2). These should be emphasized if the patient's symptoms last less than 1 week because severe PMS usually lasts 10 to 14 days. The patient's individual acceptance of this approach helps determine whether it is a viable option in her situation. Some are much more interested than others in nonpharmacologic approaches. This therapy consists of an overall healthier diet, including vitamins if desired, increased exercise, and stress reduction.

There have not been any foods specifically shown to be beneficial in the treatment of PMS, but recommendations have been made for an overall healthier diet. Vitamin and mineral supplements are often strongly suggested to improve PMS symptoms. Calcium (1000 mg elemental daily) and magnesium (360 mg Mg ion) have been shown to improve negative mood, pain, and fluid retention in the late luteal phase with an unknown mechanism of action.[25–27] Vitamin B_6 (pyridoxine), the most extensively studied, has weak support for its effect on PMS symptoms but is also widely used.[28] Interestingly, vitamin B_6, calcium, and magnesium are all cofactors in neurotransmitter

Scott B. Ransom, D.O., F.A.C.O.G., C.H.E.
Division of Obstetrics and Gynecology
Eastern Region
Grosse Pointe Farms, Michigan

HEALTH SYSTEM

PMS
MANAGEMENT
PROGRAM

MONTH _____

PATIENT NAME _____

MEDICAL RECORD NUMBER: _____

CYCLE DAY	1	2	3	4	5	6	7	8	9	10	11	12	13	14	15	16	17	18	19	20	21	22	23	24	25	26	27	28	29	30
DAY OF MONTH																														
CHECK DATE FOR MENSES																														
RECORD WEIGHT																														

PLEASE GRADE YOUR SYMPTOM INTENSITY EACH DAY FROM 0 TO 3 FOR EACH CATEGORY

	1	2	3	4	5	6	7	8	9	10	11	12	13	14	15	16	17	18	19	20	21	22	23	24	25	26	27	28	29	30
BREAST TENDERNESS																														
EXTREMITY SWELLING																														
CRAMPING																														
ABDOMINAL BLOATING																														
JOINT PAIN																														
GENERAL ACHES/ PAINS																														
HEADACHES																														
POUNDING HEART																														
HOT FLASHES																														
DIZZINESS																														
INSOMNIA																														
FATIGUE																														
NERVOUS TENSION																														
MOOD SWINGS																														
IRRITABILITY																														
ANXIETY																														
DEPRESSION																														
CRYING EPISODES																														
FORGETFULNESS																														
CONFUSION																														
NAUSEA																														
CONSTIPATION																														
DIARRHEA																														
URINARY FREQUENCY																														
CRAVING SWEETS																														
CRAVING SALTS																														
INCREASED APPETITE																														
INCREASED THIRST																														
CRAVING ALCOHOL																														
SKIN BLEMISHES/ACNE																														

This journal is designed for you to keep an accounting of changes that you may experience as you go through a two month period of requested record keeping. With this information, we will then be allowed to make a more accurate assessment for your personal care. Please maintain this form as accurately as possible for two months in a row, then return it to us. When the form is reviewed, we would appreciate a follow-up visit with you to discuss the best approach in meeting your personal needs. Should you have any questions or concerns regarding this form, please do not hesitate to call. (D. TOLFORD 3/96)

Figure 15–1. Record for patient charting of premenstrual syndrome symptoms.

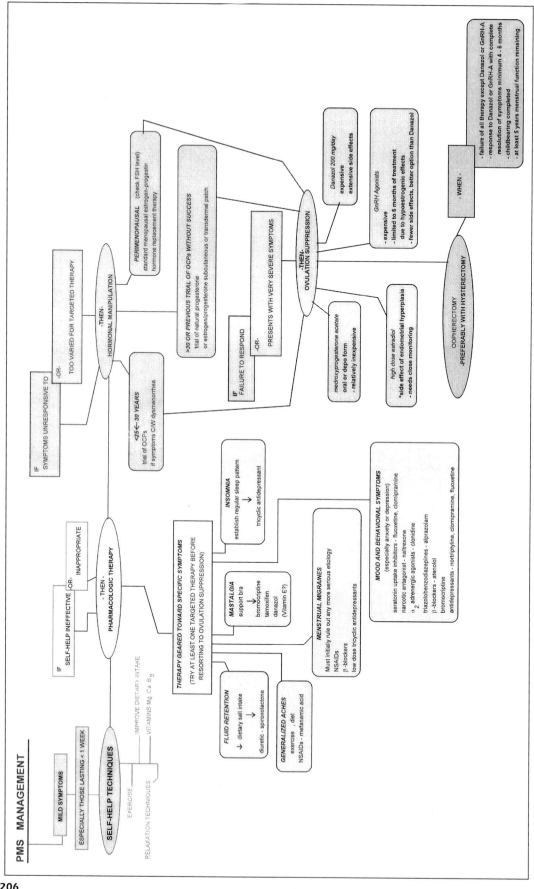

PMS MANAGEMENT

MILD SYMPTOMS
ESPECIALLY THOSE LASTING < 1 WEEK

SELF-HELP TECHNIQUES
EXERCISE
IMPROVE DIETARY INTAKE
VITAMINS Mg Ca B₆
RELAXATION TECHNIQUES

IF
SELF-HELP INEFFECTIVE -OR- INAPPROPRIATE

- THEN -
PHARMACOLOGIC THERAPY

THERAPY GEARED TOWARD SPECIFIC SYMPTOMS
(TRY AT LEAST ONE TARGETED THERAPY BEFORE
RESORTING TO OVULATION SUPPRESSION)

FLUID RETENTION
→ dietary salt intake
diuretic - spironolactone

GENERALIZED ACHES
exercise , diet
NSAIDs - mefanamic acid

MENSTRUAL MIGRAINES
Must initially rule out any more serious etiology
NSAIDs
β-blockers
low dose tricyclic antidepressants

MASTALGIA
support bra
bromocriptine
tamoxifen
danazol
(Vitamin E?)

INSOMNIA
establish regular sleep pattern
→ tricyclic antidepressant

MOOD AND BEHAVIORAL SYMPTOMS
(especially anxiety or depression)
seratonin uptake inhibitors - fluoxetine, clomipramine
narcotic antagonist - naltrexone
α₂ adrenergic agonists - clonidine
triazolobenzodazepines - alprazolam
β-blockers - atenolol
bromocriptine
antidepressants - nortriptyline, clomipramine, fluoxetine

IF
SYMPTOMS UNRESPONSIVE TO
-OR-
TOO VARIED FOR TARGETED THERAPY

-THEN-
HORMONAL MANIPULATION

PERIMENOPAUSAL (check FSH level)
standard menopausal estrogen-progestin
hormone replacement therapy

<25 ← 30 YEARS
trial of OCPs
if symptoms C/W dysmenorrhea

>30 OR PREVIOUS TRIAL OF OCPs WITHOUT SUCCESS
trial of natural progesterone
or estrogen/progesterone subcutaneous or transdermal patch

IF
FAILURE TO RESPOND
-OR-
PRESENTS WITH VERY SEVERE SYMPTOMS

-THEN-
OVULATION SUPPRESSION

Danazol 200 mg/day
expensive
extensive side effects

GnRH Agonists
- expensive
- limited to 6 months of treatment
due to hypoestrogenic effects
- fewer side effects, better option than Danazol

medroxyprogesterone acetate
oral or depo form
- relatively inexpensive

high dose estradiol
*side effect of endometrial hyperplasia
- needs close monitoring

OOPHERECTOMY
-PREFERABLY WITH HYSTERECTOMY

-WHEN -
- failure of all therapy except Danazol or GnRH-A
- response to Danazol or GnRH-A with complete
resolution of symptoms minimum 4 - 6 months
- childbearing completed
- at least 5 years menstrual function remaining

synthesis, such as tryptophan to serotonin, with this link further supporting the role of serotonin deficiency as a possible cause of PMS symptoms. Of note, if multivitamins are taken to obtain the recommended dose of the above-mentioned vitamins, it could lead to unsafe levels of other vitamins and minerals. Vitamin B_6 can cause neurotoxicity at doses as little as 200 mg daily; therefore the recommended daily dose is less than or equal to 100 mg/day.

Exercise has not been tested directly for its effectiveness in therapy for PMS. Women who exercise, however, have fewer luteal-phase symptoms compared with those who do not.[29] The goal as part of PMS treatment is regular, moderate aerobic exercise individualized to the woman's capabilities. Stress has not been shown to be a direct cause of PMS, yet a change in stressors can decrease intensity of symptoms, and relaxation techniques have been shown to reduce the mood symptoms of PMS.[30] This approach is especially important and effective in women who are able to identify their stressors and the effect on their symptoms.

If self-help strategies are ineffective or inappropriate for a patient, medical therapy should be considered. There are a few general principles of which clinicians and patients should be clear about before drug therapy is initiated. First, no drug is approved by the Food and Drug Administration for the treatment of PMS. Next, birth control is an important consideration of treatment if pregnancy is not desired because drugs are given in the luteal phase and could potentially affect the fetus should conception occur. Therefore, amenorrhea experienced during treatment should be addressed promptly. Also, the therapy for PMS is usually on a long-term basis and in most cases leads to reduction versus elimination of symptoms. Finally, drug costs and possible side effects can be significant and should be clearly discussed up front before starting any new drug therapy.

Pharmacotherapy should be geared to-

Table 15–2. Symptom Based Treatment of Premenstrual Syndrome

Fluid retention
  Diuretic—spironolactone
Generalized aches
  NSAIDs—mefenamic acid, ibuprofen
Mastalgia
  Bromocriptine
  Tamoxifen
  Danazol
  Vitamin E?
Menstrual migraines
  NSAIDs
  β-blockers
  Low-dose tricyclic antidepressants
Insomnia
  Tricyclic antidepressant
Mood and behavioral symptoms
  Serotonin uptake inhibitors—fluoxetine, clomipramine
  Narcotic antagonist—naltrexone
  α_2-adrenergic agonists—clonidine
  Triazolobenzodiazepines—alprazolam
  β-blockers—atenolol
  Bromocriptine
  Antidepressants—nortriptyline, clomipramine, fluoxetine
Dysmenorrhea
  Oral contraceptives
  Estrogen/progestin hormone replacement therapy
  Natural progesterone
  Estrogen/progestin subcutaneous or transdermal patch
Severe symptoms
  Medroxyprogesterone acetate
  High-dose estradiol
  Danazol
  GnRH agonists

NSAIDs = Nonsteroidal anti-inflammatory drugs; GnRH = gonadotropin-releasing hormone.

ward the specific symptoms the patient is experiencing (Table 15–2), and at least one type of targeted treatment should be tried before resorting to ovulation suppression. There is no experimental evidence to show that women with PMS actually retain fluid, but this symptom can often be treated. Reduction in dietary salt intake should be the first step. If a diuretic is still needed, spironolactone is the

Figure 15–2. Management of premenstrual syndrome. NSAIDs = Nonsteroidal anti-inflammatory drugs; OCPs = oral contraceptive pills; FSH = follicle-stimulating hormone; GnRH-A = gonadotropin-releasing hormone agonist.

drug of choice because it is a weaker diuretic with less risk of dependence, and it spares potassium, thus reducing the risk of rebound edema attributed to thiazides when discontinued.[31] Diuretic abuse can actually cause edema because of decreased sodium, stimulating the renin-angiotensin-aldosterone system to promote sodium retention. Diuretics are best initiated at the onset of the sensation of fluid retention and continued until the onset of menses, when resolution usually occurs.

Mastalgia may first be approached conservatively by use of a support bra and a trial of reduced caffeine intake. For those unresponsive with severe symptoms, bromocriptine, tamoxifen, and danazol have all been shown to reduce pain.[32–34] Patients experiencing insomnia, waking in the middle of the night, and fatigue should be encouraged to establish a regular sleep pattern and avoid physical or dietary stimulation before bedtime. Alcohol should be avoided because it disrupts sleep cycles. If pharmacologic therapy is still needed, a tricyclic antidepressant taken 1 to 2 hours before bedtime may prove helpful.[24] Benzodiazepines should be avoided because they are intended for short-term use only and can lead to physical dependence. Nonsteroidal anti-inflammatory drugs (NSAIDs), specifically mefenamic acid (Ponstel), have been shown to improve a variety of PMS symptoms, including mastalgia, backache, lower abdominal/pelvic pain, general aches, and headache.[25–37] This medication should be started just before the onset of pain symptoms and continued until the onset of menses. In patients suffering from dysmenorrhea, therapy may be continued until menstruation ceases if necessary. Although mefenamic acid has been shown to be effective for these symptoms in clinical trials, many different NSAIDs may be attempted before one is found that relieves a patient's symptoms with tolerable side effects.

Menstrual migraines must have their association to menses confirmed in the late luteal or early menstrual phase with other causes ruled out. The advantage to menstrual migraines is that their pattern is somewhat predictable, and prophylactic treatment may be effective. This is usually accomplished with NSAIDs, which can be used as prophylactic or abortive therapy. If NSAIDs fail, β-adrenergic blockers such as propranolol in daily divided doses or low-dose tricyclic antidepressants at bedtime may be tried. If first-line therapies are found to be ineffective, referral to a consultant should be considered before further trials are made to rule out a more serious underlying pathology. Hormonal therapies using low-dose estrogen alone or ovulation suppression with estradiol, danazol, or gonadotropin-releasing hormone (GnRH) agonists have also been suggested after first-line treatment has proven ineffective.[24] It is important to remember that migraine prophylaxis is not 100% effective and should not be considered a failure based on occasional recurrences.

If the patient's most severe symptoms cannot be treated adequately with the specific therapies mentioned, hormonal manipulation is generally the next step in treatment. Women at the extremes of menstrual years may have different types of symptoms, requiring different treatments, with their age reinforcing the need for individualized approaches.[24] Younger women tend to have symptoms occurring more in the menstrual than in the luteal phase, suggesting dysmenorrhea as a larger component of these symptoms. OCPs are a reasonable approach in this situation considering that this age group is usually in need of contraception and OCPs are an effective treatment for dysmenorrhea. Adding to their popularity as an initial approach in this group are OCPs' relative safety and inexpensiveness. OCPs are a controversial treatment for PMS symptoms. Women in their 30s typically have more characteristic PMS symptoms and have often already had an unsuccessful trial of OCPs before presentation. These factors suggest a different hormonal option. Perimenopausal women with PMS symptoms and associated irregular menses should have an FSH level drawn to rule out the possibility of menopause. The challenge in treating these women with the diagnosis of PMS includes the difficulty of predicting the onset of the luteal phase in their irregular cycles and adequately preventing symptoms. The duration of treatment in this group is most likely to be relatively short, so it is often reasonable to go directly to ovulation suppression with daily medroxyprogesterone acetate. If the FSH level is elevated, the standard combined estrogen-progestin hormone replacement therapy is recommended.

In considering the range of hormonal treatment options, progesterone was the leading choice for many years. It is most important to make a distinction between natural and synthetic progestins. Natural progesterone is secreted by the corpus luteum starting with ovulation and peaking at around day 21 to 23 of the menstrual cycle and prepares the lining of the uterus for the fertilized ovum and maintains the pregnancy. Progesterone also promotes pregnancy by affecting the contractile function of the fallopian tubes as well as thickening the consistency of the vaginal mucus and slightly raising the body temperature. Its production falls until menses occurs, and after stimulation of the endometrium, this withdrawal of the hormone promotes menstrual bleeding. Synthetic progestogens, such as those used in OCPs or medroxyprogesterone acetate are chemical analogues and derivatives of the naturally produced progesterone and androgens. The difference in their chemical structure is minimal, but the effects on the body are distinct, and they should not be used interchangeably. Although progesterone causes a secretory endometrium, progestogens enhance the endometrial glandular response leading to secretory exhaustion, making this a useful treatment in endometriosis and menorrhagia but actually contraindicated for PMS. Synthetic progestogens have also been shown to lower plasma concentrations of progesterone.

Interestingly, PMS has never been proven to be associated with a progesterone deficiency, and studies show its effectiveness in PMS to be no better than placebo.[38] Studies have shown that patients with PMS who have had a hysterectomy and bilateral oophorectomy did not exhibit symptoms of PMS when placed on continuous estrogen replacement therapy but did develop PMS symptoms when progesterone or progestins were added to the estrogen regimen.[39] A similar study with medroxyprogesterone acetate added as the progestin to the estrogen regimen did not exacerbate PMS symptoms.[40] Because of such contradicting studies and the extensive history of progesterone use for PMS, it is important to discuss the theoretical basis of its ineffectiveness to prevent future misuse of this therapy. The use of synthetics, such as medroxyprogesterone acetate, noresethindrone, *d*-norgestrel, and dydrogesterone, has been shown to be associated with exacerbation of PMS symptoms, especially depression, headaches, and water retention.[41] Again, in line with the progesterone controversy, studies have shown the converse with medroxyprogesterone acetate improving PMS symptoms.[42,43] This information may be useful, for example, in the perimenopausal woman who experiences PMS symptoms, and a natural progesterone may be considered for use with estrogen in hormone replacement therapy versus a synthetic progesterone. If a patient is already taking synthetic progestogens, a 1- to 2-month treatment-free period should be considered because their action may interfere with the therapeutic effect of natural progesterone. This period may allow for an improvement in symptoms if they had been exacerbated by the synthetic progestin use. This is true of withdrawing younger PMS patients off of synthetic progestogen therapy, as in OCPs or medroxyprogesterone acetate, helping to establish a true baseline of symptoms. In this situation, it is often helpful to extend the washout period up to as long as 6 months if possible. The use of the natural progesterone has shown positive response for some clinicians.[41] Some believe that the controversy over its efficacy is due to the misunderstanding of the differences between natural progesterone and synthetic progestogens as well as a lack of adequate double-blind studies supporting the efficacy of natural progesterones. In addition, oral micronized forms of natural progesterones are now available that may alleviate previous difficulties with vaginal and rectal absorption. In fact, Freeman and associates[44] performed a study using a vaginal form of natural progesterone and found it no more effective than placebo for the treatment of PMS. More recently, in a small series, oral micronized natural progesterone was shown to have an immediate alerting effect on the brain, consistent with positive clinical results noted in these PMS patients.[45] Thus, although the vast majority of literature does not support progesterone as an effective treatment for PMS, there are some who still advocate its use with the previously stated arguments in opposition to the literature, continuing the controversy and confusion over this treatment option.

OCPs are another rather debatable form of hormonal therapy in PMS. Their effect on PMS is poorly defined in the literature because few studies have specifically addressed this treatment, especially with the more current OCP formulations being used. Those studies that have been completed show little if any effect on PMS symptoms with OCP use. Many studies focusing on other aspects of OCP use in women also report their effects on PMS symptoms, without the study specifically designed to evaluate PMS prospectively. These reports can often be misleading because these women have not been appropriately, prospectively diagnosed with PMS. Therefore, conclusions are based on patients not necessarily with PMS but with PMS-like symptoms. Many of these women may have dysmenorrhea, molimenal symptoms, or luteal phase/menstrual symptoms, all of which have clearly been shown to improve with the use of OCPs, with the results, of course, claiming the effectiveness of this therapy. If adequate criteria have not been met to diagnose PMS in these patients, before treatment with OCPs, the majority of these women probably do not have PMS based on the fact that they responded to this treatment. The results of such studies should be closely evaluated. Also, results may simply reflect symptoms similar to those of PMS that were brought on by use of the OCPs, which again may be indistinguishable from PMS symptoms if an accurate prospective diagnosis was not made before the clinical trial. Overall, experience has shown that most severe PMS symptoms are not improved with OCPs, and claims of their effectiveness in PMS should be critically reviewed.[46–48]

Estrogen suppression of ovarian cyclicity has also been evaluated as a treatment for PMS with positive results; however, replication of trials is needed before this option is established as effective. The estradiol subcutaneous implant, with monthly cyclic norethisterone, showed improvement in symptoms over placebo. In a follow-up study, the addition of cyclic progestin, regardless of dosage or type, caused PMS-like side effects in more than half of the patients. Transdermal estradiol patches were also evaluated with positive results, although 10% of the women in the study had to discontinue use because of skin irritation.[49,50] Another notable side effect is the occasional onset of PMS symptoms in the first week of the cycle, after the patch has been placed, presumably because of the rapid induction of pharmacologic levels of estradiol, an effect that can similarly be seen with the initiation of OCP therapy.

Ovulation suppression is usually reserved for cases that have been refractory to one or more nonsuppressive therapies or those that present with extremely severe disruptive symptoms. They are also used when the prospectively recorded symptom pattern is confusing. Suppressive therapy may assist in further evaluating symptoms, enabling a more accurate diagnosis and management plan. Also, in rare cases, this limited therapy may aid in restoring psychological health and personal relationships of women who are rapidly deteriorating because of their symptoms by allowing a symptom-free period of 6 months, showing the woman and her family that there is indeed a biologic basis underlying her problems. This can be especially important when the patient herself or those closely involved in her life have attributed her problems to a personality or psychiatric disorder. Finally, in women with severe symptoms undergoing hysterectomy for another gynecologic disorder, the potential benefit of performing bilateral oophorectomy simultaneously can be determined by first performing medical castration and evaluating symptomatic improvement before definitive therapy is undertaken.

There are essentially four methods of ovulation suppression to choose from, with no strict rules or criteria established for method. Each treatment has potential disadvantages that leads to the requirement of an individualized approach in the decision-making process. Oral medroxyprogesterone acetate, which can then be switched to depo form after several months of effective therapy, is an inexpensive drug relatively free of major side effects. This option is a recent addition to this group of drugs for treatment with limited studies to evaluate its effectiveness. Financial considerations often make this the appropriate choice in many situations.

High-dose estradiol has the relatively serious potential side effect of endometrial hyperplasia requiring close monitoring, which may include the extra cost and inconvenience of endometrial biopsy should irregular bleeding become a problem. Also, there is limited information on the long-term side effects of the recommended dose of 0.2 mg/day. Many clinicians understandably have concern about administering high-dose unopposed estrogen therapy with the limited information on its use available, when other treatment options are available.

The next ovulation suppressant option is danazol, which through a variety of mechanisms produces an anovulatory, androgenic, hypoestrogenic environment. Studies have shown danazol to be effective therapy in PMS; however, the side effects associated with this drug cause many patients to discontinue therapy. The optimal therapeutic dose with the fewest side effects appeared to be 200 to 400 mg/day, with the greatest benefit reported to be with mastalgia.[51–53] Danazol's significant disadvantages are its high cost and extensive side effect profile. Danazol's specific hypoestrogenic side effects include amenorrhea, irregular bleeding, decreased breast size, and hot flashes. Androgenic changes are even more troublesome to the patients, including acne, oily skin from increased sebum production, hirsutism, deepening of the voice, and changes in libido. Additional effects that are presumably due to danazol's progesterone-like activity can mimic PMS symptoms, such as depression, weight gain, and bloating sensation. Additionally, there is the risk of in utero virilization of female fetuses if conception occurs during therapy as well as decreased bone mass and the theoretical risk for accelerated cardiovascular disease from lowered high-density lipoprotein and elevated low-density lipoprotein

cholesterol concentrations secondary to prolonged hypoestrogenism. Overall, danazol is reported to be a successful therapy for PMS by several investigators, even in severe cases. Its use is usually limited by its expense and extensive short-term and potentially long-term side effects.

The final option available for ovulation suppression are GnRH agonists. These can be administered as nasal spray, subcutaneous injections, or intramuscular injections. Initially the pituitary-gonadal axis is activated for 1 to 2 weeks (the flare response) after which time the pituitary produces gonadotropins with little or no biologic activity. The majority of studies with GnRH agonists in PMS support their effectiveness, and, in contrast to danazol, they act specifically on the gonadotrophs resulting in many fewer side effects.[54,55] Success of this treatment seems to be most evident in patients with true, severe PMS symptoms. The disadvantage of GnRH agonist therapy, besides expense, is that the duration of treatment is limited, usually to 6 months, because of development of hypoestrogenic effects after approximately 2 to 3 months. These effects include the potential for osteoporosis. Loss of bone mass has been demonstrated after only 6 months of therapy, with partial recovery seen with discontinuation of therapy and return of menstrual cyclicity.[56] There is a place for short-term therapy, as previously discussed, to confirm or clarify the diagnosis of PMS or as a trial before possible definitive surgical castration. If the objective is to extend medical therapy, the potential does exist with the addition of indefinite estrogen-progesterone add-back therapy. This approach has been effective, resulting in a level of symptoms intermediate between baseline and GnRH agonist alone, which is acceptable to most patients.[57] Danazol and GnRH agonist appear to be the most effective of the hormonal suppressive therapies and with roughly equivalent cost. Most patients are therefore better served with GnRH agonist because of the bothersome androgenic side effects of danazol.

Thus far, two pharmacologic treatment approaches have been reviewed, including symptomatic relief of specific complaints and suppression of the menstrual cycle. The last logical general treatment approach would ideally be designed at correcting the underlying cause of the disorder, which is obviously difficult in PMS because the cause has not clearly been established. There does appear to be a major mood and behavioral component to PMS, however, which varies among individual patients. For those experiencing symptoms such as mood lability, irritability, anxiety, or depression as a major component of PMS symptoms, psychotropic medications may provide a reasonable treatment option. Some studies suggest that changes in neuropeptide or neurotransmitter physiology occurs during the menstrual cycle in PMS patients that differ from controls.[58-61] Although no specific or consistent change on neurotransmitters has been identified, studies have suggested a few that are mentioned with their available treatment plans.

Serotonin uptake inhibitors, such as fluoxetine and clomipramine, have been found effective in double-blind trials at improving premenstrual psychological symptoms.[62-64] Serotoninergic drugs treat PMS by increasing central nervous system neuroendocrine response to the ovary. Naltrexone, a narcotic antagonist, and clonidine, a central α_2-adrenergic presynaptic autoreceptor agonist, have both shown improvement, possibly by modulation of β-endorphin levels, over placebo on premenstrual psychiatric symptoms.[21,65,66] The use of triazolobenzodiazepines, such as alprazolam, provides a relatively newer, shorter-acting and potent anxiolytic shown to improve irritability, mood lability, anxiety, fatigue, and depression.[67,68] Atenolol, with its sympatholytic action, has been used to treat premenstrual tension. Bromocriptine, as previously discussed for the treatment of mastalgia, has demonstrated positive effect on premenstrual mood symptoms.[69-71] Antidepressants, including nortriptyline clomipramine and fluoxetine, have reported improvement in the depressive symptoms of PMS.[72-76] Although most psychotropic medications have been shown to be more effective than placebo in treating the psychiatric and mood symptoms of PMS, their use is not recommended for the diagnosis of PMS.

Psychoactive medications most likely have the greatest effect on women with anxiety or depression as a major component of their PMS. A large proportion of patients presenting for PMS, after prospective recording of symptoms, do not actually have menstrual related complaints, and approximately one half of those presenting meet diagnostic criteria for a separate psychiatric disorder.[77-83] Psychoactive medications are among the most commonly prescribed agents for PMS that are often used before an accurate diagnosis is made. The Beck Depression Inventory may help in the diagnosis of depressive symptoms in PMS. By having the patient complete this test during the midfollicular and again in the late luteal phase, it acts as a screening tool to separate those suffering from chronic depression versus PMS-associated depression. This test along with prospective recording of symptoms increases the chances of obtaining the appropriate diagnosis and instituting the best treatment plan.

Oophorectomy as definitive treatment for PMS is rarely indicated, and strict criteria should be met before being performed.[84,85] The patient should have failed all therapy except danazol or GnRH agonist ovulation suppression. The response to one of these regimens must be the complete resolution of symptoms for a minimum of 4 to 6 months. The patient's childbearing must be completed with at least 5 years, and preferably 10 to 15, of menstrual function remaining. If oophorectomy is being performed solely for treatment of severe PMS, hysterectomy should also be performed; otherwise, estrogen replacement therapy also requires cyclic progesterone to prevent endometrial carcinoma, with its added risks and expense. In patients with severe PMS, progestin therapy can create PMS-like symptoms, as previously discussed, and should be avoided. Laparoscopic oophorectomy as treatment for PMS, brought into question with the continued development of endoscopic surgery, is also incomplete treatment for the same reason. Endometrial ablation, although supported by an uncontrolled study,[86] and hysterectomy without oophorectomy are also inappropriate

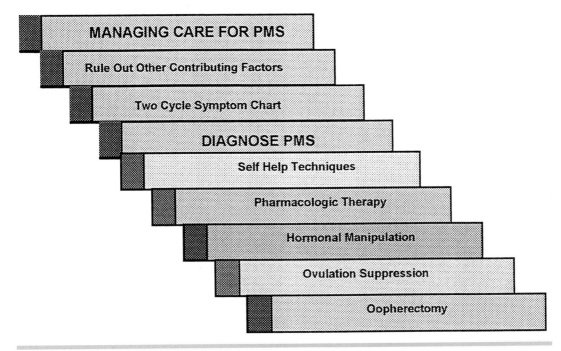

Figure 15–3. Managing care for premenstrual syndrome (PMS).

surgical therapies because ovarian function is left intact.

Therapy options in PMS appear overwhelming, but with accurate, prospective recording of symptoms, an individualized treatment plan can be developed for each patient (Fig. 15–3). Patients with mild symptoms or those lasting less than 1 week should be encouraged to try self-help techniques. Specific physical or behavioral/mood symptoms should be treated with the appropriate directed medical therapy if unresponsive to or too severe for self-help approaches. For a wider range of symptoms, hormonal therapy is usually more effective. Especially with younger patients, this can be initially approached with OCPs, which offer a reasonable cost-to-benefit ratio, with cost often being an important factor in the final decision-making process of treatment options. Because other hormonal therapies are controversial in their proven effectiveness yet still popular in use and requested by patients, many trials of different regimens may be required before an effective choice is found or the patient is convinced that this therapy is appropriate for their particular symptoms. Progesterone is seldom an indi-

cated or effective treatment for PMS, but because of its extensive history of use, it is still requested by many patients. It is not unreasonable to proceed with a trial of progesterone with continued symptom charting. In this type of unique situation, in which the patient plays a significant role in treatment choice, with obvious great optimism about its outcome, it is even more important to continue symptom recording for an extended period of time (up to 4 to 6 months) while undergoing therapy because of the increased chance of placebo effect in the first month or two and the need for objective results to review with the patient in evaluating the drug's true efficacy. Patients with severe symptoms or those who have failed other pharmacologic therapies are best served with ovulation suppression. After considering the more extensive side effect profile of danazol, GnRH agonists are usually the choice for initial therapy in this class of agents. When the symptoms are predominantly psychological or the patient has PMS secondary to a primary psychiatric disorder, psychoactive agents are obviously the correct treatment choice. During any of these pharmacologic treatment courses, the importance of contraception must be emphasized to the patient because of the potential adverse drug effects on a developing fetus.

FOLLOW-UP

An aspect of therapy that is just as important as the treatment choice is appropriate patient follow-up after a treatment plan or medication has been chosen and instituted. It should be clear to the patient that symptom recording, although laborious, does not end with the diagnosis and that it must continue as an important and necessary part of the treatment plan. If efficacy of a pharmacologic agent is established by symptom recording, the symptom calendars should be continued at least every other cycle. This recording identifies a decrease in effectiveness or development of side effects of the agent and allows for early and appropriate adjustments. It may take a combination of therapies to establish efficacy. The first cycle or two may have improved symptoms because of placebo (or attention) effect. A cycle in which symptoms flare may occur unrelated to therapy. For both of these reasons, it is best not to change therapy on the basis of one or two symptomatic cycles. If initial therapy remains effective over the first three cycles, it is reasonable to reevaluate the patient on a more extended scheduling basis. Regardless of therapy effectiveness, if the patient initially presented with more severe symptoms, especially if psychological symptoms play a large part and underlying depressive disorder is suspected, more frequent visits are recommended until effective treatment is instituted and diagnosis is clearly resolved.

Once treatment effectiveness is established and side effects are acceptable to the patient, timing of follow-up visits can be extended. If the patient's therapy includes only self-help techniques or NSAIDs, yearly visits may be sufficient. For other treatments, a 3- to 4-month follow-up is appropriate initially and can be extended to 6 months if the patient remains stable. Consultation with a psychiatrist is necessary for any patient with risk of suicide or overdose and should be seen frequently with limited, if any, refills prescribed on psychoactive medications. These, of course, are only loose guidelines and should be individualized to the patient's presenting symptoms profile, specific drug therapy, and personal requests.

Total duration of therapy varies greatly. Most therapeutic regimens continue anywhere from months to years, until the onset of menopause. Any patient on medication with duration-related side effects should be monitored closely and a plan developed for alternative therapy should the current one need to be discontinued.

REFERENCES

1. Johnson SR: The epidemiology and social impact of premenstrual symptoms. Clin Obstet Gynecol 1987; 30:367–376.
2. Van Keep PA, Lehert P: The premenstrual syndrome—an epidemiologic and statistical exercise. *In* Van Keep PA, Utian WH, eds: The Premenstrual Syndrome. Lancaster, England, MTP Press Limited, 1981.
3. Andersch B, Wenderstram G, Hahn L, et al: Premenstrual complaints: Prevalence of premenstrual symptoms in a Swedish urban population. J Psychosom Obstet Gynaecol 1986; 5:39.
4. U.S. Bureau of the Census: Statistical Abstract of the United States, 111th ed. 1991.
5. Reid RL: Premenstrual syndrome. Curr Probl Obstet Gynecol Fertil 1985; 8:1.
6. Mortola JF, Girton L, Beck L, Yen SSC: Diagnosis of premenstrual syndrome by a single prospective, and reliable instrument: The calendar of premenstrual experiences. Obstet Gynecol 1990; 76:302.
7. Hamilton JA, Parry B, Alagna S, et al: Premenstrual mood changes: A guide to evaluation and treatment. Psychiatr Ann 1984; 14:426.
8. Mortola JF: Issues in the diagnosis and research of premenstrual syndrome. Clin Obstet Gynecol 1992; 35:591.
9. Rubinow DR, Hoban C, Roy-Byrne P, et al: Premenstrual syndromes: Past and future research strategies. Can J Psychiatry 1985; 30:469.
10. Harrison WM, Rabkin JG, Endicott J: Psychiatric evaluation of premenstrual changes. Psychosomatics 1985; 296:789.
11. Yuk VJ, Jugdutt AV, Cumming CE, et al: Towards a definition of PMS: A factor analytic evaluation of premenstrual

change in noncomplaining women. J Psychosom Res 1990; 34:439.

12. Gise LH, Lebovits AH, Paddison PL, et al: Issues in the identification of premenstrual syndromes. J Nerv Mental Dis 1990; 178:228.

13. American Psychiatric Association: Diagnostic and Statistical Manual of Mental Disorders, 3rd ed rev. Washington, DC, American Psychiatric Association, 1987; pp 367–369.

14. Smith S, Schiff I: The premenstrual syndrome—diagnosis and management. Fertil Steril 1989; 52:527.

15. Andersch B, Hahn L: Premenstrual complaints: II. Influence of oral contraceptives. Acta Obstet Gynaecol Scand 1981; 60:579.

16. Herzberg B, Coppen A: Changes in psychological symptoms in women taking oral contraceptives. Br J Psychiatry 1970; 116:161.

17. Rubinow DR, Hoban MC, Grover GN, et al: Changes in plasma hormones across the menstrual cycle in patients with menstrually related mood disorder and in control subjects. Am J Obstet Gynecol 1988; 158:5.

18. Reid RL: Premenstrual syndrome (editorial). N Engl J Med 1991; 324:1208.

19. Freeman EW, Sondheimer S, Weinbaum PJ, et al: Evaluating premenstrual symptoms in medical practice. Obstet Gynecol 1985; 65:500.

20. Schmidt PJ, Neiman LK, Grover GN, et al: Lack of effect of induced menses on symptoms in women with premenstrual syndrome. N Engl J Med 1991; 324:1174.

21. Backstrom T: Neuroendocrinology of premenstrual syndrome. Clin Obstet Gynecol 1992; 35:612–628.

22. Muse KN, Cetal NS, Futterman LA, et al: The premenstrual syndrome: Effects of "medical ovariectomy." N Engl J Med 1984; 311:1345.

23. Casson P, Hahn PM, Van Vogt DA, et al: Lasting response to ovariectomy in severe intractable premenstrual syndrome. Am J Obstet Gynecol 1990; 162:99.

24. Johnson SR: Clinician's approach to the diagnosis and management of premenstrual syndrome. Clin Obstet Gynecol 1992; 35:638.

25. Thys-Jacob S, Ceccarelli S, Bierman A: Calcium supplementation in premenstrual syndrome: A randomized crossover trial. J Gen Intern Med 1989; 4:183.

26. Alvir JM, Thys-Jacobs S: Premenstrual and menstrual symptom clusters and response to calcium treatment. Psychopharmacol Bull 1991; 27:145.

27. Facchinetti F, Borela P, Sances G, et al: Oral magnesium successfully relieves premenstrual mood changes. Obstet Gynecol 1991; 78:177.

28. Kleijnen J, Ter Riet G, Knipschild P: Vitamin B6 in the treatment of the premenstrual syndrome: A review. Br J Obstet Gynaecol 1990; 97:847.

29. Prior JC, Vigna Y, Sciarretta D, et al: Conditioning exercise decreases premenstrual symptoms: A prospective, controlled 6-month trial. Fertil Steril 1987; 47:402.

30. Goodale IL, Domar AD, Benson H: Alleviation of premenstrual syndrome symptoms with the relaxation response. Obstet Gynecol 1990; 75:649.

31. Friedlander MA: Fluid retention: Evaluation and use of diuretics. Clin Obstet Gynecol 1987; 30:431.

32. Blichert-Toft M, Andersen AN, Henriksen OB, Mygind T: Treatment of mastalgia with bromocriptine: A double-blind cross-over study. Br Med J 1979; 1(6158):237.

33. Fentiman IS, Caleffi M, Brame K, et al: Double-blind controlled trial of tamoxifen therapy for mastalgia. Lancet 1986; 8476:287.

34. Watts JF, Butt WR, Edwards RL: A clinical trial using danazol for the treatment of premenstrual tension. Br J Obstet Gynaecol 1987; 94:30.

35. Budoff PW: Use of prostaglandin inhibitors in the treatment of PMS. Clin Obstet Gynecol 1987; 30:453.

36. Budoff PW: The use of prostaglandin inhibitors for the premenstrual syndrome. J Reprod Med 1983; 28:469.

37. Jakabowicz DL, Godard E, Dewhurst J: The treatment of premenstrual tension with mefanemic acid: Analysis of prostaglandin concentrations. Br J Obstet Gynaecol 1984; 91:78.

38. Osofsky HJ: Efficacious treatments of PMS: A need for further research (editorial). JAMA 1990; 264:387.

39. PMS O'Brien: Helping women with premenstrual syndrome. Br Med J 1993; 307:1471.

40. Kirkham C, Hahn P, Vugt D, et al: A randomized, double-blind, placebo-controlled, cross-over trial to assess the side effects of medroxyprogesterone acetate in hormone replacement therapy. Obstet Gynecol 1991; 78:93.

41. Martorano JT, Ahlgrimm M, Myers D: Differentiating between natural progesterone and synthetic progestogens: Clinical implications for premenstrual

syndrome management. Compr Ther 1993; 19:97–98.

42. Helberg D, Claesson B, Nilsson S: Premenstrual tension: A placebo-controlled efficacy study with spironolactone and medroxyprogesterone acetate. Int J Gynaecol Obstet 1991; 34:243.

43. DeLia JE, Keye W: Preliminary report on the effects of depo-medroxyprogesterone acetate on premenstrual tension syndrome (abstract). International Symposium on Premenstrual Tension and Dysmenorrhea, Kiawa Island, South Carolina, 1983.

44. Freeman E, Rickels K, Sondheimer S, et al: Ineffectiveness of progesterone suppository treatment for premenstrual syndrome. JAMA 1990; 264:349–353.

45. Martorano J: Case study: The use of the CEEG in treating premenstrual syndrome. J Integrative Psychiatry 1991; 7:63–64.

46. Kutner SJ, Brown WL: Types of oral contraceptives, depression, and premenstrual symptoms. J Nerv Ment Dis 1972; 155:153.

47. Fleming O, Seager CP: Incidence of depressive symptoms in users of the oral contraceptive. Br J Psychiatry 1978; 132:431.

48. Herzberg B, Coppen A: Changes in psychological symptoms in women taking oral contraceptives. Br J Psychiatry 1970; 116:161.

49. Magos AL, Brincat M, Studd JWW: Treatment of the premenstrual syndrome by subcutaneous oestradiol implants and cyclical oral norethisterone: Placebo controlled study. Br Med J 1986; 292:1629.

50. Watson N, Studd J, Savvas M, Baber RJ: The long term effect of oestradiol implant therapy for the treatment of premenstrual syndrome. Gynecol Endocrinol 1990; 4:99.

51. Halbreich U, Rojansky N, Palter S: Elimination of ovulation and menstrual cyclicity (with danazol) improves dysphoric premenstrual syndromes. Fertil Steril 1991; 56:1066.

52. Gilmore DH, Hawthorn RJS, Hart DM: Danazol for premenstrual syndrome: A preliminary report of a placebo-controlled double-blind study. J Int Med Res 1985; 13:129.

53. Watts JF, Butt WR, Edwards RL: A clinical trial using danazol for the treatment of premenstrual tension. Br J Obstet Gynaecol 1987; 94:30.

54. Muse KN, Cetel NS, Futterman LA, Yen SSC: The premenstrual syndrome: Effects of "medical oophorectomy." N Engl J Med 1984; 311:1345.

55. Hammarback S, Backstrom T: Induced anovulation as treatment of premenstrual tension syndrome: A double-blind cross-over study with GnRH-agonist versus placebo. Acta Obstet Gynaecol 1988; 67:159.

56. Johansen JS, Riis BJ, Hassager C, et al: The effect of a gonadotropin-releasing hormone agonist analog (Nafarelin) on bone metabolism. J Clin Endocrinol Metab 1988; 67:701.

57. Mortola JF, Girton L, Fischer U: Successful treatment of severe premenstrual syndrome by combined use of gonadotropin-releasing hormone agonist and estrogen/progestin. J Clin Endocrinol Metab 1991; 71:252A-F.

58. Giannini AJ, Martin DM, Turner CE: Beta-endorphin decline in late luteal phase dysphoric disorder. Int J Psychiatry Med 1990; 20:279.

59. Facchinetti F, Genazzani AD, Martignoni E, et al: Neuroendocrine correlates of premenstrual syndrome: Changes in the pulsatile pattern of plasma LH. Psychoneuroendocrinology 1990; 15:269.

60. Bancroft J, Cook A, Davidson D, et al: Blunting of neuroendocrine responses to infusion of L-tryptophan in women with premenstrual mood change. Psychol Med 1991; 21:305.

61. Odink J, Van Der Ploeg HM, van den Berg H, et al: Circadian and circatrigintan rhythms of biogenic amines in premenstrual syndrome (PMS). Psychosom Med 1990; 52:346.

62. Rapkin AJ: The role of serotonin in premenstrual syndrome. Clin Obstet Gynecol 1992; 35:629–636.

63. Menkes DB, Ebrahim T, Mason PA, et al: Fluoxetine treatment of severe premenstrual syndrome. Br Med J 1992; 305:346–347.

64. Wood SH, Mortola JF, Chan YF, et al: Treatment of premenstrual syndrome with fluoxetine: A double-blind, placebo-controlled crossover study. Obstet Gynecol 1992; 80:339–344.

65. Giannini AJ, Sullivan B, Sarachene J, Loiselle RH: Clonidine in the treatment of premenstrual syndrome: A subgroup study. J Clin Psychiatry 1988; 49:62.

66. Chuong CJ, Coulam CB, Bergstralh EJ, et al: Clinical trial of naltrexone in premenstrual syndrome. Obstet Gynecol 1988; 72:332.

67. Harrison WM, Endicott J, Nee J: Treat-

ment of premenstrual dysphoria with alprazolam: A controlled study. Arch Gen Psychiatry 1990; 47:270.

68. Smith S, Rinehart JS, Ruddock VE, Schiff I: Treatment of premenstrual syndrome with alprazolam: Results of a double-blind, placebo-controlled, randomized crossover clinical trial. Obstet Gynecol 1987; 70:37.

69. Benedek-Jaszmann LF, Hearn-Sturtevant MD: Premenstrual tension and functional infertility: Aetiology and treatment. Lancet 1976; 1:1095.

70. Ylostalo P, Kauppila A, Puolakka J, et al: Bromocriptine and norethisterone in the treatment of premenstrual syndrome. Obstet Gynecol 1982; 59:292.

71. Elsner CW, Buster JE, Schindler RA, et al: Bromocriptine treatment of premenstrual tension syndrome. Obstet Gynecol 1980; 56:723.

72. Harrison WM, Endicott J, Nee J: Treatment of premenstrual depression with nortriptyline: A pilot study. J Clin Psychiatry 1989; 50:139.

73. Eriksson E, Lisjo P, Sundblad C, et al: Effect of clomipramine on premenstrual syndrome. Acta Psychiatry Scand 1990; 81:87.

74. Jacobson JN: Premenstrual syndrome treatments. J Clin Psychiatry 1989; 50:393.

75. Metz A: Fluoxetine treatment of premenstrual syndrome. J Clin Psychiatry 1990; 51:260.

76. Pies RW: Fluoxetine treatment of premenstrual syndrome. J Clin Psychiatry 1990; 51:348.

77. Endicott J, Halbreich U, Schacht S, Nee J: Premenstrual changes and affec-

tive disorders. Psychosom Med 1981; 43:519.

78. DeJong R, Rubinow D, Roy-Byrne P, et al: Premenstrual mood disorder and psychiatric illness. Am J Psychiatry 1985; 142:1359.

79. Stout AL, Steege JF, Blazer DG, George LK: Comparison of lifetime psychiatric diagnoses in premenstrual syndrome clinic and community samples. J Nerv Ment Dis 1986; 174:517.

80. Halbreich U, Endicott J: Relationship of dysphoric premenstrual changes to depressive disorders. Acta Psychiatr Scand 1985; 71:331.

81. Gise LH, Lebovits AH, Paddison PL, Strain JJ: Issues in the identification of premenstrual syndromes. J Nerv Ment Dis 1990; 178:228.

82. Endicott J, Halbreich V: Psychobiology of premenstrual change. Psychopharmacol Bull 1982; 18:109.

83. Metcalf MG, Hudson SM: The premenstrual syndrome: Selection of women for treatment trials. J Psychosom Res 1985; 29:631.

84. Casson P, Hahn PM, Van Vugt DA, Reid RL: Lasting response to ovariectomy in severe intractable premenstrual syndrome. Am J Obstet Gynecol 1990; 162:99.

85. Casper RF, Hearn MT: The effect of hysterectomy and bilateral oophorectomy in women with severe premenstrual syndrome. Obstet Gynecol 1990; 162:105.

86. Lefler HT, Lefler CF: Endometrial ablation: Improvement in PMS related to the decrease in bleeding. J Reprod Med 1992; 37:596–598.

CHAPTER 16

Urinary Tract Disorders

Lisa J. McIntosh

The two functions of the lower urinary tract are the storage and expulsion of urine from the bladder. Abnormalities in storage or release can lead to incontinence or voiding disorders. Pain during voiding with or without infection is a common complaint. This chapter addresses major categories of urinary tract disorders: urinary incontinence, urinary tract infection (UTI), sensory disorders, and emptying disorders.

URINARY INCONTINENCE

Urinary incontinence represents a large medical, social, psychological,[1] and economic problem.[2] A *Clinical Practice Guideline* published by the U.S. Department of Health and Human Services targeted urinary incontinence in adults because of its prevalence and toll on physical and psychological health.[3]

Genuine stress urinary incontinence is the condition in which urinary leakage occurs in the absence of a detrusor contraction as intravesical pressure during stress exceeds urethral pressure.[4] Detrusor overactivity is characterized by involuntary detrusor contractions during filling. Overactive detrusor function in the absence of a known neurologic abnormality is called *unstable detrusor;* overactivity because of disturbance of the nervous control mechanisms is termed *detrusor hyperreflexia.*

The basic evaluation of urinary incontinence includes a history and physical examination, urinalysis and culture, assessment of urethral angulation, a simple cystometrogram, and urinary diary.

History and Physical Examination

An important step in the evaluation of the incontinent patient is a complete history and physical examination. Medications, disease processes, and social behavior affect the continence mechanism. Certain *red flags* should alert the physician to potential problem patients: previous surgery that has failed to correct the urinary leakage, multiple complaints in all organ systems, dementia or mental impairment, significant neurologic problems (multiple sclerosis, stroke, back trauma), and an inconsistency between severity of symptoms and reported leakage.

The major urinary complaint should be elicited along with a detailed description of onset, duration, frequency, amount, and previous therapy for the problem. A description of incontinence type should be obtained, including its relation to coughing, sneezing, laughing, exercise, lifting, straining, urgency, or sexual intercourse. Further questions include whether the urgency increases during cold weather or is precipitated at the sound of running water. Symptoms of dysuria, frequency, hematuria, incomplete voiding, fecal incontinence, nocturia, or enuresis should be sought.

Antihypertensives, antidepressants, antipsychotics, hypnotics, caffeine, muscle relaxants, antihistamines, diuretics, and hormones (estrogen, thyroid) produce pharmacologic effects that can change urethral pressure, prevent effective bladder emptying, produce urinary retention, or challenge the bladder with an excessive fluid load.[5] A study exploring drug use by elderly incontinent female nursing home residents found 454 drugs taken by the 84 subjects, with 70% of the subjects taking drugs having the potential to cause urinary incontinence.[6] It is important to assess the necessity for the different medications and whether the patient is taking the medications as directed.

History alone does not enable the physician to make a diagnosis. If stress incontinence is the sole complaint, without any hint of frequency, nocturia, or urgency, there is approximately an 80% chance that the patient has genuine stress incontinence; however, the vast majority of patients with genuine stress urinary incontinence have other urologic complaints.[7-9] Women with detrusor instability complain of a wide variety of symptoms, and complaints of frequency and urgency did not correlate with cystometric indices.[10]

The physical examination begins with assessment of the patient's mobility. It is important to note whether she is ambulatory, uses a walker, or is confined to a wheelchair or bed. This is important in identifying those who may have normal detrusor and urethral function but are unable to make it to the toilet in time. Adjusting the patient's environment may relieve her urinary incontinence.

A pelvic examination should be performed to evaluate the vagina and urethra for evidence of estrogen deficiency.

An atrophic vagina or urethra is thought to contribute to lower urinary tract symptoms, by decreasing urethral pressure and producing a noncompliant urethra, showing urodynamic and symptomatic improvement with estrogen therapy.[11,12]

The existence of concomitant gynecologic pathology, such as cystocele, rectocele, enterocele, or uterine prolapse, can influence the management of a patient.[13] Reduction of a prolapse in some patients relieves urethral obstruction, rendering a continent patient incontinent. A pessary is the only conservative treatment for women with prolapse and is also useful in predicting those who require urethrovesical neck suspension if the prolapse is treated surgically.

The neurologic evaluation consists of assessment of perineal sensation (S-2, S-3, S-4), continuity of the sacral reflex centers, and lower limb strength. The rectal reflex is tested by gently stroking the perianal region and watching for the wink or contraction of the rectal sphincter. The bulbocavernosus reflex, elicited by tapping or lightly touching the clitoris, produces contraction of the rectal sphincter. These reflexes may be absent in older patients and difficult to elicit in the obese patient. Further neurologic tests or referral requires individualization based on history and physical findings.

An evaluation of muscle function and use is then performed to determine the tone and strength.[14] The urethra is normally attached to the levator ani muscle. Contraction of the pelvic floor muscles leads to an elevation of the urethra. Urinary incontinence can be significantly decreased by training that strengthens and educates the patient to use these muscles during stress.[15,16] Training of the pelvic floor is accomplished through various methods, including biofeedback, electrical stimulation, and vaginal cones, which enhance the standard muscle contraction exercises.[17]

Laboratory Tests

A urinalysis should be performed in all women presenting with urinary incontinence. It is not unusual for both urinary symptoms and positive urodynamic findings to regress after adequate treatment of an infection. In a study of 20 patients with acute UTI, 45% exhibited an unstable bladder. After appropriate treatment, 60% regained bladder stability, and 30% of stress incontinent patients became continent.[18] The presence of hematuria in the absence of a documented UTI requires urethrocystoscopy.

Laboratory tests such as electrolytes, blood urea nitrogen, creatinine, thyroid-stimulating hormone, thyroxine, calcium, and glucose should be performed as clinically indicated. Electrolyte abnormalities and elevated calcium can cause confusion that impairs toileting. Hyperglycemia and subsequent osmotic diuresis can aggravate incontinence. Hypothyroidism has been associated with detrusor instability.

Assessment of Urethral Mobility

The assessment of urethral mobility is used to define therapeutic options. Downward urethrovesical junction movement can be assessed by palpation, the Q-tip test, ultrasound, and fluoroscopy. The Q-tip test is performed by placing a lubricated Q-tip at the urethrovesical junction and measuring deflection from the horizontal with an orthopedic goniometer. Patients without urethral mobility are poor urethrovesical suspension candidates but with concomitant low urethral pressure may be helped by periurethral bulking agents.

Simple Cystometrogram

The simple cystometrogram is performed to answer four vital questions.[19–21] (1) Can the patient empty her bladder completely? (2) Does the patient have normal bladder function? (3) Is there evidence of an unstable bladder? (4) Can the urinary leakage be documented?

After obtaining a clean voided urine specimen, the patient is catheterized and the remaining urine measured. Residual urine is defined as greater than 50 mL of urine in the postvoid bladder. Residual urine alerts the physician to serious urethral/vesical dysfunction such as outlet obstruction, multiple sclerosis, occult spina bifida, peripheral neuropathy, autonomic neuropathy, or spinal cord injury. Detrusor hyperactivity with impaired contractile function is a subset of detrusor hyperreflexia in which the bladder is overactive but empties ineffectively, leaving a significant amount of residual urine.[22]

The bladder is then filled with saline using a 60-mL catheter tip syringe, noting the volume of first bladder sensation, fullness, and maximum capacity. Under normal conditions, the bladder is capable of increasing fluid storage without an increase in bladder pressure. The patient should have a first sensation between 90 and 200 mL, fullness at 350 mL, and a maximum capacity around 500 mL. The patient should not experience severe urgency or bladder pain. Painful bladder syndrome or sensory urgency is suggested by severe urgency or pain at low bladder volume without demonstration of a detrusor contraction. A patient with an areflexic bladder has little or no sensation of fullness at high bladder volumes, such as greater than 600 mL.

The water level in the syringe is observed during filling. Detrusor instability is defined as objective detrusor contractions occurring during filling cystometry when the patient is actively trying to inhibit micturition.[23] In the absence of increased intra-abdominal pressure (respiration, coughing, or bearing down), an elevation of water height occurring simultaneously with the sensation of urgency is diagnostic of an unstable bladder. In a study of 170 geriatric patients (mean age 80), the finding of detrusor instability (64%) was compared by multichannel and simple cystometry (sensitivity 75%, specificity 79%, positive predictive value 85%).[22]

With the bladder full and the patient in the sitting position, a stress test is performed. The patient is asked to cough and strain while the perineum is visualized to document urine leakage occurring simultaneously with stress. The use of pyridium or methylene blue to color the urine in conjunction with a pad test can help to delineate the source of the leakage.[24] The provocative stress test had a sensitivity of 91% and a specificity of 100% to detect incontinence in a group of 108 women.[25]

Urinary Diary

It is not unusual for a patient with lower urinary tract dysfunction either to exaggerate or to underestimate the severity of the incontinence problem. A voiding diary can be kept from 24 hours up to a week to obtain an accurate assessment of voiding time, volumes voided, incontinence episodes, severity of leakage, and diurnal/nocturnal frequency. Occasionally, patients are found voiding greater than 3000 mL daily. Patients may be infrequent voiders, using the bathroom once or twice daily and voiding volumes of 1200 mL. Simple behavior intervention encouraging decreasing fluid intake or more frequent voiding can reduce leakage. This diary can serve as a baseline before beginning bladder drill therapy.[26]

Treatment

At the conclusion of the initial evaluation, therapy can be initiated in many patients. The atrophic vagina can be treated with estrogen cream, medications can be changed, fluid intake can be decreased, caffeine can be stopped, alterations can be made in voiding habits, and pelvic floor muscle exercises can be initiated. Although adequate data are present to start therapy under these circumstances, before surgery the physician should carefully consider further testing (Table 16–1).

A major shortcoming of the core investigation is that a number of patients with detrusor instability and mixed incontinence are missed. In an attempt to circumvent this shortcoming, empiric therapy, including anticholinergic medication, bladder drills, and pelvic floor muscle exercises, has been recommended. Because cure rates from anticholinergic therapy range from 50% to 80%, with a large placebo effect, results of therapy—success or failure—do not establish the diagnosis. Anticholinergic medications should be used judiciously because of a high rate of undesirable side effects.

If a patient complains only of stress incontinence, has a normal simple cys-

Table 16–1. Indications for Urodynamic Laboratory Testing of the Incontinent Woman

Failed continence surgery
Symptoms of mixed incontinence
Poor urethral mobility
No objective demonstration of urine leakage
Abnormal neurologic evaluation
Prior pelvic irradiation
Prior radical pelvic surgery

tometrogram, and has a positive stress test and urethral descensus from the symphysis pubis is documented (angle >30 degrees), no further testing may be necessary before therapeutic intervention. Retropubic surgical success rates average 90% at 5 years; long-term success is not as well established. Pelvic floor rehabilitation success averages 50% to 70%, but long-term success also is not established.[27]

URINARY TRACT INFECTION

UTI and asymptomatic bacteriuria are common in women of all ages and increase in frequency as the population ages.[28] During their lifetime, 20% of women develop a UTI, with 6% of women developing one or more infections yearly.[29] UTIs are much more common in women than in men because of a number of predisposing factors. In women, continuous contamination of the distal one third of the urethra by pathogens from the vagina and rectum and a shorter urethra enables easier access of bacteria into the bladder. The ease in which bacteria can enter the bladder has been documented by bacterial count studies obtained after massage of the urethra and sexual intercourse.[30,31]

Postmenopausal women have higher rates of UTI because of decreased estrogen. The epithelium of the urethra, trigone, and vagina is estrogen dependent. Decreased estrogen lowers the glycogen content of vaginal epithelium, resulting in less nutrients for the lactobacilli to metabolize lactic acid, thereby increasing the pH of vaginal secretions. Change in pH is responsible for a change in the vaginal and introital bacterial flora that increases the prevalence of uropathogens.[32]

In a controlled trial of 93 postmenopausal women with recurrent UTI, the intravaginal administration of estriol significantly reduced the incidence of UTIs.[33]

Incomplete emptying because of neuropathy, spinal cord lesions, trauma, and tumor can predispose to UTI. Uterine prolapse or large cystocele formation can predispose to UTI by producing a kinking mechanism at the urethrovesical junction.[34]

Diagnosis

Symptoms commonly include abrupt onset of frequency, urgency, dysuria, and suprapubic pain. The traditional method of diagnosing UTI is the presence of greater than 100,000 cfu/mL in a symptomatic patient. A false-negative diagnosis is common using these classic criteria. Lower quantitative yields may result from increased fluid consumption, contamination of urine with antimicrobial cleansing solution, previous antibiotic therapy, improper transportation of sample, or failure to use organism-specific culture medium.[35] In symptomatic women, lowering the threshold to 100 cfu/mL significantly improves sensitivity without lowering specificity.[36] It is cost-effective to diagnose bladder infections in low-risk symptomatic patients with biochemical tests (nitrate and leukocyte esterase). Urine cultures are helpful in patients at increased risk for developing a complicated UTI (Table 16–2). The most frequent pathogen isolated in urine is *Escherichia coli,* but other aerobic gram-negative bacilli and enterococci are commonly encountered.

Table 16–2. High-Risk Group for Complicated Urinary Tract Infection

Recent hospitalization
Catheterization or instrumentation
Antibiotic therapy
Diabetes mellitus
Recent urinary tract infection
Pregnancy
Immunosuppression
Prolonged duration of symptoms

Treatment

Simple UTI can be treated with single-dose or short 3-day course of trimethoprim, trimethoprim-sulfamethoxazole, or nitrofurantoin.[37] Patients at increased risk for developing a complicated UTI should not be treated with single or short-course therapy. Patients should be reevaluated in 4 to 7 days and a repeat urinalysis performed. In complicated UTI, urine cultures should be obtained and long-term therapy (7 to 10 days) initiated.[38] Fluoroquinolones have been advocated for the treatment of UTI because of their high serum and urine levels, good tissue penetration, broad spectrum of activity against common pathogens, and long half-life.[39]

URETHRITIS

It is important to differentiate between external and internal dysuria. Burning on urination can be secondary to *Trichomonas vaginalis, Candida albicans, Chlamydia* or painful vulvar syndrome.[40] Pelvic examination is essential in differentiating between external and internal dysuria. In the geriatric population, atrophy has been reported to produce urethritis in the absence of an infection.

SENSORY DISORDERS

Painful bladder syndrome is a group of disorders that present as pain associated with the bladder or voiding. Ninety percent of all reported cases of interstitial cystitis occur in women. The majority of cases diagnosed occur between the ages of 30 and 50 years. This is the more classic form of interstitial cystitis. These patients are generally older and have reduced bladder capacity with fibrosis of the bladder musculature.

There is another group of patients who are younger, whose bladder capacities are not yet diminished under anesthesia but who have symptoms and cystoscopic finding of interstitial cystitis. Whether these are two separate entities or whether one is an early form of the other is unclear.

A number of factors have been associated with painful bladder syndrome.

There is no direct positive relationship between infectious organisms and painful bladder syndrome. Marked elevation of certain anticapsid antigen antibodies in the blood to *Epstein-Barr virus* of 150 patients with painful bladder syndrome has been reported.[41] One investigator, postulating an autoimmune cause, found antibladder antibodies present in 75% of women with painful bladder syndrome versus 40% controls.[42] It has been demonstrated that bladders in patients with painful bladder syndrome were more permeable than controls.[43] Another author reported a greater number of nerve fibers within the detrusor muscle of patients with painful bladder syndrome than normal women, suggesting a role for increased sensitivity to external stimuli.[44] Patients with painful bladder syndrome demonstrate psychopathology similar to those with chronic illness, requiring physicians to treat not only the physical symptoms, but also underlying psychological or psychiatric problems.[45]

Diagnosis

Symptoms include urgency, frequency, nocturia, and voiding small amounts both day and night. The patients report they void frequently because of severe pressure or suprapubic pain. The suprapubic pain is typically relieved by voiding. Incontinence is usually not seen in contrast to patients with unstable bladders. Often, there are associated symptoms of dyspareunia and concomitant diagnoses of painful vulvar syndrome and endometriosis.

The diagnosis of painful bladder syndrome is established in a symptomatic patient by a negative urine culture and a typical cystoscopic appearance. In the early stage of the disease, small discrete, submucosal hemorrhages or glomerulations have been reported.[46] Linear cracking and ulceration (Huhner's ulcers) may be seen. It has been suggested that non-ulcerative and ulcerative painful bladder syndrome are distinct clinical entities and the clinical response is different. Histologic findings in painful bladder syndrome may consist of nonspecific inflammation, vasodilatation, and edema of the bladder submucosa. A subset of patients demonstrate detrusor mastocytosis (>28 mast cells/mm²).[47] Cytologic screening or random bladder biopsy should be performed to rule out carcinoma in situ.

Treatment

Various therapies for painful bladder syndrome have been proposed, including dimethylsulfoxide (DMSO), amitriptyline, bladder drills, hydrodilation under anesthesia, infiltration of the bladder wall with steroids, transurethral resection, fulguration of the bladder, laser of the bladder mucosa, bladder denervation, and cystoplasty. DMSO has anti-inflammatory effects, breaks down collagen, and blocks conduction of peripheral nerves. Satisfactory symptomatic relief has been reported in 80%, with no systemic or local toxicity.[48] Amitriptyline with dosages starting at 10 mg before bedtime and increasing to 75 mg every hour of sleep has been useful in patients with painful bladder syndrome.[49] Bladder drills were shown to decrease symptoms significantly in up to 70% of patients.[50] Even with the improvement in symptoms, however, there is no significant alteration in the endoscopic or morphologic appearance of the bladder after treatment.

EMPTYING DISORDERS

The normal bladder must not only store urine, but also expel it in a controlled fashion. Emptying disorders are categorized as acute and chronic urinary retention.[51]

Diagnosis

Acute urinary retention in women is less common than in men. Acute urinary retention can be precipitated by an acute stressful event: medical, surgical, or psychological. Table 16–3 lists the common causes of acute urinary retention. The retention may be related to the discomfort associated with a procedure or illness and recumbency. Workup usually does not reveal any neurologic or mechanical cause for the retention.[52]

Table 16–3. Causes of Acute
Urinary Retention

Acute inflammation
  Genital herpes[67]
  Urinary tract infection
  Urethral diverticulum
Postoperative
  Levator spasm
    Posterior colporrhaphy
    Episiotomy
  Anesthesia
  Obstruction
    Anti-incontinence procedures
    Vaginal packing
Medications
Psychogenic

Acute urinary retention can be seen as an acute or early manifestation of a neurologic abnormality affecting sacral nerves such as multiple sclerosis or herniated disks.[53] Urethral obstruction in women is quite rare but can occasionally occur postoperatively or be seen in patients with significant pelvic floor prolapse.[54,55] Acute retention can also rarely be caused by urethral or bladder outlet obstruction owing to stricture, stenosis, tumors, and urethral stones.[56]

Postoperative urinary retention is a fairly common occurrence. Anesthesia can affect urinary retention.[57] There is an increased rate of retention in patients with anesthesia for more than 60 minutes, in patients ventilated, in patients relaxed and reversed by atropine and neostigmine, and in patients who had opiate analgesia.

Other factors that may contribute to urinary retention are bladder overdistention and overcorrection of the urethrovesical angle. To prevent bladder overdistention, patients should be checked to ensure adequate voiding after removal of catheters postoperatively or before discharge from ambulatory surgical settings. Acute overdistention of the bladder can produce a temporary paralysis of detrusor activity, which can take days or weeks to resolve.

It is important in anti-incontinence surgery to avoid overcorrection of the urethral-vesical angle. Unfortunately, there are no criteria available to assist the physician in adequately gauging the proper elevation necessary to cure incontinence yet prevent urinary retention. Voiding dysfunction occurs in 20% of patients after retropubic urethropexy with marked decrease in maximum flow and increase in urethral resistance.[58]

In women who develop chronic retention, there is evidence to suggest a higher incidence of spina bifida occulta related to tethered cord.[59] Decreased bladder sensation can be seen with peripheral neuropathy secondary to diabetes mellitus, vitamin deficiency, hypothyroidism, or alcoholism. It is important to realize that in the majority of elderly diabetics, involuntary bladder contractions are a more common finding than urinary retention.[60] Anticholinergic agents, ganglionic blockers, tricyclic antidepressants, anticonvulsants, α-adrenergic agonists, and phenothiazines may produce voiding dysfunction.

Treatment

The most effective form of therapy in the management of acute urinary retention is *tincture of time.* Patients can be discharged home with a suprapubic catheter and be reassured that typically normal voiding resumes shortly. If voiding is delayed, patients can be taught self-catheterization. Intermittent self-catheterization is probably the most effective overall therapy for patients whether the retention is secondary to neurologic or other etiologic factors.[61,62]

Medical therapy of urinary retention has proven to be of little benefit. The majority of the studies are uncontrolled and end point criteria not given.[63] In one controlled study of postpartum patients, urinary retention was not significantly altered by the routine administration of bethanechol. α-Adrenergic blockers have been used to prevent postoperative urinary retention and improve flow in patients with urethral obstruction. In several studies, phenoxybenzamine has been shown to be significantly more effective than placebo in preventing prolonged micturition problems in patients with postoperative urinary retention.[64]

For urinary retention secondary to anti-incontinence surgery that does not resolve with time or conservative therapy, several surgical alternatives have been described. These have included loosening or takedown of sutures.[65,66]

REFERENCES

1. Wyman JF, Harkins SW, Choi SC, et al: Psychosocial impact of urinary incontinence in women. Obstet Gynecol 1987; 70:378–381.
2. Hu TW: Impact of urinary incontinence on health-care costs. J Am Geriatr Soc 1990; 38:292–295.
3. Urinary Incontinence Guideline Panel: Urinary Incontinence in Adults: Clinical Practice Guideline. AHCPR Pub. No. 92-0038. Rockville, MD, Agency for Health Care Policy and Research, Public Health Service, U.S. Department of Health and Human Services, 1992.
4. The standardization of terminology of lower urinary tract function: Produced by the International Continence Society Committee on Standardization of Terminology. Scand J Urol Nephrol 1988; 114 (suppl):5–19.
5. Creighton SM, Stanton SL: Caffeine: Does it affect your bladder? Br J Urol 1990; 66:613–614.
6. Keister KJ, Creason NS: Medications of elderly institutionalized incontinent females. J Adv Nurs 1989; 14:980–985.
7. Bergman A, Bader K: Reliability of the patient's history in the diagnosis of urinary incontinence. Int J Gynaecol Obstet 1990; 32:255–259.
8. Fischer-Rasmussen W, Hansen RI, Stage P: Predictive values of diagnostic tests in the evaluation of female urinary stress incontinence. Acta Obstet Gynaecol Scand 1986; 65:291–294.
9. Ramsay IN, Hilton P, Rice N: The symptomatic characterization of patients with detrusor instability and those with genuine stress incontinence. Int Urogynecol J 1993; 4:23–26.
10. Wiskind AK, Miller KF, Wall LL: One hundred unstable bladders. Obstet Gynecol 1994; 83:108–112.
11. Fantl JA, Cardozo L, McClish DK: Estrogen therapy in the management of urinary incontinence in post-menopausal women: A meta-analysis. First report of the hormones and urogenital therapy committee. Obstet Gynecol 1994; 83:12–18.
12. Bhatia NN, Bergman A, Karram MM: Effects of estrogen on urethral function in women with urinary incontinence. Am J Obstet Gynecol 1989; 160:176–181.
13. Richardson DA, Bent AE, Ostergard DR: The effect of uterovaginal prolapse on urethrovesical pressure dynamics. Am J Obstet Gynecol 1983; 146:901–905.
14. McIntosh LJ, Mallett VT, Frahm JD, Richardson DA: Abdominal and perineal muscle reaction to an increase in intra-abdominal pressure. Int Urogynecol J 1994; 5:90–93.
15. Burgio KL: Behavioral training for stress and urge incontinence in the community. Gerontology 1990; 36:27–34.
16. Ferguson KL, McKey PL, Bishop KR, et al: Stress urinary incontinence: Effect of pelvic muscle exercise. Obstet Gynecol 1990; 75:671–675.
17. Peattie AB, Plevnik S, Stanton SL: Vaginal cones: A conservative method of treating genuine stress incontinence. Br J Obstet Gynaecol 1988; 95:1049–1053.
18. Bergman A, Bhatia NN: Urodynamics: Effect of urinary tract infection on urethral and bladder function. Obstet Gynecol 1985; 66:366–371.
19. Dennis PJ, Rohner TJ, Hu TW, et al: Simple urodynamic evaluation of incontinent elderly female nursing home patients: A descriptive analysis. Urology 1991; 37:173–179.
20. Ouslander J, Leach G, Abelson S, et al: Simple versus multichannel cystometry in the evaluation of bladder function in an incontinent geriatric population. J Urol 1988; 140:1482–1486.
21. Sand PK, Brubaker LT, Novak T: Simple standing incremental cystometry as a screening method for detrusor instability. Obstet Gynecol 1991; 77:453–457.
22. Resnick NM, Yalla SV: Detrusor hyperactivity with impaired contractile function: An unrecognized but common cause of incontinence in elderly patients. JAMA 1987; 257:3076–3081.
23. The standardization of terminology of lower urinary tract function. Produced by the International Continence Society Committee on Standardization of Terminology. Scand J Urol Nephrol 1988; 114 (suppl):5–19.
24. Wall LL, Wang K, Robson I, Stanton SL: The Pyridium pad test for diagnosing urinary incontinence: A comparative study of asymptomatic and incontinent women. J Reprod Med 1990; 35:682–684.
25. Swift SE, Ostergard DR: Evaluation of current urodynamic testing methods in the diagnosis of genuine stress incon-

tinence. Obstet Gynecol 1995; 86:85–91.

26. Fantl JA, Wyman JF, McClish DK, et al: Efficacy of bladder training in older women with urinary incontinence. JAMA 1991; 265:609–613.

27. McIntosh LJ, Frahm JD, Mallett VT, Richardson DA: Pelvic floor rehabilitation in the treatment of incontinence. J Reprod Med 1993; 38:662–666.

28. Dontas AS, Kasviki-Charvati P, Papanayiotou PC, et al: Bacteriuria and survival in old age. N Engl J Med 1981; 304:939.

29. Kraft JK, Stamey TA: The natural history of symptomatic recurrent bacteriuria in women. Medicine (Baltimore) 1977; 56:55–60.

30. Bran JL, Levison ME, Kaye D: Entrance of bacteria into the female urinary bladder. N Engl J Med 1972; 286:626.

31. Buckley RM, McGuckin M, MacGregor RR: Urine bacterial counts after sexual intercourse. N Engl J Med 1978; 298:321–324.

32. Mattsby-Blatzer I, Hanson LA, Olling S, Kaijser B: Experimental *Escherichia coli* ascending pyelonephritis in rats: Active peroral immunization with live *Escherichia coli*. Infect Immunol 1982; 35:647–653.

33. Raz R, Stamm WE: A controlled trial of intravaginal estriol in postmenopausal women with recurrent urinary tract infections. N Engl J Med 1993; 329:753–756.

34. Richardson DA, Bent AE, Ostergard DR: The effect of uterovaginal prolapse on urethrovesical pressure dynamics. Am J Obstet Gynecol 1983; 146:901–905.

35. Richardson DA: Dysuria and urinary tract infections. Obstet Gynecol Clin North Am 1990; 17:881–887.

36. Stamm WE, Counts GW, Running KR, et al: Diagnosis of coliform infection in acutely dysuric women. N Engl J Med 1982; 307:463–468.

37. Stamm WE, Hooton TM: Management of urinary tract infections in adults. N Engl J Med 1993; 18:1328–1334.

38. Thomas S, Bhatia NN: New approaches in the treatment of urinary tract infections. Obstet Gynecol Clin North Am 1989; 16:897–909.

39. Rocco F, Franchini V: Antimicrobial therapy for treatment of UTI in the elderly. Eur Urol 1991; 19:7–15.

40. Komaroff AL: Acute dysuria in women. N Engl J Med 1984; 310:368–375.

41. Gillespie L, Said J, Sostrin S, Kleiwer K: Immunofluorescent and histochemical staining confirm the identification of the many diseases called interstitial cystitis. Br J Urol 1990; 66:265–273.

42. Anderson JB, Parivar F, Lee G, et al: The enigma of interstitial cystitis—an autoimmune disease? Br J Urol 1989; 63:58–63.

43. Parsons CL, Lilly JD, Stein P: Epithelial dysfunction in nonbacterial cystitis (interstitial cystitis). J Urol 1991; 145:732–735.

44. Christmas TJ, Rode J, Chapple CR, et al: Nerve fibre proliferation in interstitial cystitis. Virchows Arch Pathol Anat Histopathol 1990; 416:447–451.

45. Keltikangas-Jarvinen L, Auvinen L, Lehtonen T: Psychological factors related to interstitial cystitis. Eur Urol 1988; 15:69–72.

46. Holm-Bentzen M, Jacobsen F, Nerström B, et al: Painful bladder disease: Clinical and pathoanatomical differences in 115 patients. J Urol 1987; 138:500–502.

47. Lynes WL, Flynn SD, Shortliffe LD, Stamey TA: The histology of interstitial cystitis. Am J Surg Pathol 1990; 14:969–976.

48. Barker SB, Matthews PN, Philip PF, Williams G: Prospective study of intravesical dimethyl sulfoxide in the treatment of chronic inflammatory bladder disease. Br J Urol 1987; 59:142–144.

49. Hanno PM, Buehler J, Wein AJ: Use of amitriptyline in the treatment of interstitial cystitis. J Urol 1989; 141:846–848.

50. Parsons CL, Koprowski PF: Interstitial cystitis: Successful management by increasing urinary voiding intervals. Urology 1991; 37:207–212.

51. Preminger GM, Steinhardt GF, Mandell J, et al: Acute urinary retention in female patients: Diagnosis and treatment. J Urol 1983; 130:112.

52. Wheeler JS, Walter JS: Urinary retention in females: A review. Int Urogynecol J 1992; 3:137–142.

53. Sandri SD, Fanciullacci F, Politi P, Zanollo A: Urinary disorders in intervertebral disc prolapse. Neurourol Urodyn 1987; 6:11–19.

54. Richardson DA, Bent AE, Ostergard DR: The effect of uterovaginal prolapse on urethrovesical pressure dynamics. Am J Obstet Gynecol 1983; 146:901.

55. Delaere KPJ, Moonen WA, Debruyne FMJ, et al: Anterior vaginal repair, cause of troublesome voiding disorders. Eur Urol 1979; 5:190.

56. Axelrod SL, Blaivas JG: Bladder neck

obstruction in women. J Urol 1987; 137:497.

57. Stallard S, Prescott S: Postoperative urinary retention in general surgical patients. Br J Surg 1988; 75:1141–43.

58. Lose G, Jorgensen L, Mortensen SO, et al: Voiding difficulties after colposuspension. Obstet Gynecol 1987; 69:33.

59. Fidas A, MacDonald JL, Elton RA, et al: Neurological defects of the voiding reflex arcs in chronic urinary retention and their relation to spina bifida occulta. Br J Urol 1989; 63:16–20.

60. Starer P, Libow L: Cystometric evaluation of bladder dysfunction in elderly diabetic patients. Arch Intern Med 1990; 150:810–813.

61. Kornhuber HH, Schutz A: Efficient treatment of neurogenic bladder disorders in multiple sclerosis with initial intermittent catheterization and ultrasound-controlled training. Eur Neurol 1990; 30:260–267.

62. Wheeler JS Jr, Culkin DJ, Walter JS, Flanigan RC: Female urinary retention. Urology 1990; 35:428–432.

63. Finkbeiner AE: Is bethanechol chloride clinically effective in promoting bladder emptying? A literature review. J Urol 1985; 134:443.

64. Livne PM: Prevention of post-hysterectomy urinary retention by alpha-adrenergic blocker. Acta Obstet Gynaecol Scand 1983; 62:337.

65. Araki T, Takamoto H, Hara T, et al: The loop-loosening procedure for urination difficulties after Stamey suspension of the vesical neck. J Urol 1990; 144:319–323.

66. Webster GD, Kreder KJ: Voiding dysfunction following cystourethropexy: Its evaluation and management. J Urol 1990; 150:810–813.

67. Greenstein A, Matzkin H, Kaver I, Braf A: Acute urinary retention in herpes genitalis infection: Urodynamic evaluation. Urology 1988; 31:453–456.

CHAPTER 17

Sexuality

Sally A. Kope

A woman's sexual response has been viewed from a sociologically different perspective since the advent of reliable birth control, the pioneering work of Masters and Johnson in the study of human sexual response, and the survey of human sexual behavior conducted by the Kinsey Institute. As practitioners enter the next millennium, they draw from an ever evolving body of medical and psychological knowledge about how women function and respond in sexually.

Masters and Johnson delineated the human sexual response cycle in their research of the 1960s. This delineation remains useful for the primary care practitioner as a framework for determining treatment interventions when problems occur. Sexual problems are organized into two categories: sexual dysfunction and paraphilic behavior. Sexual dysfunction is medically, trauma, or psychologically based.[1] Paraphilic behavior refers to sexual arousal to stimulus considered to be outside of the psychological norms. Paraphilias have been "characterized by arousal to objects or situations that are not considered reasonable or appropriate for psychologically normal adults. They may interfere with the establishment of reciprocal, pleasurable, adult sexual activity. Paraphiliac behav-

ior may have psychogenic bases and can cause psychological distress."[2] Paraphilic behavior requires specialized evaluation and treatment and is not addressed here.

SEXUAL RESPONSE CYCLE

An overview of female sexual response and factors that can cause problems is not easily condensed. This chapter focuses on disorders of the sexual response cycle (desire, arousal, orgasm) and on the impact of pain and trauma on sexual functioning.

The sexual response cycle is summarized in Figure 17–1. The *desire phase* of human sexual response refers to a woman's energy, positive or negative, for her sexuality. One specific descriptor refers to her interest to engage in sexually stimulating activity, alone or with a partner, and her motivation to follow through on that interest. A more subtle contributor to the desire phase and its disorders is the comfort or discomfort a woman experiences living in her adult or adolescent body. Of significant influence to this phase is a woman's general sense of well-being in her world of relationships, sexual or not.

FEMALE SEXUAL RESPONSE

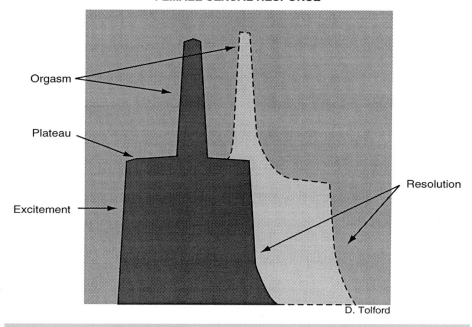

Figure 17–1.   Female sexual response.

The *arousal* and *orgasm phases* of sexual response refer to the physiologic and psychological response to sexually stimulating activity. Therapists watch for discrepant reports of objective and subjective experiences. For example, a patient may say, "I have no difficulty lubricating, but I certainly don't feel any great excitement when my partner is stroking me."

Pain and trauma, not necessarily to be viewed collectively, can have a profound effect on sexual response. The biochemical response of an individual recalling a past trauma can be experienced as if the trauma were occurring all over again. Usual therapeutic modalities may be of limited help in modifying this automatic and autonomic response.[3] Vaginal or vulvar pain, vaginismus, or pelvic pain can be daunting to a woman and to her partner. A pain response to an activity that is normally expected to be pleasurable can set up a cycle of anticipatory fear and avoidance.

DESIRE PHASE

The desire phase of sexual response is inclusive of a woman's adaptability to de-

velopmental changes; her body image; expectations of sex and of her partner; and her experience of intimacy, present and past. These aspects are fundamental to the robustness of her desire for sexually stimulating activity.

Sexual desire phase disorders generally present to the clinician within the context of a relationship because a desire discrepancy may prompt the couple to seek outside intervention. Many women who are not currently in a relationship also seek assistance if they believe their sexual drive and interest are low, absent, or aversive.

Hypoactive Sexual Desire

Hypoactive sexual desire is also called low sexual desire or inhibited sexual desire. Women who experience hypoactive sexual desire describe a lack of sexual interest or a widely sporadic sexual desire.[2] This low sexual desire persists beyond common circumstantially based low sexual interest, such as recovering from an illness. Low sex drive tends to be the most commonly referred sexual complaint, and hypoactive sexual desire is known to be multifactorial.[4]

Hormonal Factors

Seagraves[5] summarizes research on the effects of endocrine function on sexual desire in women in three areas: cyclic changes in libido such as during the menstrual cycle; the use of exogenous hormones in specific situations such as treatment of disease, hormone replacement therapy, and oral contraceptives; and the changes in sexual desire women report after changes in endogenous hormone production, such as menopause or surgically induced menopause. He reported no association between sexual desire and cyclic changes in hormones through the menstrual cycle and stated, "Natural and surgical menopause are events of considerable psychological significance for most women. From the available evidence it is impossible to ascertain whether the decrease in libido associated with menopause is endocrinologically based or related to other factors."[5] Androgens are important in both female and male libido. Ovaries and the adrenal glands produce androgens, and changes in ovarian function can affect that output.[6] Studies have suggested that a reduction of testosterone below physiologic levels reduces libido; however, it is unclear whether variations in female androgens within the normal physiologic range are related to libido.[5]

Medical Illness and Treatment

Chronic illness and medical treatment tends to be the most prevalent secondary cause of low sexual desire.[7] A discussion here cannot be comprehensive, but the treating clinician should be aware of and communicate the effects on sexual function of medications, invasive treatments, and the disease process. For example, an individual suffering from diabetic neuropathy may find it reassuring to discuss the changes related to libido with her physician or support group.

The question of when to address anticipated changes is a dilemma facing medical practitioners. At the time of diagnosis and treatment decisions, a patient may be preoccupied by concerns of the medical intervention, the disruption to life and relationships, and concerns about long-term effects. In the midst of this anxiety, it may be gratuitous to discuss the changes she may incur with sexual function (e.g., vaginal dryness from the effects of chemotherapy). Therapists facing this dilemma of timing often find it effective to lay the groundwork: "I anticipate that you will have questions some time in the future about effects of this (treatment, surgery, medication) on sexual functioning. I want you to know that we will discuss these questions when you're ready."

Depression and other mental health disorders left untreated may have a predictably negative effect on sexuality. Pain disorders of any origin tend to affect sexual desire. In fact, the presence of pain may affect a woman's choice about whether to engage in a sexual activity more than depression.[8] This is understandable if one considers that pain is invisible in its intensity and that to have the experience of pain be consistently valid to others around the patient, she may need to "hold onto" its presentation and not be distracted for fear of being discounted about the tenacity of her pain.

Iatrogenic Factors

Occasionally, medical intervention actually causes psychogenic sexual dysfunction. This is strikingly seen with patients who are undergoing treatment for infertility. After the experience of having their reproductive systems and sexual practices scrutinized and frequently categorized as pathology, some women report that they develop a "flashback" during sex in which they vividly recall being in stirrups or subjected to an uncomfortable procedure.[9] A poignant example of an iatragenically caused sexual problem is the case of a 47-year-old woman, several years out from aggressive, although successful, treatment for vaginal cancer. When she was going through her treatment, which included vaginal radiation implants, she kept up a light dialogue, almost banter, with the treatment team. She and her partner did not resume sexual activity for some months after her recovery from treatment, and when they did, she began to have feelings of terror and seemingly unrelated crying episodes. This led to a deliberate avoidance of any situation that she could imagine might lead to the expectation of sexual stimulation or penetration. With therapy, she was able to disentangle her sexual life with her husband from her experiences as a cancer patient.

In treating disease, the treatment cannot be sacrificed to the psychosexual concerns. The sensitive clinician may instruct the patient that aversive reactions could occur and that those reactions are normal to the circumstances. Frequently, physicians and medical practitioners are concerned that dwelling on invasive aspects of medical interventions may actually cause the disordered response. In the author's experience at the Sexual Health Counseling Services at University of Michigan, patients integrate their experiences of distressing or painful treatment more readily if they know what to anticipate.

Body Image

Sex therapy practices abound with women who exempt themselves from feeling desirable because they anguish about their less than perfect bodies. This can be true for women who become overly focused about minor flaws as well as for women who are adjusting to aging, pregnancy, surgery, or disability altered bodies. *Beauty* and *sexuality* are both commonly misunderstood as some transcendant inevitable fact; falsely interlocking the two makes it seem doubly true that a woman must be *beautiful* to be *sexual.* That, of course, is not true. The definitions of both *beautiful* and *sexual* constantly change to serve the social order, and the connection between the two is a recent invention.[10] This statement addresses one pervasive social construction about the relationship of beauty to a woman's sense of self in a sexual context.

One definition of *self* includes a sense of body integrity and mastery.[11] This can be compromised in numerous ways. A retired violinist grieved because her hands had become gnarled with arthritis. Not only was she unable to hold her bow and play her violin, but also she had a significantly altered sense of self as lover to her partner because of her stiff and deformed fingers. Body image can be negatively affected by physical disorders that are invisible, such as epilepsy. A woman may view herself as less than desirable resulting in lower self-esteem and avoidance behavior.

Person of the Patient

Each patient presents with her own set of values, cultural influence, ethnicity, personality structure, developmental stage, sex education, socioeconomic state, and roles she is occupying in her world. These issues can compete with each other and frequently create dilemmas for the individual. For example, a patient was confronted with a moral struggle when in therapy. The therapeutic suggestions were carefully made, within the context of areas of her sexual life she wanted to improve. It was recommended that she explore her body through masturbation. She felt a conflict between her wish to overcome her sexual symptom (in this case vaginismus) and her religious proscriptions against masturbation. Since living in a university town 2000 miles away from her country, she felt entrapped within her dilemma. After seeking the counsel of a priest, she was able to overcome her distressing symptom.

Multiple role demands tend to be an ongoing problem for women. Overwork and exhaustion do not mean a woman is avoidant of sexual intimacy, but this is frequently a secondary effect. Expectations about sexual desire happening spontaneously in the midst of such a busy life continue to lead women to experience disappointment about their sexual life. Unfortunately, traditional sex education and the media do nothing to challenge this unlikely expectation.

Relationships

Most complaints about sexual difficulty come from women who are in relationships. The quality of the relationship is significant to determine the course of treatment. For example, if a woman complains of no sexual interest in her partner whatsoever but frequent sexual interest in others outside of her relationship, the relationship, not the partner, may be the problem. Unaddressed issues of violence, alcoholism, or other destructive family secrets can manifest in sexual desire problems. A 50-year-old woman, married to a man with active alcoholism for three decades, was slow to heal following a hysterectomy. This was surprising because she was in good general health and had been athletic and active before her surgery. Furthermore, her symptoms seemed unrelated either to sex or to recovery from her hysterectomy. She developed chronic vomiting 6 weeks after surgery. It was finally determined that the patient's vomiting began when her husband approached her for sex after surgery. The hiatus from her home life—she had spent several weeks recovering at her sister's home—made her aware of the intolerability of her situation. "I just couldn't stomach him coming at me smelling drunk and disgusting," she said.

Education and encouragement for patients to assume responsibility is an ongoing conjunctive aspect of medical treatment. In regard to intervention for women seeking help with low sexual desire, the persistence and scope of the problem offer some indication whether the concern can be handled effectively with patient education or whether a referral for sex or couple therapy is more appropriate. Although it is tempting to offer behavioral change suggestions, such as "get a babysitter and go out for an evening," the most effective behavior changes come when women face their own dilemmas, struggle with the conflicts they present (no time/work overload/partner intimacy), and consider their own solutions. The patient's willingness to assume responsibility for actively seeking solutions for her own dilemmas is a good predictor for a positive outcome. This can be true whether the conflict is role overload or sexual boredom. Entrenched anger toward partner; resistance to any suggestion of personal responsibility for change; and aversion to genitals, her own or her partner's, may be indicators that a more systematic and therapeutic approach to the problem is indicated.

Hyperactive Sexual Desire

Hyperactive sexual desire is often paired with difficulty in making discriminating decisions about sexual partners, number of partners, and places where sexual activity may occur. When this manifests in women, it is much more likely to have its roots in an anxiety disorder than in the woman being physiologically insatiable for sex.[2,12] The individual may manage anxiety through compulsive sexual activity or obsessive thoughts pertaining to sex. The term *sexual addiction* has been used in conjunction with this disorder.

Sexual Aversion

Sexual aversion goes beyond indifference to, low interest in, or sporadic interest in sexual activity. It takes on a quality of fear and avoidance behavior.[13] This may be characterized by mild behaviors, such as a woman dreaming about sexual experience in a pleasurable context but actively avoiding sexual interaction or masturbation because she feels "nothing." At the other end of the continuum, the woman may experience an adrenal response: fight/flight/fear. She may exhibit symptoms of stress far beyond the "danger" the present circumstances warrant. This is explored more fully under trauma.

SEXUAL AROUSAL PHASE

The sexual arousal phase refers to the physiologic and psychological responses a woman experiences in fantasy, dreams, or through sexual stimulation. Vasocongestion is evident with engorgement of the genitalia with the upper portion of the vagina beginning to balloon out. Transudation occurs on the walls of the vagina, lubricating the vaginal tract and the vaginal opening. As stimulation and excitement continue, the uterus and genitals continue to engorge. The clitoris enlarges and becomes extremely touch sensitive. The uterus moves forward.[14] The woman may experience a generalized neuromuscular tension, and her nipples may become erect.

Sexual arousal disorders (pain disorders are considered separately) tend to be related to a lack of lubrication, vasocongestion, and physiologic sign of arousal, with no psychological experience of feeling sexually stimulated. Initially, evaluation of the problem should ascertain the woman's desire to be in the sexually stimulating situation in the first place. Determining her desire and motivation is crucial to any intervention regarding arousal phase problems.

Physiologic changes related to aging, illness, medications, and medical treatments should be assessed. For example, a lactating mother may complain of vaginal dryness, which may be remedied through education, reassurance, and vaginal lubrication. Frequently the lack of physical response in arousal is due to a misunderstanding or miscommunication about how and when sexual activity should proceed. Despite this being an era of overabundant self-help, it is not uncommon for a woman to be unaware of or uncommunicative about her need for sustained stimulation to achieve arousal. When a patient describes physical signs of arousal such as the presence of lubrication and blood engorgement but denies any correlating sensation, the practitioner should attempt to decipher the origin of the difficulty.

Arousal can be affected or interrupted if the individual has a concern about birth control efficacy, or sexually transmitted disease. It is a given that S.T.D.'s inclusive of H.I.V. are a serious health concern: primary care providers and specialists continue to disseminate vital information to women about these health risks, often including innovative outreach. Condom use, spermicides, and vaginal dams are being used by women to thwart transmission of H.I.V. and other sexually transmitted diseases. Because the employment of these devices often means an interruption in the pace of sexual activity, many couples are learning to incorporate the application of a condom, for example, into their sensual and sexual play.

ORGASM PHASE

The orgasm phase of the sexual response cycle refers to the release of accumulated sexual tension, optimally through an orgasmic response. This response has been evasive to discrete description because it is an *experience of sensation*. Striated muscles of the pelvic floor and the genital and anal areas involuntarily, rhythmically contract. This is sometimes described as waves of sensual pleasure focused in the genitals. The pudendal nerve transmits messages of stimulation to the spinal cord and to the brain where it is interpreted as pleasurable.[7,14]

The experience of orgasm is subjective and contextual, frequently it is most intensely experienced through masturbation but often most satisfactorily experienced with a partner.[15] Michael and associates' research for *Sex in America*[16] showed few differences in orgasmic frequency for women by education, religion, race, or ethnicity, but the relationship between being married and experiencing orgasms was significant, with many more married women reportedly being consistently orgasmic.

It is not considered to be a sexual dysfunction if a woman is nonorgasmic through intercourse but is able to achieve orgasm in some manner with her partner.[2] A careful evaluation of, and sometimes reframing of, a woman's perception about her orgasmic experience is important. In cases of lifelong anorgasmia, the factors discussed in the desire phase section must be considered.

PAIN DISORDERS

Conditions associated with dyspareunia are summarized in Table 17–1. Dyspareunia may be classified as introital or with deep thrust.

Vulvar Disorders

Patients present with chronic vulvovaginal pain, often years in duration. Frequently, their experience includes numerous treatment attempts that have been unsuccessful. Although the primary symptom may be pain during attempts at intercourse, women also complain of painful symptoms at other times. The most common descriptive term tends to be *burning*.[18] Experiencing intense pain with attempts at penetration has a dramatic effect on a couple's sexual functioning, particularly when the symptoms remain unrelieved for years. The effect of intermittent, sporadic, unpredictable pain can cause sexual dysfunction.

Table 17-1. Causes of Dyspareunia (Pain Disorders)

Introital Dyspareunia	Deep Thrust Dyspareunia
Anatomic abnormalities (partial or complete hymenal obliteration)	Cystitis
Bartholin's gland cyst/abscess	Endometriosis
Dermatitis	Fibroid uterus
External genital infections	Genital prolapse
Human papillomavirus	Interstitial cystitis
Lichen sclerosus	Ovarian cyst
Urethritis	Pelvic inflammatory disease
Vaginal atrophy	Vaginismus
Vaginismus	
Vulvar vestibulitis	
Vulvodynia	

Patients with vulvar pain scored more highly on general stress and anxiety symptoms than patients with other vulvar disorders, according to a study from University of Toronto.[19] The researchers noted, however, that the findings did not establish a psychosomatic cause for the disorder, and the increased stress may result from the patient having chronic symptoms of pain.

Sexual desire can be strongly affected during acute phases of vulvar vestibulitis or vulvodynia. Couples at the University of Michigan Medical Center for Vulvar Disease are questioned about the quality of their sexual interaction before the onset of the symptoms. Anecdotally, unless other pathology is present, most couples report a dramatic, negative change.[20] This change frequently manifests in avoidance behaviors. This is understandable because the couple's attempts at solving the problem, including achieving medical control of the pain, have not worked: Their usual coping skills are not effective against this challenge.

Effective Interventions for Dyspareunia

A thorough physical examination and treatment of organic disease is an integral part of managing vulvar pain. Establishing a working alliance is imperative. Frequently the starting place for this alliance is a validation of pain the patient is experiencing. This does not mean overriding clinical judgment, being insincerely supportive or falsely reassuring. The fact is many of these patients have believed or been led to believe that their problem is entirely psychological. Even if this is the final clinical judgment, the patient is experiencing pain, the pain is interfering with her sexual pleasure, and she has not yet come up with an effective strategy against it. Pain-based sexual dysfunction, even if completely secondary to a disease process, has a psychological impact. The reasons are basic: Her pain affects her partner directly, sexuality is a part of primary identity and its compromise is injurious to that identity, and pain is isolating her from a libidinal pleasure. Normalizing the experience for the couple is helpful. Simply reassuring an individual or couple that their avoidance of sexual activity or their frustration in dealing with the symptom would be a circumstantially expected response can help them feel less isolated.

The most effective therapeutic strategy to employ with women or couples dealing with vulvar pain is to facilitate their expansion of their sexual repertoire. This may include discussion of alternative ways of achieving or providing sexual pleasure. The couple may benefit from a discussion about incorporating into their sexual experience sensual pleasuring other than orgasm-oriented activities. Unfortunately, many women with vulvar disorders experience physical pain with physiologic arousal. This is especially challenging and not easily amenable to cognitive behavioral recommendations.

Secondary vaginismus may be related to vulvar pain and may not remit when the vulvar pain is eliminated.

Vaginismus

Vaginismus is the involuntary spasm of musculature in the pelvic floor and near the vaginal introitus that makes penetration painful or impossible. It can be primary or secondary. It can remit and recur. It is generally described as a burning pain, often of severe intensity.[17] Women with vaginismus may have sexual desire and orgasmic capacity intact; however, they simply cannot achieve intercourse, at least without serious pain. The cause of this symptom has many factors. A careful medical evaluation and psychosocial evaluation are indicated in cases of vaginismus. The treatment of vaginismus is multimodal, including education, desensitization of the spasming muscles, relaxation techniques, and therapy.[21]

Effective Interventions for Vaginismus

Employing the use of vaginal dilators is effective in the desensitization portion of treatment. Vaginal dilators are smooth plastic, cylinder-shaped objects with rounded tips, resembling a tampon, although longer. They come in graduated circumference sizes from extra small, approximately the size of a tampon, to a large size, which is about the size of an erect penis. Dilators were originally developed for women who had experienced vulvar/vaginal reconstructive surgery or treatment. Their use, however, translates well to the patient with vaginismus. The patient must understand that the goal of dilator therapy is not to stretch her vagina, but to gain control of the spasm response. Instructions for dilator therapy should be specific, including the purpose of the therapy; the need for regularity in working with dilators; specifics about relaxation techniques before beginning each dilator session; the course of dilator therapy (when she will switch to another size, what to do if problems occur, anticipating setbacks); assessing motivation for this aspect of treatment, and anticipating issues that may impede therapy,

such as wavering motivation and lack of privacy. The errors that are made in prescribing dilator therapy seem to be related to vague instructions and lack of follow-up at intervals of no more than 2 weeks.

Repeated instruction to the patient and her partner is essential. A tenacious symptom such as vaginismus can lead to a distorted sense of anatomy and self. It is common for even educated patients to fear that their vaginas are too small or that the dilator (or speculum or penis) will "hit something." Some patients do not understand the pelvic skeletal muscle structure. Most patients do not know what is happening in their bodies when they have vaginismis.

Treatment for vaginismus should be geared toward the woman assuming responsibility for the resolution of her symptom, in conjunction with her treating clinician. It is important to establish clearly that therapy is not effective or appropriate if the patient is not motivated for reasons of her own. Otherwise the therapist is in the unreasonable position of colluding to have the patient have sex she does not want to have. Finally, it is important to address the issue of birth control with vaginismic patients. Sometimes the fear of pregnancy can keep the symptom static.

When dilator therapy progresses and the patient is ready to proceed, treatment moves toward allowing penile-vaginal intercourse. This tends to be a "crisis" time in treatment because the focus has moved from being specifically within the patient's control to the inclusion of another person.[23] The entire process of moving treatment toward sexual intercourse is slow and incremental in small steps.

TRAUMA-BASED SEXUAL PROBLEMS

It has long been known that trauma, whether a single, overwhelming event such as rape or a series of events such as repeated incestual abuse of a child, has permanent effects on the individual survivor of the experience.[24] van der Kolk[3] discussed the psychobiology of an overwhelming and uncontrollable experience. He refers to the disturbance in the way such experiences are stored as memory. Instead of being stored in declarative memory, such experiences seem to be stored as visceral sensations such as anxiety or visual images such as nightmares and flashbacks. Further, this appears to be a normal response to overwhelming experiences. For some people, this *posttraumatic stress* response fades over time, but for others it remains vivid. Unfortunately, one's response, which can be as intense as the feeling of the original event happening all over again, can be excessive to the dangers at hand. The body's emotional response then cannot be relied on to give signals about how to act. For example, a woman who was grabbed from behind, overpowered, and sexually assaulted may have an emotional response, body memories, and terror about that event when her partner lovingly approaches her from behind, with only the intention of giving her an affectionate hug. van der Kolk explains: "Excessive stimulation of the central nervous system at the time of trauma may result in permanent neuronal changes that have a negative effect on learning, habituation, and stimulus discrimination." He goes on to describe available mechanisms to deal with such a response: remembering too much (hypermnesia) or too little (amnesia), hyperresponsiveness to stimuli, or avoidance and numbing.

Although memory is ordinarily an active and constructive process, in PTSD [posttraumatic stress disorder] failure of declarative memory may lead to organization of the trauma on a somatosensory level (as visual images or physical sensations) that is relatively impervious to change. The inability of people with PTSD to integrate traumatic experiences is related to their tendency to continuously relive the past which is mirrored physiologically and hormonally in the misinterpretation of innocuous stimuli as potential threats. Animal research suggests that intense emotional memories are processed outside of the hippocampally mediated memory system and are difficult to extinguish. Cortical activity can inhibit the expression of these subcortically based emotional memories. The effectiveness of this inhibition depends, in part, on physiological arousal and neurohormonal activity. These formulations have implications for both the psychotherapy and the pharmacotherapy of PTSD.[3]

van der Kolk's work and the work of others study the intricacies of neurobiology treatment strategies for individuals who are paralyzed in the throes of their trauma experiences. Psychopharmacology may play a more significant role in the management of intrusive symptoms. *Survivor* psychotherapy treatment includes the goal of improved patient understanding and mastering the trauma from her current, more empowered position. Treatment strategies that both acknowledge and explore the ramifications of traumatic events and equally focus on the present moment and the present relationship and choices have been shown to be effective.[25]

The effects of traumatic events involving physical endangerment, such as sexual assault, sexual exploitation, and abuse at any age, or physical abuse can have an impact on one's present-day sexual experience. Being in a situation reminiscent of the original trauma, even though the present-day situation is desired, can evoke the original feelings. Odors, gestures, lighting, touch, and background music can trigger a flashback or emotional response. In books, videos, and workshops, Maltz[26] focuses on a step-by-step process to stop old behaviors such as emotionally shutting down (psychic numbing) or emotionally overreacting (hyperresponsivity). She encourages partners, who are often equally bewildered as to how to react, to participate in the process she calls the "sexual healing journey."[26] Behaviors may include sexual aversion and avoidance or negative sexual behaviors with a compulsive component. These behaviors are then addressed within the context of the individual, her (or his) relationships, with concentration on adaptive choices. This intervention may begin with gentle touch exercises, perhaps guided hand-to-hand touch. The process of integrating new responses to painful past experiences is complex and requires determined effort and commitment that many women accomplish successfully.

REFERENCES

1. American Psychiatric Association: Sexual and Gender Identity Disorders. *In* Quick Reference to the Diagnostic and Statistical Manual of Mental Disorders: DSM IV. Washington, DC, American Psychiatric Association, 1994; pp 233–249.
2. Foley SM: Psychogenic sexual dysfunction. *In* Lechtenberg R, Ohl D, eds. Sexual Dysfunction: Neurologic, Urologic and Gynecologic Aspects. Philadelphia, Lea & Febiger, 1994; pp 189–193.
3. van der Kolk B: The body keeps the score: Memory and the evolving psychobiology of posttraumatic stress. Harvard Rev Psychiatry 1994; 1:253–255.
4. LoPiccolo J, Friedman J: Broad spectrum treatment of low sexual desire: Integration of cognitive, behavioral and systemic therapy. *In* Lieblum SR, Rosen RC, eds: Sexual Desire Disorders. New York, Guilford Press, 1988; pp 108–111.
5. Seagraves T: Hormones and libido. *In* Lieblum SR, Rosen RC, eds: Sexual Desire Disorders. New York, Guilford Press, 1988; pp 273–307.
6. Lectenberg R, Ohl D, eds: Sexual dysfunction: neurologic, urologic and gynecologic aspects. Philadelphia, Lea & Febiger, 1994; p 14.
7. Schover L, Jensen S: sexuality and chronic illness: A comprehensive approach. New York, Guilford Press, 1988.
8. Maruta T, Osborne D, Swanson D, Halling J: Chronic pain patients and spouses: Marital and sexual adjustment. Mayo Clin Proc 1992; 56:307.
9. Zoldbrod A: Men, women and infertility. New York, Lexington Books, 1993.
10. Wolf N: The beauty myth: How images of beauty are used against women. New York, Doubleday, 1991.
11. Greenberg J, Mitchell S: Object relations in psychoanalytic theory. Massachusetts, Howard Press, 1983.
12. Levine SB: Intrapsychic and individual aspects of sexual desire. *In* Leiblum SR, Rosen RC, eds: Sexual Desire Disorders. New York, Guilford Press, 1988; pp 42–43.
13. Kaplan HS: Disorders of sexual desire and other new concepts and techniques in sex therapy. New York, Brunner/Mazel, 1979.
14. Kaplan HS: The new sex therapy: Active treatment of sexual dysfunctions. New York, Brunner/Mazel, 1974.
15. Kitzinger S: Woman's experience of sex: The facts and feelings of female sexuality at every stage of life. New York, Penguin, 1983.
16. Michael R, Gagnon J, Laumann E, Kolata G: Sex in America: A Definitive Survey. Boston, Little, Brown, 1994.
17. Sarrel P, Sarrel L, Nadelson C: Dyspareunia and vaginismus. *In* Lief H, et al, eds: Treatments of Psychiatric Disorders. Washington, DC, American Psychiatric Association, 1989; pp 2291–2295.
18. Jones KD, Tyler-Lehr S: Vulvodynia: Diagnostic techniques and treatment modalities. Nurse Pract 1994; 19:34.
19. Stewart D, Reicher A, Gerulath A, Boydell K: Vulvodynia and psychological distress. Obstet Gynecol 1994; 84(4 part 1):587.
20. Lynch P: Vulvodynia: A syndrome of unexplained vulvar pain, psychologic disability and sexual dysfunction. J Reprod Med 1986; 31:773.
21. Scholl G: Prognostic variables in treatment of vaginismus. Obstet Gynecol 1988; 72:2.
22. Kaplan HS: Sexual Aversion, Sexual Phobias and Panic Disorder. New York, Brunner/Mazel, 1987.
23. Kope S: Treating vaginismus: If treatment is so simple why is the symptom so tenacious? Presentation, National Meeting of American Association of Sex Educators, Counselors and Therapists, Colorado, 1993.
24. Terr L: Too Scared to Cry: Psychic Trauma in Childhood. New York, Harper & Row, 1990.
25. Maltz W: The Sexual Healing Journey: A Guide for Survivors of Sexual Abuse. New York, Harper Collins, 1991.
26. Maltz W, Holman B: Incest and Sexuality: A Guide to Healing and Understanding. Lexington, MA, Lexington Books, 1992.

CHAPTER 18

Pregnancy Complications During the First Trimester

Deborah Hamby

Scott B. Ransom

S. Gene McNeeley, Jr.

Pregnancy complications are common in the first trimester. Although some complications that occur in the first trimester may not be serious, other conditions pose serious health risks to the mother and may cause loss of the pregnancy. This chapter reviews common complications of pregnancy that occur in the first trimester (Table 18–1).

SPONTANEOUS ABORTION (MISCARRIAGE)

Spontaneous abortion is the most common complication of the first trimester of pregnancy. Approximately 15% of fertilized ova are lost before implantation with the pregnancy not generally recognized clinically. An additional 15% of conceptions are lost before 8 weeks' gestation. Once a pregnancy achieves viability as evidence by cardiac motion, the likelihood of abortion is less than 5% after 8 weeks' gestation.

The most common symptoms seen with spontaneous abortion consist of cramping and vaginal bleeding. The degree of symptoms varies from mild cramping and minimal spotting to frank hemorrhage, with the duration of symptoms quite variable. In the woman with threatened abortion, the cervix appears normal with scant bloody discharge often present. Mild uterine tenderness may be present.

When the diagnosis of threatened abortion is made, patient reassurance and confirming the viability of the pregnancy via rising human chorionic gonadotropin (hCG) levels or pelvic ultrasound is indicated. The patient should be instructed in pelvic rest and avoid intercourse and tampons.

For patients who appear to have passed all tissue, observation is a viable option. For a woman with an incomplete abortion, suction dilation and curettage is indicated and may be performed under local anesthesia with intravenous sedation. Blood should be drawn to determine the patient's blood type and immune globulin administered as clinically indicated. It is commonplace for a short course of doxycycline prophylaxis to be administered; however, the efficacy of this practice has not been convincingly presented. Patients who experience miscarriage or who have undergone dilation and curettage should refrain from intercourse, douching, and tampons for 2 weeks after the procedure.

Table 18–1. Definitions of Early Complications in Pregnancy

Abortion	Termination of pregnancy before 20 weeks' gestation or the delivery of a fetus weighing <500 g
Complete	Spontaneous expulsion of all fetal and placental tissues before 20 weeks' gestation
Incomplete	Passage of some but not all of the products of conception
Inevitable	Uterine bleeding, rupture of membranes, and cervical dilation before 20 weeks' gestation
Missed	Fetal death before 20 weeks without expulsion of the products of conception
Threatened	Uterine bleeding without cervical effacement or dilation before 20 weeks' gestation
Hyperemesis gravidarum	Vomiting before 20 weeks' gestation associated with weight loss, dehydration, and electrolyte imbalance
Hydatidiform mole	Placental growth shown with trophoblastic hyperplasia, loss of fetal blood vessels, and swollen placental villi
Ectopic pregnancy	Pregnancy occurring outside the endometrial cavity

Conditions Associated with First-Trimester Abortion

The most common causes of first-trimester abortion are noted in Table 18–2. Approximately 50% of first-trimester abortuses and 20% of second-trimester abortuses contain chromosomal abnormalities. Autosomal trisomies are the most common chromosomal defects in spontaneous abortion and are associated

Table 18–2. Causes of Habitual Abortion

Chromosomal abnormalities
Collagen vascular disease
Diabetes
Luteal phase defect
Infection
Congenital anomalies of uterus

with increasing maternal age. Chromosomal rearrangements (i.e., translocations and mosaicisms) are also associated with spontaneous abortions. Most translocations in parents are balanced but may result in an unbalanced fetal karyotype and subsequent abortion.[11] Women with X chromosome mosaicism have a high incidence of abortion, probably secondary to fetal monosomy XO.

Collagen Vascular Disease

Autoimmune factors are an important cause of recurrent spontaneous abortion. Lupus anticoagulant and anticardiolipin are two antibodies targeted for negatively charged phospholipids. These may cause recurrent abortion by thrombosis or infarction within the placental bed. Women with recurrent spontaneous abortion (three or more) should be tested for lupus anticoagulant, anticardiolipin antibody, and antinuclear antibody. Women who test positive for antiphospholipid syndrome may have an improved pregnancy outcome if treated with (baby) aspirin and heparin (5000 units subcutaneously twice a day).[20]

Diabetes

Diabetes alone is rarely associated with an increased incidence of spontaneous abortion; however, poor glycemic control is associated with major congenital malformations. There may also be a glycemic threshold over which there is an increased incidence of spontaneous abortion at approximately 12% to 13% glycohemoglobin (at conception).[13] There may be a relationship between spontaneous abortion and duration of disease. In a study by Miodovnik and colleagues,[7] White's classification D patients had significantly higher abortion rates than class C (D = onset <10 years of age or duration >20 years; C = onset 10 to 20 years of age or duration 10 to 20 years).

Luteal Phase Defect

Luteal phase defect or inadequacy may be a cause for (recurrent) spontaneous abortion. This refers to an insufficient quantity of progesterone synthesis during the luteal phase of the menstrual cycle and a decreased secretion by the corpus luteum that helps maintain the gestation until 10 weeks.[2] A decrease in progesterone can cause a lag in the development of the endometrium in relationship to ovulation, rendering it inadequate for implantation or support of an early gestation.

Approximately 20% to 30% of normal cycles have a lag in endometrial development, and approximately 5% have repetitive lags in subsequent cycles. Whether this is clinically significant is unclear; however, luteal phase defect must lag 3 days behind, on two or more cycles. Luteal phase serum progesterone levels between 2 and 10 ng/mL and serum progesterone less than 15 ng/mL in the first 10 weeks of gestation is diagnostic for corpus luteal dysfunction.[3] A luteal phase defect should be suspected in those with recurrent spontaneous abortion, in those with infertility with normal cycles, and in those who reveal a short luteal phase on basal body temperature charts.

Treatment for luteal phase defect includes clomiphene citrate 50 mg for 5 days starting day 3, 4, or 5 of the menstrual cycle. Another option of treatment is progesterone vaginal suppositories 25 mg twice a day starting 3 days after ovulation and continuing until pregnancy is diagnosed for those with infertility. For those with recurrent spontaneous abortion and luteal phase defect or threatened abortion, progesterone vaginal suppositories until 10 weeks of gestation may be indicated.

Uterine Factors

Alterations in the anatomy of the uterus can be associated with pregnancy loss. These changes may cause crowding of the fetus, cause growth inhibition, and act as a foreign body, resulting in expulsion of the fetus. Uterine fibroids are a rare cause of infertility and occur in 30% of women with the highest incidence in the 40s. Subserosal myomas may distort the uterine cavity or cause crowding, and submucosal myomas may act as a foreign body preventing implantation of the fetus. Similarly, endometrial polyps within the uterine cavity may act as a foreign body, causing an inflammatory reaction preventing implantation of the gestation. Women with an abnormally shaped uterus, for instance, secondary to maternal exposure to diethylstilbestrol (DES), exhibit similar difficulties maintaining pregnancy. Diagnosis by hysterosalpingogram or laparoscopy and hysteroscopy may lead to surgical repair and subsequent successful pregnancy outcome.

Infection

Mycoplasma may play a role in the cause of habitual abortions. Colonization of the cervix is common and may represent normal vaginal flora; however, colonization of the endometrium is more frequent among habitual aborters and infertility patients.[14] Treatment consists of a course of doxycycline, erythromycin, or azithromycin.

Evaluation of Recurrent Abortion

Table 18–3 lists diagnostic studies for recurrent abortion. It is not generally necessary to investigate the cause of miscarriage unless the patient has had three consecutive abortions or if she is at high risk for one of the problems mentioned previously. As previously noted, spontaneous abortion is common, and by chance alone it is not unusual for a woman to have two consecutive spontaneous abortions with an 80% chance of subsequently having a normal pregnancy.

Table 18–3. Diagnostic Studies for Recurrent Abortion

Karyotype of husband and wife
Hysterosalpingogram
Antinuclear antibody
Anticardiolipin antibody
Thyroid-stimulating hormone
ABO, RH, and antibody screen
Rapid plasma reagin
Lupus anticoagulant

HYPEREMESIS GRAVIDARUM

Morning sickness is common in the first trimester of pregnancy and is characterized as mild nausea and vomiting. It occurs most frequently at 8 to 12 weeks' gestation and usually subsides near the end of the first trimester. It is usually felt to be a nuisance or an uncomfortable inconvenience of early pregnancy; however, it can become much more serious and interfere with food intake and hydration. Hyperemesis gravidarum is a condition characterized by vomiting that occurs for the first time before the 20th week of gestation associated with weight loss, dehydration, and electrolyte imbalances.[18]

Hyperemesis gravidarum affects approximately 0.5 to 10 per 1000 pregnancies with an unknown cause.[18] Some believe there is a relationship between hCG and hyperemesis gravidarum because the level of hCG is highest during those weeks in which hyperemesis occurs. Similarly, hCG is higher in twin gestations and molar pregnancies, as is the incidence of hyperemesis in these conditions. Nutritional factors may play a role in hyperemesis, especially a deficiency in vitamin B_6, although this mechanism is unclear. Psychological or social factors may play a role, such as a conflict with spouse or family regarding the pregnancy.

The diagnosis is made by history, physical examination, and laboratory findings. Women usually present in the first trimester with complaints of intractable nausea and vomiting. On physical examination, the patient may be orthostatic and dehydrated with an increased pulse, dry mucous membranes, and evidence of weight loss. Laboratory findings may include ketonuria and elevated hematocrit and blood urea nitrogen, owing to dehydration. Electrolyte abnormalities such as hyponatremia and hypokalemia are secondary to intractable emesis with metabolic alkalosis often present.

Treatment consists of correction of electrolyte imbalances and ketosis with intravenous hydration and electrolyte supplementation. The patient should not be fed until ketonuria has resolved. When attempting to start the patient on a diet, initially give sips of water, then work up to a dry diet consisting of such things as bread and crackers, then advance the diet as tolerated. Fatty or greasy foods should be avoided. Antiemetics may be indicated. Rarely the patient is not able to tolerate food and requires total parenteral nutrition. Because nutritional deficiencies may be severe, and thiamine deficiency can lead to Wernicke's encephalopathy, those with severe hyperemesis gravidarum should be given daily supplementation of thiamine 100 mg intravenously or intramuscularly. A psychological or social component to the illness should be investigated, and referral to a counselor may be indicated.

Pregnancy outcome is not threatened by hyperemesis gravidarum. On the contrary, studies indicate the risk of spontaneous abortion before 20 weeks is decreased if nausea and vomiting are present early in pregnancy.[18] Historically, hyperemesis gravidarum was a rare cause of maternal death because of hepatorenal failure. Total parenteral nutrition has significantly decreased the rate of maternal morbidity and mortality with occasional complications from line placement and line sepsis.

Hydatidiform Mole

A hydatidiform mole represents an abnormal pregnancy with the potential to become a serious illness for the patient. It is caused by abnormal fertilization at conception. There are two types, complete and incomplete or partial mole.

A complete mole is the result of fertilization of essentially an empty egg or one with no maternal genetic information. After fertilization, the chromosomes from the sperm duplicate, causing the genetic component of the complete mole to be 46XX completely paternal in origin. The complete mole is more common than an incomplete and has a greater risk of malignant transformation. Approximately 8% of patients with complete hydatidiform moles require subsequent chemotherapy for gestational trophoblastic tumor.[19] An incomplete or partial mole occurs after dispermic fertilization resulting in 69XXY.

Risk factors for molar pregnancy include increasing maternal age and low socioeconomic status; the latter may represent a nutritional component. Other risk factors include a history of prior hydatidiform mole, fetal wastage, and ABO blood group relationship in which maternal blood type is A and paternal is O.

Hydatidiform mole is frequently diagnosed in the first trimester of pregnancy. Patients occasionally complain of passing tissue that looks like grape clusters. Vaginal bleeding, as seen with threatened abortion, is a more common presenting complaint. Nausea and vomiting are common and may progress to hyperemesis. Occasionally, patients present with symptoms of hyperthyroidism or preeclampsia. On x-ray, the uterus may or may not be larger than expected for gestational age, and fetal heart tones are absent.

Ultrasound is an excellent tool for diagnosing hydatidiform mole. Usually, there is no fetus, and the tissue within the uterine cavity has a snowstorm-like appearance from the swollen villi. In the case of a partial mole, a gestational sac may be visualized but without an embryo or fetal heart tones. In a normal pregnancy, the concentration of hCG peaks at 10 to 14 weeks and usually does not exceed 100,000 mIU/mL. With a molar pregnancy, the hCG concentration in a molar pregnancy is usually greater than 100,000 mIU/mL and may exceed 1 million mIU/mL.[25,26] The hCG level of complete moles is usually higher than beta hCG than incomplete moles. A chest film should be obtained to evaluate for metastatic disease. Other helpful tests are noted in Table 18–4. The treatment of molar pregnancy is surgical removal by dilation and curettage. If the patient has clinical signs and symptoms of hyperthyroidism, she should be treated with β-blockers preoperatively to prevent thyroid storm.

The histopathology report must always be reviewed to determine the type of mole (i.e., complete or incomplete or a more serious condition, choriocarcinoma). Depending on the findings, the patient may require further surgical intervention or chemotherapy. These patients need to be followed carefully postoperatively to insure the quantitative beta hCG decreases and eventually disappears. Because a new subsequent pregnancy soon after dilation and curettage would mask persistent or recurrent trophoblastic disease, contraception is a must for at least 1 year.

Table 18–4. Preoperative Evaluation of Suspected Hydatidiform Mole

Hemoglobin
Type and screen
Chest film
Thyroid-stimulating hormone
Pelvic ultrasound

ECTOPIC PREGNANCY

Despite advances in the early diagnosis and improved methods for treating ectopic pregnancy, it still remains a common cause of maternal mortality. The incidence of ectopic pregnancy is approximately 16.1/1000, with the rate of ectopic pregnancy increased nearly fourfold over the last 20 years.[1]

Ectopic pregnancy is defined as a pregnancy occurring in some place other than the endometrial cavity. The most common site is in the ampullary portion of the fallopian tube with fimbrial, interstitial, cornual, abdominal, cervical, and ovarian locations following in occurrence. Anything that obstructs or delays the passage of the embryo can cause an ectopic pregnancy. Because tubal pregnancies are the most common type of ectopic pregnancy, the discussion is limited to them.

After release, the oocyte migrates into the fallopian tube through the fimbriated aspect and is fertilized. It is subsequently transported by peristaltic movements of the tube as well as by wavelike motions of the cilia lining the inner aspect of the tube. Along its path, the pregnancy continues to divide and grow. Tubal transport takes approximately 3 to 4 days, after which the embryo reaches the uterine cavity and undergoes implantation about 3 days later.

The most common contributing factor in ectopic pregnancy is a history of pelvic inflammatory disease. Approximately 1% of sexually active women develop pelvic inflammatory disease, and of those, 5% eventually experience an ectopic pregnancy.[1] Damage to the tubal architecture by inflammation during the infection and healing process increases the likelihood of an ectopic pregnancy. Such damage may include incomplete blockage of the tube so that sperm can pass through, but the blastocyst is too large and be-

Table 18–5. Causes of Ectopic Pregnancy

Pelvic inflammatory disease
Endometriosis
Prior ectopic pregnancy
Previous tubal ligation
Infertility
Congenital anomalies
Diethylstilbestrol exposure
Cigarette smoking
Intrauterine device
Progesterone-based contraception

comes trapped in the tube. Inflammation may damage the cilia impairing peristalsis so that the blastocyst is not effectively transported. Risk factors are noted in Table 18–5.

Diagnosis and Treatment

A woman with an ectopic pregnancy usually presents with amenorrhea followed by abnormal bleeding (Table 18–6). Pain, if present, is described as "soreness" and "colicky" and may be unilateral or bilateral. Other symptoms of pregnancy are common, including breast tenderness and nausea. With a more advanced gestation, bleeding and cramping may increase, and passage of tissue (a decidual cast) may be mistaken for placental and fetal tissue. In the case of rupture with hemoperitoneum, orthostatic symptoms and shoulder pain are common because of acute hemorrhage into the abdominal cavity. A complete history and physical examination should be performed with careful attention paid to vital signs and orthostatic tendencies. Abdominal examination may vary from minimal tenderness to rebound depending on the clinical circumstances. Adnexal tenderness, unilateral or bilateral, is frequently present. An adnexal mass is palpable in approximately 50% of women. Laboratory tests include a quantitative beta hCG, complete blood count with platelets, and type and screen. The concentration of beta hCG can vary and does not necessarily correlate with the gestational age. With a normal intrauterine pregnancy, one sees doubling of the beta hCG level approximately every 48 hours.

Figure 18–1 shows common sites for ectopic pregnancy. Pelvic ultrasound is essential if one is to diagnose an ectopic pregnancy before rupture. In general, a gestational sac is seen on transabdominal ultrasound if the quantitative beta hCG exceeds 6000 mIU/mL. An intrauterine pregnancy should be seen on transvaginal ultrasound with the beta hCG greater than 1500 mIU/mL.[21] In early pregnancy, before the hCG reaches 1500 mIU/mL, one must repeat the hCG at regular intervals to insure an appropriate rise. Reasons for the abnormal rise in the beta hCG include ectopic pregnancy, intrauterine fetal demise, and incomplete abortion.

Culdocentesis may be helpful in determining if hemoperitoneum is suspected. Under sterile conditions with the patient in dorsal lithotomy position, an 18-gauge spinal needle is inserted into the posterior cul-de-sac and fluid or blood withdrawn. Nonclotting blood indicates fibrinolysis, which suggests intraperitoneal bleeding associated with ectopic pregnancy whereby surgical therapy should not be delayed. The clinician must keep in mind that a ruptured corpus luteum cyst in early pregnancy can produce similar findings.

Table 18–6. Symptoms of Ectopic Pregnancy

Amenorrhea
Irregular vaginal bleeding
Pelvic pain
Nausea/vomiting
Breast tenderness
Passage of decidual cast
Fainting
Dizziness
Urge to defecate

Medical Management

Until the late 1980s, the management of ectopic pregnancy was exclusively surgical. In selected patients, medical treatment with methotrexate has been shown to be an equally effective treatment. General guidelines for using medical management include unruptured ectopic tubal pregnancy, ectopic size less than 3.5 cm, and absence of fetal cardiac activity on ultrasound. A history of hepatic, renal, or

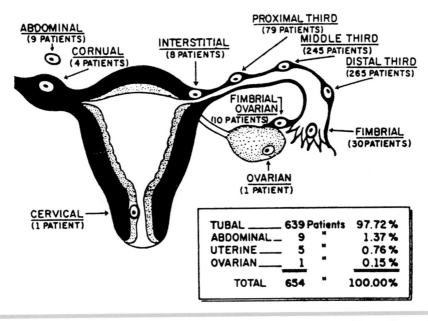

Figure 18–1. Incidence of ectopic pregnancy by anatomic site. (From Breen JL: A 21-year study of 654 ectopic pregnancies. Am J Obstet Gynecol 1970; 106: 1004.)

peptic ulcer disease precludes medical management. A single intramuscular dose of methotrexate (50 mg/m^2) is administered for medical treatment.[22] The quantitative hCG should be repeated in 7 and 14 days with 50% decline in the hCG expected in 2 weeks. It is common for mild abdominal or pelvic discomfort to occur 3 to 5 days after the administration of methotrexate. This is likely due to the beginning of placental separation from the tubal mucosa. Women who do not have a permanent address and those who do not have a telephone or immediate access to health care are not candidates for methotrexate treatment. Women with interstitial, cornual, and cervical pregnancies are not candidates for single-dose methotrexate treatment. Single-dose methotrexate has been shown to be 70% to 90% effective in treating ectopic pregnancy.[23] In addition to avoiding the morbidity associated with surgery, Stovall and colleagues[23] suggest improved reproductive potential in women treated medically when compared to those treated surgically.

Surgical Management

Not all patients with hemoperitoneum require a laparotomy. Laparoscopy is the surgery of choice in patients who are hemodynamically stable. Removal of the gestation may be completed in several ways, including salpingotomy, salpingostomy, and salpingectomy. Salpingotomy is an incision made on the tube with the pregnancy removed and the tube closed, whereas the incision in a salpingostomy is not closed. It is believed that closure of the tissue may result in more tissue destruction and scarring with an increased risk of future ectopic pregnancy; therefore, salpingostomy is the procedure of choice.[24] Salpingectomy may be completed if the tube is severely damaged or if hemostasis is unobtainable. In the authors' experience, surgery is generally completed on an outpatient basis with the woman being discharged home from the recovery room. Laparotomy is reserved for unstable patients with hemoperitoneum or with conditions in which laparoscopy is not practical.

Patients undergoing salpingostomy require postoperative follow-up similar to those receiving methotrexate. Beta hCG levels are determined weekly until negative. As with other pregnancy complications, immune globulin should be administered as indicated. Long-term sequelae resulting from ectopic pregnancy include infertility in 50% and recurrence rate for ectopic pregnancy approaching 20%. It is important to counsel patients with ectopic pregnancy to obtain early prenatal care in the future to confirm an intra-uterine pregnancy.

REFERENCES

1. Leach RE, Montgomery-Rice V: New options for the diagnosis and treatment of ectopic pregnancy. Female Patient 1993; 18:31.
2. Wintz C: Endocrine aspects of recurrent early fetal wastage: The role of luteal phase inadequacy. Eur Fertil 1992; 23:263.
3. Hensleigh PA, Fainstat T: Corpus luteum dysfunction: Serum progesterone levels in diagnosis and assessment of therapy for recurrent and threatened abortion. Fertil Steril 1979; 32:396.
4. Harder JH, Archer DF, Marches SG, et al: Etiology of recurrent pregnancy losses and outcome of subsequent pregnancies. Obstet Gynecol 1983; 63:574.
5. Jones HW Jr: Uterine factors in repeated miscarriage. Eur Fertil 1992; 23:271.
6. Cowchock S, Dehoratius RD, Warner RJ, Jackson LG: Subclinical autoimmune diseases and unexplained abortion. Am J Obstet Gynecol 1984; 150:367.
7. Miodovnik M, Lavin JP, Knowles HC, et al: Spontaneous abortion among insulin-dependent diabetic women. Am J Obstet Gynecol 1984; 150:372.
8. Kimball AC, Kean BH, Fuchs F: The role of toxoplasmosis in abortion. Am J Obstet Gynecol 1971; 111:219.
9. Popp LW, Colditz A, Gaetje R: Management of early ectopic pregnancy. Int J Gynecol Obstet 1994; 44:239.
10. Van Leeuwen I, Branch WD, Scott JR: First trimester ultrasonography findings in women with a history of recurrent pregnancy loss. Am J Obstet Gynecol 1993; 168:111.
11. Sachs ES, Jahoda MG, VanHemel JO, et al: Chromosome studies of 500 couples with two or more abortions. Obstet Gynecol 1985; 65:375.
12. Kalter H: Diabetes and spontaneous abortion: A historical review. Am J Obstet Gynecol 1987; 156:1243.
13. Rosenn B, Miodovnik M, Combs AC, et al: Glycemic thresholds for spontaneous abortion and congenital malformations in insulin-dependent diabetes mellitus. Obstet Gynecol 1994; 84:515.
14. Stray-Pedersen B, Eng J, Reikvam T, Mannsaker : Uterine T-mycoplasma colonization in reproductive failure. Am J Obstet Gynecol 1978; 130:307.
15. Harger JH, Rabin BS, Marchese SG: The prognostic value of antinuclear antibodies in women with recurrent pregnancy losses: A prospective controlled study. Obstet Gynecol 1989; 73:419.
16. Poland BJ, Miller JR, Jones DC, Trimble BK: Reproductive counseling in patients who have had a spontaneous abortion. Am J Obstet Gynecol 1977; 127:685.
17. March CM, Israes R: Hysteroscopic management of recurrent abortion caused by septate uterus. Am J Obstet Gynecol 1987; 156:834.
18. Hod M, Orvieto R, Kaplan B, et al: Hyperemesis gravidarum: A review. J Reprod Med 1994; 39:605.
19. Fesheer RA, Newlands ES: Rapid diagnoses and classification of hydatidiform moles with polymerase chain reaction. Am J Obstet Gynecol 1993; 168:563.
20. Carp H: Discussion. In Beard RW, Sharp F, eds: Early Pregnancy Loss: Mechanisms and Treatment. Ashton-under-Lyne, England, Peacock Press, 1988, pp 403–406.
21. Nyberg DA, Mack LA, Laing FC, Jeffrey RB: Early pregnancy complications: Endovaginal sonographic findings correlated with human chorionic gonadotropin levels. Radiology 1988; 167:619.
22. Tanaka T, Hyashi H, Kutsuzawa T, et al: Treatment of interstitial ectopic pregnancy with methotrexate: Report of a successful case. Fertil Steril 1982; 37:851.
23. Stovall TG, Ling FW, Buster JE: Reproductive performance after methotrexate treatment of ectopic pregnancy. Am J Obstet Gynecol 1990; 162:1620.
24. Shapiro BS, Cullen M, Taylor KJW, De Cherney AH: Transvaginal ultrasonography for the diagnosis of ectopic pregnancy. Fertil Steril 1988; 50:425.
25. Romero R, Horgan JC, Korhorn KL, et al: New criteria for the diagnosis of gestational trophoblastic disease. Obstet Gynecol 1985; 66:553.
26. Kosasa TS: Measurement of human chorionic gonadotropin. In Goldstein DP, Berkowitz RS, eds: Gestational Trophoblastic Neoplasms: Clinical Principles of Diagnosis and Management. Philadelphia, WB Saunders, 1982.

CHAPTER 19

Pediatric and Adolescent Gynecology

David Muram

Most physicians are aware of the various gynecologic disorders that may affect female infants, children, and adolescents and incorporate a limited gynecologic evaluation into the well-child examination. Such an approach permits an early detection of infections, labial adhesions, congenital anomalies, and even genital tumors.

The reproductive tract in children differs in structure and in function from the genital organs of women, and the physician caring for young patients should be familiar with these differences. Moreover, the anatomic differences require the use of specially designed equipment (e.g., vaginoscope, virginal vaginal specula) if the examination is to be completed without causing undue discomfort and subsequent anxiety about future examinations. This chapter reviews some of the common gynecologic disorders that the primary care provider may encounter in the pediatric and adolescent age group.

GYNECOLOGIC EVALUATION OF THE NEWBORN

Immediately following birth and during the first few weeks of life, the female newborn responds to maternal estrogens. The effects of such stimulation may be seen for perhaps 6 weeks and sometimes even longer. The most obvious sign, breast budding, occurs in nearly all children born at term. Sometimes the breast enlargement is marked and may be accompanied by a discharge from the nipples. This breast enlargement requires no treatment, and repeated examinations may lead to bruising of the breast tissue or an infection.

During the first few weeks of life, the female newborn is affected by estrogens transferred across the placenta. The vagina at birth is about 4 cm long. The uterus is enlarged, measures 4 cm in length, and has no axial flexion; the ratio between cervix and corpus is 3:1. The external genitalia are affected as well: The labia majora are bulbous; the labia minora are thick and protruding. The clitoris in the newborn appears relatively large. Vaginal discharge is frequently seen (Fig. 19–1). The ovaries, which arise from the T_{-10} level, are abdominal organs in early childhood and are not palpable on pelvic or rectal examination.

EXAMINATION OF THE YOUNG CHILD

The genital tract receives little estrogen stimulation during early childhood. The

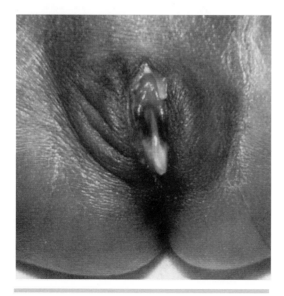

Figure 19–1. The external genitalia of a newborn female. Note the hypertrophy and turgor of the vulvar tissue. Note the large amount of vaginal secretions.

labia majora are flat, and the labia minora and hymen are extremely thin (Fig. 19–2). The clitoris is relatively small. The vagina is slightly longer than in the female newborn (5 cm in length). The mu-

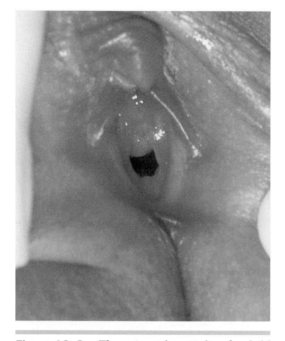

Figure 19–2. The external genitalia of a child 3 years of age.

cosa is thin and atrophic and offers little resistance to trauma and infections. The vagina has neutral or slightly alkaline secretions and is colonized with mixed bacterial flora.[1] The unstimulated uterus is small, and the cervix is flush with the vaginal vault.

Between the ages of 8 and 10 years, the external genitalia show some signs of estrogen stimulation: The mons pubis thickens, the labia majora fill out, the labia minora are rounded, and the hymen becomes thicker. The vagina elongates to 8 cm in length, and the mucosa becomes thicker. The maturation index shows mainly parabasal cells but also intermediate cells and occasionally superficial cells. The cervix is still flush with the vaginal vault. The corpus uteri grows, altering the cervix-to-corpus ratio to 1:1.

Young children are sensitive to the physician's attitude. They react positively to someone who is kind, warm, and patient. These young patients must be assured that the examination, although perhaps uncomfortable or embarrassing, will not be painful. The mother, who often accompanies the girl to the examination room, may be helpful during the examination as she provides comfort and a sense of security. Young children (≤5 years) may become apprehensive when placed on the examination table, and placing them on the mother's lap may reduce their anxiety. The mother is asked to support the child's legs, permitting an unimpaired view of the genital area (Fig. 19–3). Older children are asked to lie on the examination table, but the use of stirrups is generally not necessary. The patient is asked to flex her knees, abduct her legs, and support them by placing her hands on the dorsal aspects of the lower thighs. Asking for the child's help is of definite value because her involvement provides a sense of control over the examination and lessens the apprehension.

The examination begins with an evaluation of the child's general appearance, nutritional status, body habitus, and gross congenital anomalies. The child's breasts should be inspected and palpated. The breasts usually do not begin budding until age 8 to 9 years. At the onset of breast growth, the examiner may feel a small, firm, flat button beneath the nipple. Prominence of the nipple and

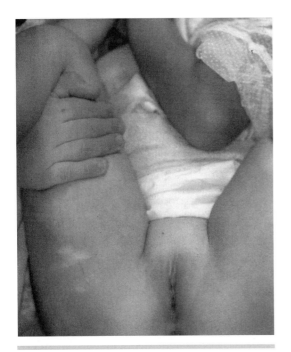

Figure 19–3. The examination of a young girl while being seated on mother's lap. The mother supports the child's legs, thereby providing an excellent view of the genital area.

breast development at an earlier age may be the first sign of sexual precocity.

The ovaries of a premenarchal child are situated high in the pelvis, and ovarian neoplasms grow toward the midabdomen. Light palpation of the abdominal wall elicits the needed information.

The examiner exposes the vulva and vestibule by exerting light lateral and downward pressure on each side of the perineum. Signs of hormonal stimulation in early childhood or their absence when they should be evident may indicate abnormal pubertal development. Enlargement of the clitoris may indicate increased androgenic stimulation and virilization. The examiner should look for skin lesions, vaginal discharge, perineal excoriations, ulcers, and tumors. In addition, the patency of the hymenal orifice should be confirmed.

It is impossible to perform a digital vaginal examination in a child if the size of the hymenal opening is normal for age. Gentle rectal digital examination, however, can be easily accomplished and should not cause pain. Nonetheless, accurate intrapelvic evaluation is often difficult because of the relatively small size

of the uterus, the size and location of the ovaries, and the firmness of the abdominal wall. If the presence of a pelvic tumor is strongly suspected, other diagnostic procedures, such as sonography, magnetic resonance imaging (MRI) or computed tomography (CT), should be performed, regardless of the rectoabdominal examination findings.

When the child is very apprehensive, sedation may be helpful. This can be achieved by using a standard pediatric cocktail such as a combination of meperidine (Demerol) 50 mg/mL, chlorpromazine (Thorazine) 12.5 mg/0.5 mL, and promethazine (Phenergan) 12.5 mg/0.5 mL. The usual dose is 1 mL for every 20 pounds (9 kg) of body weight, with a maximum 2-mL dose.

When the child is extremely apprehensive or if the child is evaluated for an acute injury, it is advisable to examine her under general anesthesia. Forceful examination is not justified. Not only is it psychologically traumatic, but also the child may be injured by the instruments as she struggles to free herself. Most children, however, can be examined without resorting to general anesthesia.

Vaginoscopy

Vaginal instrumentation is not a routine part of the gynecologic examination of young patients. It is required in some to evaluate the upper vagina, to observe and remove foreign bodies, or to assess vaginal trauma following penetrating injuries. Many instruments have been used to separate the vaginal walls: nasal specula, otoscopes, vaginoscopes, and flexible urethroscopes. If the examination is to be performed in an office setting, the patient must be relaxed and cooperative. Lidocaine (Xylocaine) jelly is placed at the vaginal introitus and on the instrument.

Before insertion, the physician shows the instrument to the girl. The child should touch the lubricated instrument, and it is pointed out to her that it feels strange, slippery, and cool. Then the instrument is placed against the inner thigh and she is reminded that it feels cool, slippery, and unusual. Only then is the instrument passed through the hymenal orifice.[2]

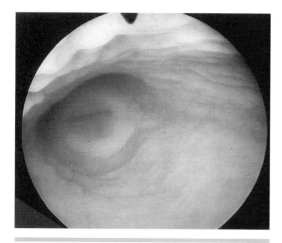

Figure 19–4. Vaginoscopy of a 2-year-old child using a water cystoscope. The vagina is distended, and the examiner has a clear panoramic view of the entire vagina and cervix.

If the aperture is too small for an instrument to be passed without discomfort or if the child is uncooperative, vaginoscopy should not be attempted without general anesthesia. Persistent manipulation of the sensitive tissues without anesthesia is traumatic and counterproductive. If the examination is performed under general anesthesia, the author uses a water cystoscope. The labia minora are compressed together to retain the water in the vagina, distend the vaginal walls, and provide a panoramic view.[2] At the same time, the water irrigates secretions, blood, and debris, which may conceal a lesion (Fig. 19–4).

EXAMINATION OF THE ADOLESCENT PATIENT

During puberty (ages 10 to 13), the vagina reaches its adult length (10 to 12 cm). It is more distensible, and the mucosa becomes thick and moist. The vaginal secretions are acidic, and lactobacilli are present. The differential growth of the uterine corpus and cervix is pronounced. The corpus is twice as large as the cervix. The cervix is clearly separated from the vaginal vault by the vaginal fornices. The ovaries descend into the true pelvis, and the external genitalia achieve adult appearance. Secondary sex characteristics develop rapidly during the late childhood period. The body habitus becomes rounded, especially in the shoulders and hips. Accelerated somatic growth (adolescent growth spurt) occurs, followed by breast development and sexual hair growth.

The adolescent's first trip to the gynecologist is often fraught with fear and apprehension. Girlfriends may have told her harrowing stories they have heard about vaginal examinations. Therefore, time spent in putting the patient at ease and winning her confidence saves time and frustration in the examining room. One must impress on the adolescent that she, not her mother, is the patient. The girl, not her mother, is asked for the pertinent medical information required for the medical record. Questions about sexual behavior and venereal diseases require a delicate approach, and, obviously, such questions should not be asked with the mother present. After the history taking, the girl is given a brief description of what the examination entails. She and her mother may need to be assured that her hymen will not be injured and that the examination, although perhaps uncomfortable or embarrassing to her, will not be painful.

The examination is performed in the presence of a female assistant who must constantly reassure the young patient. Examination of the breasts is an integral part of the physical examination of every female patient. In addition, instructions on breast self-examination and education pamphlets should be given at this time. Explanations of what is being done are given throughout the genital examination, and the physician may offer the patient a direct view of her own genitalia using a mirror or a videocolposcope.[3]

After an inspection of the external genitalia, a speculum is inserted into the vagina. The hymenal orifice of most virginal adolescents is about 1.0 cm in diameter and admits a narrow speculum without difficulty. The long-bladed Huffman-Graves speculum is specifically designed to reach the cervix and is preferable to the short-bladed pediatric speculum. In a patient with a large hymenal opening, bimanual examination is done by inserting a finger into the vagina. Those who have a hymenal orifice too small for digital examination should undergo a rectoabdominal examination.

Following the examination, the girl is given an opportunity to talk privately with the examiner. This is a prime opportunity to form a secure patient-physician relationship. The adolescent should be assured that she may discuss intimate issues and that her confidence will be respected. The examination and findings are discussed with the parent(s) only after the physician and the patient have completed their discussion and have agreed on what should be held in confidence. Under no circumstances should the physician violate the patient's request for privacy. If the physician believes the parents should be aware of certain details, the patient must be so advised and persuaded that for her own benefit this information should be released to the parents.

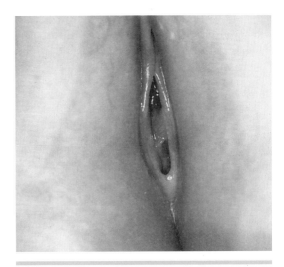

Figure 19–5. The genitalia of a 5-year-old girl with vulvovaginitis. The inflammation extends laterally from the vestibule to the thighs and posteriorly to the anus.

COMMON DISORDERS IN THE PREMENARCHEAL CHILD

Vulvovaginitis

Vulvovaginitis is the most common gynecologic disorder in children.[4] In young children, perineal hygiene is often less than adequate, and contamination by stool and other debris is common. The vaginal mucosa is thin and atrophic because of the lack of estrogen and is therefore less resistant to infectious organisms.[5]

Vulvovaginitis can be divided into three major etiologic groups:

1. *Nonspecific vulvovaginitis:* a polymicrobial infection associated with disturbed local homeostasis (caused by contamination, e.g., poor perineal hygiene, foreign body).
2. *Secondary inoculation:* denotes infections with a specific organism that causes a primary infection elsewhere (i.e., pharyngitis, strep throat). Infection of the vagina occurs following bacteremia or inoculation with the patient's hands.
3. *Specific infections:* specific primary vaginal infection, most commonly sexually transmitted (e.g., gonorrhea).

The symptoms of vulvovaginitis vary from minor discomfort to relatively intense perineal pruritus, a sensation of burning, and a foul-smelling discharge. Vaginal discharge may vary from minimal to copious. The irritating discharge inflames the vulva and may cause the child to scratch the area to the point of bleeding. Acute vulvovaginitis may denude the thin vulvar or vaginal mucosa, but bleeding is usually minimal, merely staining the vaginal secretions. Inspection of the vagina usually reveals an area of redness and soreness, which may be minimal or may extend laterally to the thighs and posteriorly to the anus (Fig. 19–5).

Evaluation of the secretions should include:

1. Smears for Gram stain.
2. Bacterial cultures and, in selected patients, cultures for mycotic organisms.
3. Wet preparation for:
   a. Mycotic organisms (potassium hydroxide [KOH] preparation).
   b. White and red blood cells.
   c. Vaginal epithelial cells (determining estrogen effect).
   d. Trichomonas.
   e. Parasitic ova.

In children in whom an infection is documented for the first time, vaginoscopy can be delayed. Vaginoscopy is indicated in children with recurrent vaginal infections, when the infection is refractory to treatment, or if the child has a foul-smelling or bloody discharge. A thorough vaginal inspection is necessary to exclude the presence of foreign bodies or neoplasms.

For all girls with vaginitis, regardless of the cause of the infection, the physician should pay close attention to vulvar hygiene and provide proper instructions to both mother and child. These instructions should include the use of sitz baths and anal wiping from front to back.[4] In patients with nonspecific vaginitis, these conservative measures are the treatment of choice, and the symptoms resolve within a few days in the majority of patients. In rare instances, allergic reactions to creams or chemical agents (e.g., harsh soaps) have been documented. In these cases, discontinuation of contact with the allergens alleviates the symptoms and prevents recurrences.

Before the initiation of antibiotic therapy for vulvovaginitis, the physician should determine the exact cause. If a specific organism is isolated, it should be treated with an appropriate antibiotic agent to which the organism is sensitive. Occasionally, when the patient suffers from an intense inflammatory reaction, the physician may choose to treat the patient empirically, using a broad-spectrum antibiotic agent (e.g., ampicillin 50 to 100mg/kg/day), while awaiting the results of the bacteriologic studies. A change in the antibiotic regimen may be required if the isolated organism is resistant.

In children with severe vulvovaginitis, denudation of the vaginal mucosa may occur. For these patients, a short course of topical estrogen promotes healing of vulvar and vaginal tissues. A small quantity of conjugated estrogen (Premarin) vaginal cream is applied twice daily for 5 to 7 days. Hydrocortisone cream may be necessary in patients complaining of intense pruritus to alleviate the itch. This may be given as triamcinolone 0.025% or hydrocortisone cream 1% applied to the affected area twice daily for 5 to 7 days.

Enterobiasis

Enterobiasis or pinworm infection affects individuals of all ages but is especially common in children. It affects mainly children 5 to 14 years of age. The child is infected following the ingestion of embryonated eggs, which are usually carried on fingernails, clothing, bedding, or house dust. In the stomach, the eggs hatch, and larvae migrate to the cecal region where they mature into adult worms. *Enterobius vermicularis* are small (1 cm) white worms; the gravid females migrate by night to the perianal region to deposit masses of eggs.

There are no specific syndromes caused by *E. vermicularis*. Symptomatic individuals most commonly complain of nocturnal anal pruritus and sleeplessness. Because tissue invasion does not occur in most cases of enterobiasis, diagnosis is established by either finding the parasite eggs or examining recovered worms. Eggs can easily be detected on adhesive cellophane tape after it is pressed against the perianal region early in the morning.

Drug therapy should be given to all infected and symptomatic individuals; mebendazole (single oral dose of 100 mg) is recommended. Piperazine salts or pyrvinium pamoate may also be used. Although personal cleanliness is a useful general recommendation, there is no proof that it plays a significant role in control of enterobiasis.

Sexually Transmitted Diseases in Children

The diagnosis of a sexually transmitted disease (STD) is fortunately a rare occurrence in childhood. Most survey studies estimate the incidence of STDs in children to be 1% to 5%. This section provides the clinician with a brief overview of the clinical presentation, the choice of appropriate diagnostic tests, and the treatment options.

Gonorrhea

Beyond the neonatal period, sexual contact is nearly the exclusive cause of gonococcal infections in children.[6–9] There is only one documented case of a fomite transmission of *Neisseria gonorrhoeae* to a child.[10] The most commonly infected sites are the vagina, rectum, pharynx, and conjunctiva. The vaginal epithelium of the prepubertal child may be infected if exposed to the organism. The absence of endocervical glands on the ectocervix of the prepubertal child makes the cervix more resistant to infection, and ascending genital tract infection with *N. gonorrhoeae* is rare in prepubertal children.

The symptoms appear 2 to 7 days after the inoculation. Some children may have asymptomatic colonization with *N. gonorrhoeae*,[11,12] but most girls present with vulvovaginitis accompanied by erythema, purulent vaginal discharge, and pruritus. Dysuria may result from the vulvitis or from urethritis.[13] If untreated, the purulent vaginal discharge is replaced by a serous discharge, which may persist for several months. Although pharyngitis and proctitis have been reported, most of these children are asymptomatic.[14]

Selective cultures are required to establish the diagnosis of *N. gonorrhoeae*. If a nonselective medium is used, confirmation of *N. gonorrhoeae* is necessary, using methods such as carbohydrate degradation, enzyme substrate, or immunologic testing. It is also recommended that isolates obtained from children be stored at $-70°C$ for additional confirmatory testing, should this be needed at a later date.[15]

The use of indirect testing methods for *N. gonorrhoeae* is not recommended in children; both false-positive and false-negative tests have been reported with monoclonal antibody and direct fluorescent antibody testing methods before adolescence.[15,16] DNA probes for *N. gonorrhoeae* may prove useful once clinical trials in children are completed.

The Centers for Disease Control (CDC) recommends the use of ceftriaxone in children with gonococcal infections. Children with an uncomplicated infection (vulvovaginitis, urethritis, pharyngitis, or proctitis) may be treated with a single, 125-mg intramuscular dose of ceftriaxone. Spectinomycin 40 mg/kg may be used intramuscularly in children who cannot tolerate ceftriaxone. Because of the relatively high association of infection with *N. gonorrhoeae* and *Chlamydia trachomatis* in children, coverage for *C. trachomatis* should be included in treatment for children with gonococcal infection if chlamydial cultures are not available. Because of the high prevalence of a concurrent infection with *C. trachomatis*

(27%), it is recommended that children older than 8 years of age also receive a 7-day course of doxycycline (4 mg/kg/day). Children with complicated gonococcal infections (conjunctivitis, peritonitis, arthritis, or meningitis) should be given a more prolonged course of parenteral ceftriaxone. Follow-up cultures after treatment are important to document cure. Prophylactic treatment for gonococcal infection in asymptomatic children being evaluated for possible sexual abuse is not recommended.[17]

Chlamydia trachomatis

The primary modes of transmission of *C. trachomatis* involve direct contact, rather than fomite transmission. Concomitant infection with *C. trachomatis* and *N. gonorrhoeae* is fairly common (27%).[18] At birth, the neonate may be inoculated by contact with infected secretions. Vertical transmission at the time of cesarean section performed after the rupture of membranes has also been reported.[19-24]

Perinatal exposure may also result in colonization of the vagina and rectum.[25] Longitudinal studies of infants exposed to *C. trachomatis* at birth have shown carriage of the organism up to 55 weeks in the rectum and 53 weeks in the vagina.[26] A more recent study has demonstrated rectal colonization up to 2 years of age after perinatal exposure.[27] In these studies, the vast majority of the infants were asymptomatic.

Infection of the genital tract is the most common presentation in children beyond infancy.[22,28] The *atrophic,* unestrogenized vaginal epithelium may be directly infected with the organism, causing a true vaginitis. Asymptomatic colonization of the genital tract, however, may occur in up to 60% of children.[1,24] The children usually present with vaginitis, urethritis, or pyuria. Vulvar erythema, vaginal discharge, rectal pain, and vaginal bleeding are common complaints.

Cell culture, using a monolayer of susceptible cells (e.g., McCoy cells), is regarded as the optimal method. Because this organism is intracellular, it is important to obtain epithelial cells for the culture, rather than simply culturing any discharge that is present.[26] In prepubertal children, a careful vaginal or urethral culture is necessary. Use of an adequate growth or transport medium is also important. Urethral swabs of calcium alginate are often useful in obtaining cultures from children because of their small diameter. When the cultures grow *C. trachomatis,* freezing of the organism at −70°C is suggested for future forensic confirmation.

Antigen detection testing (e.g., Micro-Trak, Chlamydiazyme) has become increasingly popular in response to the expense and limited availability of cell cultures for *C. trachomatis.* The CDC recommends against the use of these testing methods in prepubertal children. The low prevalence of *C. trachomatis* infection in sexually abused children and the need to test anatomic sites other than the cervix and urethra contribute to unacceptable sensitivity and specificity rates. Up to 50% false-positive and false-negative rates have been reported with the use of antigen detection methods in children.[29]

Erythromycin (30 to 50 mg/kg/day) is the treatment of choice for genital chlamydial infections in children 8 years and younger. Doxycycline (200 mg/day) is recommended for children older than 8. *C. trachomatis* is also suspectible to sulfonamides and trimethoprim; however, this antibiotic has not been widely used because of its lack of activity against other STDs. Prophylactic treatment for *C. trachomatis* in children is not indicated. The low prevalence and the minimal risk for upper genital tract disease allows the practitioner to await culture results before instituting treatment.

Syphilis

Syphilis in a child beyond the neonatal period is usually acquired through sexual contact. Transmission during transfusion of blood, by contact with syphilitic lesions on the breast of a nursing mother, and by *nonsexual* kissing have all been described; however, these forms of transmission are rare.[30,31]

Primary syphilis has a similar presentation in the pediatric and adult population, generally appearing as a painless genital chancre at an average of 21 days after exposure. Primary lesions may also present in the oral cavity and perianal area. The clinician should obtain a dark-field examination for diagnosis.[32] Secondary syphilis often presents as a skin rash within 1 to several months after exposure. A relatively high index of suspicion is necessary to identify the infrequent condition of secondary syphilis in the pediatric population.[33]

The CDC currently recommends that cerebrospinal fluid samples be obtained to rule out congenital syphilis. Any child with congenital syphilis or evidence of neurologic involvement should be treated with aqueous crystalline penicillin G (200,000 to 300,000 units/kg/day) for 10 to 14 days. When congenital syphilis and neurosyphilis are ruled out, infected children should be treated with 50,000 units/kg of intramuscular benzathine penicillin, not to exceed the dose of 2.4 million units administered to adults.[17]

Genital Herpes

Herpes simplex virus (HSV) is transmitted by close contact with an individual who is shedding the virus. The virus enters the mucosal surfaces through an epithelial break.[34] Transmission by sexual contact is the most common source of childhood genital herpes.[35–39] Auto-inoculation from nongenital lesions has been documented as a source of genital herpes during childhood,[40] but casual transmission and fomite transmission have not been documented.[41] Genital herpes lesions, caused by both HSV 1 and 2, have been reported in children. The clinical presentation of primary genital herpes is similar to that described in adults. Painful vesicular lesions develop after an incubation period of 2 to 20 days.[42] These lesions are often accompanied by systemic symptoms: inguinal adenopathy, fever, malaise, nausea, and headache. The lesions later ulcerate and may become secondarily infected. Urinary retention may develop. Lesions caused by HSV 1 and 2 may be clinically indistinguishable, but HSV 2 is four times more likely to cause recurrent genital herpes. Secondary lesions are generally less severe, with less viral shedding and no systemic symptoms.[42]

The use of antigen detection testing has not been evaluated in children and therefore is not recommended. The diagnosis of genital herpes is established when the virus is isolated from suspicious lesions. False-negative cultures may occur if specimens are obtained from lesions with decreased viral shedding, such as recurrent lesions or those that are ulcerated or crusted.[42] False-positive cultures, however, may occur in children with herpes zoster because of the similar cytopathic effects of herpes simplex and herpes zoster in cell culture. Therefore, positive herpes cultures in children should be subjected to confirmatory testing.[15]

There are no treatment guidelines for children with genital herpes infection. Acyclovir has been demonstrated in adults to be effective for the treatment of primary herpes and suppressive treatment of secondary lesions.[34] Because the therapeutic safety of acyclovir during childhood has been demonstrated with neonatal herpes simplex and childhood herpes zoster, some clinicians treat children with genital herpes. Others prefer to use symptomatic treatment of the genital lesions with local care: sitz baths, topical anesthetics, and drying agents.[34,42,43]

Condyloma Acuminatum

A dramatic increase has occurred in the number of clinical cases of human papillomavirus (HPV).[44] Vertical transmission at birth, casual transmission, and sexual transmission have all been implicated as possible means of infection in children with HPV. The majority of presumed perinatally transmitted HPV cases have been reported in children less than 2 years of age,[45,46] in keeping with data suggesting an incubation period of up to 20 months in children.[47] Sexual transmission is likely to occur in older children. In series excluding children under 2, sexual transmission was documented in as many as 90% of these children.[48]

Prepubertal children are more likely to present with periurethral and perianal condylomata.[47,49,50] Studies examining the upper genital tract of prepubertal girls for the presence of HPV lesions have shown this to be unusual. HPV lesions, however, are often present in the anal canal.

Anogenital condylomata in children generally present as flesh-colored verrucous growths. These lesions are often asymptomatic and are noted by the caretaker during diaper changes or bathing. The condylomata in diaper-age children appear as pink or red fleshy growths, often with marked vascularity (Fig. 19–6). The friable and vascular nature of pediatric condylomata may result in vaginal or rectal bleeding, dysuria, vaginal discharge, or painful defecation.

The diagnosis of genital condyloma acuminatum in children is often established by careful clinical inspection. The application of 3% to 5% acetic acid on a compress for 10 to 15 minutes may elicit the classic acetowhite appearance of condylomata. Biopsy may be indicated in those cases in which the diagnosis is in question. The role of DNA typing in the assessment of pediatric genital condylomata has been examined. HPV 6 and 11 are most commonly reported, with occasional reports of HPV 2.[51] The clinical usefulness of HPV typing of pediatric lesions is still undetermined.

Although spontaneous regression of condylomata has been described, it is not

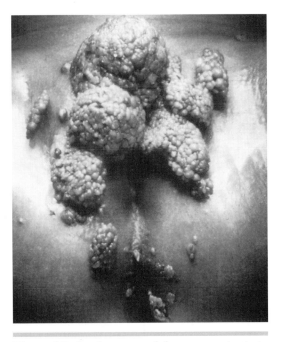

Figure 19–6. Large condyloma acuminata in a 17-month-old infant.

recommended as a treatment of choice in children. Topical agents (e.g., podophyllin, 5% to 25% solution with tincture of benzoin) have been used in the pediatric age group. The therapeutic value of topical agents is limited by the discomfort or actual pain involved in their use. An older child with a few condylomata may tolerate this treatment modality. In young children and in those with extensive disease, however, the usefulness of topical agents is limited. Interferon has been used only sporadically for the treatment of genital HPV in children.[52,53]

The use of the carbon dioxide (CO_2) laser has become increasingly popular in the treatment of genital condylomata. It allows control over depth of tissue destruction and avoids much of the scarring associated with electrosurgery. The CO_2 laser may also be used to treat lesions in the periurethral and perianal area as well as in the anal canal, where other modalities are more difficult to use. Recovery is well tolerated by children. Even so, recurrence rates of almost 30% have been reported.[54]

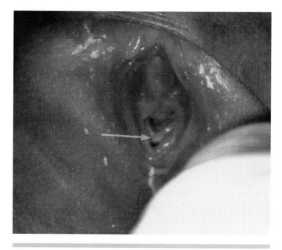

Figure 19–7. A foreign body (*arrow*) is seen in the lower vagina.

Foreign Bodies

The presence of foreign bodies in the vagina induces an intense inflammatory reaction that produces a bloody, foul-smelling discharge. In most instances, foreign bodies are lodged accidentally in the vagina, and the child does not recall the incident. Even if the girl intentionally inserted the foreign object into the vagina, she rarely admits to it.

The most commonly found objects are small pieces of toilet paper. These appear as amorphous conglomerates of grayish material, in which white and red blood cells are embedded (Fig. 19–7). They are often seen on the posterior wall in the lower third of the vagina. They can be easily seen when the labia are separated and the perineum is pushed downward. Radiographs are of little value in diagnosis because most foreign bodies are not radiopaque. Many of these objects can be irrigated and removed with warm saline. Vaginoscopy is indicated for the removal of large foreign bodies or to con-

firm that no other foreign objects are present in the upper vagina.

Occasionally, when a solid foreign body is left in the vagina for a prolonged period of time, it may become embedded in the vaginal mucosa and may even penetrate the rectovaginal or vesicovaginal septum into the rectum or bladder, creating fistulous tracts.

Lichen Sclerosus

Vulvar pruritus may be caused by any of several vulvar or perineal dermatologic disorders. These conditions are often not limited to the vulva but affect other body areas as well. Lichen sclerosus of the vulva is a hypotrophic dystrophy. Although it affects mainly women in the postmenopausal age group, it is occasionally seen in young children.[55] The symptoms consist of vulvar irritation, dysuria, and pruritus. Examination of the vulva shows flat, ivory-colored papules that may coalesce into plaques and may have pronounced vascular markings. In extreme cases, the lesion may involve the entire vulvar surface (Fig. 19–8). The lesion does not extend laterally beyond the middle of the labia majora, and it does not encroach into the vagina. Nonetheless, the clitoris, posterior fourchette, and anorectal area are frequently affected. The lesions tend to bruise easily, forming bloody blisters susceptible to secondary

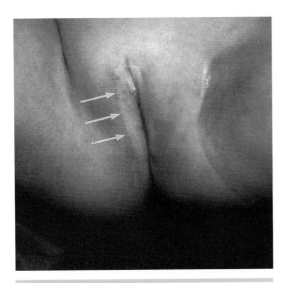

Figure 19–8. Lichen sclerosus of the vulva of a 6-year-old child. The margins of the lesion are clearly defined (*arrows*).

infections.[55] The affected skin may bleed after minor trauma, such as friction from tight-fitting jeans or riding a bike. Some children present with genital bleeding without history of trauma and are mistaken to be victims of sexual abuse.[56]

In most children, the experienced physician is able to establish the diagnosis based on the clinical features and the typical appearance of the affected skin. When the lesion is atypical or the diagnosis is in doubt, a skin biopsy is required. The histologic features are quite typical. The biopsy specimen shows flattening of the rete pegs, hyalinization of the subdermal tissues, and keratinization.

Lichen sclerosus in children has no malignant potential. Treatment consists of improved local hygiene, reduction of trauma, and the short-term use of hydrocortisone creams to alleviate the intense pruritus. Treatment may be repeated when exacerbations occur. The long-term use of estrogen or testosterone is not recommended in children because it may result in feminization or virilization, depending on the medication used.

Patients often experience a marked improvement in symptoms and appearance of the skin lesions following puberty. Review of the literature suggests that up to 50% of girls improve significantly or re-

cover during puberty, 30% to 45% experience no change in symptomatology, and in 5% to 10% of affected girls experience worsening of the disease.[55,57]

Labial Adhesions

Labial adhesions in prepubertal children are believed to be relatively common. Huffman and colleagues[58] consider girls age 2 to 6 years most likely to be affected; however, others have found the highest frequency to be in children under 2 years of age.[59] Many physicians believe that the prevalence of labial adhesions is significantly higher because many children with labial fusion are asymptomatic and remain unreported.

The cause is not known but is probably related to the low levels of estrogens in the prepubertal child. It is suggested that the thin skin covering the labia may be denuded as a result of local irritation and scratching. The labia then adhere in the midline, and as reepithelialization occurs on both sides, the labia remain fused in the midline (Fig. 19–9). Some studies re-

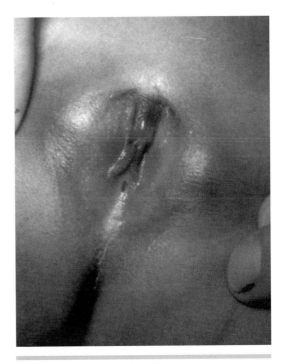

Figure 19–9. Labial adhesions in a young girl. Note the translucent vertical line in the center where the labia are fused together.

ported that labial adhesions were more prevalent in prepubertal girls who were sexually abused. It is possible that the abusive relationship causes denudation of the vulvar tissues and subsequently results in labial agglutination.[60,61]

The diagnosis of labial adhesions is made by the visual inspection of the vulva. The examiner can see a thin, avascular line of fusion in the midline. Most children with minor degrees of labial adhesion are asymptomatic. When symptoms do occur, they usually relate to interference with urination or to the accumulation of urine behind the fused labia. Dysuria and recurrent vulvar or vaginal infections are the presenting symptoms. On rare occasions, when complete occlusion is present, urinary retention may occur.[62]

If the girl is asymptomatic, a minimal to moderate degree of labial fusion does not require treatment. When the degree of fusion is significant or the child is symptomatic, a short course of treatment with Premarin cream, applied twice daily for 7 to 10 days, may separate the labia. At times, the fused labia respond only partially to the treatment with estrogen. In such cases, when the patient is cooperative, the physician can separate the labia in the office. A few minutes after the application of generous amount of 5% Xylocaine ointment to the labia, a small probe is inserted through the opening between the labia and gently passed along the line of fusion, teasing them apart. If medical treatment fails or if severe urinary symptoms exist, surgical division of the fused labia is indicated.[63]

Recurrence of labial adhesions is common because the estrogen-deficient state exists until puberty. Improved perineal hygiene and removal of irritants from the vulva may prevent recurrences. The condition usually resolves spontaneously following puberty.[63]

Urethral Prolapse

The urethral mucosa protrudes through the meatus and forms a hemorrhagic, tender vulvar mass that bleeds quite easily (Fig. 19–10). The cause of this condition is unknown. Capraro and associates[64] suggested that there is redundancy of the urethral mucosa associated with some laxity of the support of the urethra. This predisposition is further aggravated by an increase in the intra-abdominal pressure caused by coughing, sneezing, or straining.[64] Although the lack of estrogenic effect has been considered to be a contributing factor, hormonal studies failed to show differences between affected and nonaffected girls.[65]

The diagnosis is often made by the typical appearance and location of the mass, which is separated from the vagina. In most girls, the urethral orifice can be identified in the center of the mass. When the lesion is small and urination is unimpaired, a short course of topical estrogens is beneficial.[66] Resection of the prolapsed tissue should be considered if urinary retention is present, the lesion is large and necrotic, or the child is examined under anesthesia.[65,67]

Genital Tumors

Although uncommon, genital tumors must be considered whenever a girl is found to have a chronic genital ulcer, a nontraumatic swelling of the external genitalia, tissue protruding from the vagina, foul-smelling bloody discharge, abdominal pain, genital enlargement, virilization, or premature sexual maturation. Despite their rarity, virtually every type of genital neoplasm reported in adults has also been found in girls under 14 years, and about half of these are found to be malignant.

Most benign tumors of the vagina in children are unilocular cystic remnants of the mesonephric duct. Other benign neoplasms include teratomas, hemangiomas, simple cysts of the hymen, retention cysts of the paraurethral ducts, benign granulomas of the perineum, and condylomata acuminata.

Small cysts of the mesonephric (Gartner's) duct do not require surgery when asymptomatic. Large cysts, however, may interfere with urination or vaginal drainage thereby requiring surgical treatment. The cyst is opened, most of the accessible cyst wall is removed, and the edges are marsupialized to prevent future reaccumulation of fluid. Obstruction of a paraurethral duct may form a relatively large cyst, distorting the urethral orifice.

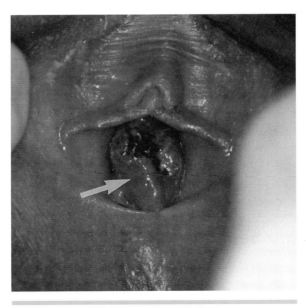

Figure 19–10. Urethral prolapse in a 6-year-old child.

Simple excision or marsupialization is again the recommended treatment. Teratomas usually present as cystic masses arising from the midline of the perineum. Although a teratoma in this area is often benign, local recurrences may occur. Therefore, a generous margin of healthy tissue should be excised about its periphery. Capillary hemangiomas usually disappear as the child grows older and require no therapy. In contrast, cavernous hemangiomas are composed of vessels of considerable size, and injury to them may cause serious hemorrhage. For this reason, cavernous hemangiomas are best treated surgically.

Embryonal carcinoma of the vagina (botryoid sarcoma) is seen most commonly in the very young age group (<3 years old). In these young children, the tumor is often situated in the lower vagina, whereas in an older child (>10 years old), the tumor more often affects the upper vagina or the cervix. The tumor arises from the lamina propria (from undifferentiated mesenchyme); spreads rapidly beneath the vaginal epithelium, infiltrating the vaginal wall; and forces the wall to bulge into a series of polypoid growths that contain abundant edematous stroma and dilated blood vessels. The loose, myxomatous nature of the matrix gives it the characteristic soft, grape-like appearance (Fig. 19–11). The growths

may be hemorrhagic or ulcerated. The neoplasm may also infiltrate nearby pelvic structures (e.g., bladder, rectum, pelvic cavity).

The diagnosis is confirmed by histologic examination of a biopsy specimen. Microscopically, these masses contain poorly differentiated round or spindle-shaped cells, the rhabdomyoblasts. The cambium layer, described as a cell-dense zone of primitive cells just beneath the overlying basement membrane of the epithelium, is another histologic feature.

The management and prognosis of childhood pelvic rhabdomyosarcoma have undergone a remarkable change for the better over the last three decades, evolving from a position of primary radical excision with no adjuvant treatment to a combined treatment modality using chemotherapy with subsequent limited surgery or radiotherapy. Survival has not been compromised in the process. Initial treatment of embryonal carcinoma consists of combination chemotherapy, usually vincristine, actinomycin D, and cyclophosphamide. Following the course of chemotherapy, the tumor is reexamined, and another biopsy is performed. Complete resolution may be seen in some patients. If the neoplasm persists, further therapy is indicated. If it is amenable to surgical removal, radical hysterectomy and vaginectomy with preservation of the

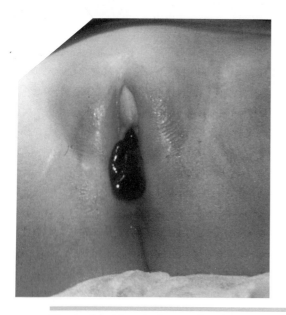

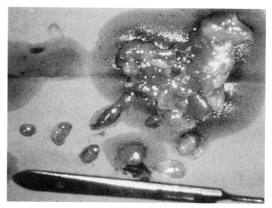

Figure 19–11. *A,* Botryoid sarcoma presenting as a hemorrhagic growth extruding from the vagina. *B,* Note the appearance of the lesion. The cystic structures are loosely connected and appear as grapes. This appearance is the origin for the name *sarcoma botryoides.*

ovaries is performed. If the tumor is still unresectable following chemotherapy, radiotherapy is employed to assist further in shrinking and controlling tumor growth. Exenteration is not recommended, although it may be required in some patients who do not respond to other treatment modalities.[68]

Several studies suggest that favorable prognosis in rhabdomyosarcoma is governed by site and histologic type and clinical group.[69] Genitourinary rhabdomyosarcoma has the best prognosis because most of these neoplasms are of the embryonal variety, which carries a favorable prognosis when compared to the alveolar, pleomorphic, or mixed variants.[70] Because of the communicative nature of the genitourinary tract, these lesions tend to produce symptoms quite early.

Genital Trauma

Prepubertal girls often sustain genital injuries. Young children are adventuresome and often take unnecessary risks. Accidental injuries usually occur as a result of a fall and result in hematomas, lacerations, or even penetrating injuries. Such injuries often affect the external genitalia and the perineum. Because the perineum and vulva are extremely vascular and the subcutaneous tissues are loosely arranged, an injury may cause blood vessels underneath the perineal skin to rupture. Blood accumulates under the skin and forms a hematoma, producing a rounded, tense, and tender swelling, the size of which depends on the amount of bleeding (Fig. 19–12). A contusion of the vulva does not usually require treatment. A small vulvar hematoma can usually be controlled by pressure with an ice pack. A large hematoma or one that continues to increase in size should be incised, the clotted blood removed, and bleeding points ligated. If the source of the bleeding cannot be found, the cavity should be packed with gauze and a pressure dressing applied. The pack is removed in 24 hours. The prophylactic use of broad-spectrum antibiotics is advisable. The vulva should be kept clean and dry. When the urethra is obstructed by the hematoma, it is necessary to insert a suprapubic catheter. Pelvic x-ray may be indicated in a few patients to rule out a fracture of the pelvis.

Most vaginal injuries occur when an object penetrates the vagina through the hymenal opening. Such penetration

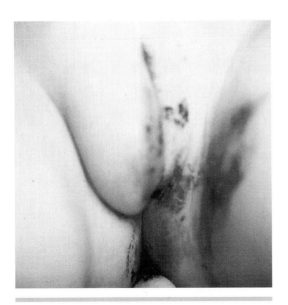

Figure 19–12. A vulvar hematoma in a 12-year-old girl caused by a straddle injury.

causes a laceration or a tear of the hymenal ring. Hymenal injuries are often seen in girls who are victims of sexual abuse. The tearing of the hymen occurs as the vagina is entered by a blunt object, usually following digital or penile penetration. Because the unestrogenized hymen has only limited elasticity, the shearing force causes the hymen to tear, and the tear may then extend to the vaginal wall or to the perineum (Fig. 19–13).[71] The

hymenal tissue is thin, poorly vascularized, and easily stretched. Bleeding is often minimal, and the patient has no acute symptoms. Penetration in the very young patient, however, is often associated with a significant vaginal injury. The thin vaginal mucosa with its limited distensibility often lacerates with the hymen. Penile pressure on the introitus is directed toward the posterior vaginal wall, the hymen tears from its posterior aspect, and then the laceration secondarily enlarges to involve the posterior vaginal wall. With further penetration, the rectovaginal septum is torn, and the tear extends into the rectum. A detailed examination is necessary in patients with acute hymenal injuries to exclude injuries to the upper vagina. Most vaginal wounds involve the posterior wall. The blood loss is relatively minimal, and the child does not have much pain.[71]

Injuries of the vagina or rectum may present surgical difficulties because of the small caliber of the organs involved. Small instruments are required as well as proper exposure and assistance. Vaginal lacerations should be repaired in a single layer. Care must be taken to begin the repair from the apex of the tear. A continuous locking suture (polyglactin 910 [Vicryl] 3–0) is often satisfactory to approximate the tissues and to control the bleeding. The perineal tear and the anal sphincter are approximated only on

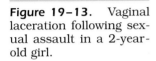

Figure 19–13. Vaginal laceration following sexual assault in a 2-year-old girl.

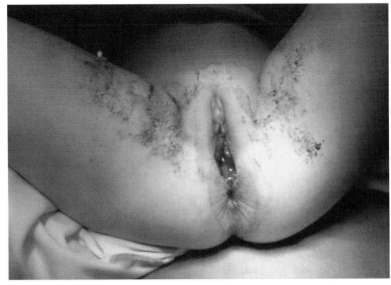

completion of the vaginal repair. This delay affords the surgeon better access into the narrow vagina.

If the laceration extends to the vaginal vault, surgical exploration of the pelvic cavity is necessary to rule out extension into the broad ligament or peritoneal cavity and injuries to intraperitoneal organs. Bladder and bowel integrity must be confirmed by inspection, catheterization, and rectal palpation.

The appearance of accidental sharp penetrating injuries has been reported.[72] Penetrating sharp injuries have a typical appearance that is significantly different than that caused by blunt penetrating trauma. Penetration by a sharp object, whether accidental or intentional, may cause hymenal or even vaginal injury, with minimal or no disruption of the hymenal edge. One series described four patients who sustained a sharp penetrating injury to the hymen. In all patients, the hymenal injury was left to heal by secondary intention, although a vaginal laceration was repaired surgically in one patient. In the three patients in whom the injury was surrounded entirely by hymenal tissue, fenestration of the hymen was seen following the healing process. In the fourth patient, who required surgical repair of an accompanying vaginal laceration, the hymenal defect was no longer visible, possibly as a result of the surgical repair.

CONGENITAL MALFORMATIONS

Anomalies of the genitalia may be divided into two major categories: those that suggest sexual ambiguity (intersex problems) and those that do not. This section discusses some of the more common congenital abnormalities affecting the external and internal genitalia. For a more detailed discussion of the various anomalies and their management, the reader is referred to other sources.[73–75]

Ambiguous Genitalia

Ambiguous genitalia denotes a partial or incomplete virilization of the external genitalia (Fig. 19–14). Ambiguous geni-

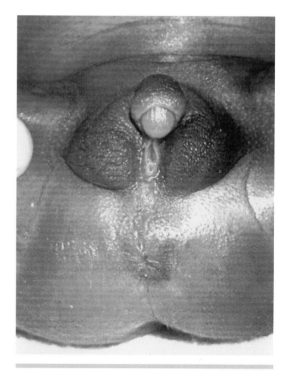

Figure 19–14. Ambiguous genitalia of a female child caused by congenital adrenocortical hyperplasia.

talia may be seen in genetic females who were virilized in utero, in undervirilized males, or in true hermaphrodites. In general, exposure to androgens after 12 weeks of gestation leads only to clitoral hypertrophy. Examination of the genitalia reveals an enlarged clitoris with a normal vestibule, urethra, and vagina. The labia majora are altered by redundancy, wrinkling, and skin pigmentation. Exposure at progressively earlier stages of embryologic development also leads to clitoral hypertrophy as well as to retention of the urogenital sinus and to fusion of the labioscrotal folds. In these severely virilized individuals, the labia are fused in the midline to form a median raphe. The area of fusion may be partial or extend the entire distance from the perineum to the phallus. When extensive, the fused labia form a wrinkled, pouchlike structure that resembles the scrotum in a male with cryptorchidism. The vaginal opening is absent. Instead, a single opening is present, which extends to a common passage connecting the urethra and vagina. Müllerian and gonadal development remain unaffected because neither is androgen dependent. The medical management and surgical correction of genital ambiguity are beyond the scope of the primary care provider. A multidisciplinary team approach is best suited for the comprehensive management of these patients.

Anomalies of the Vulva and Labia

As in any other part of the body, minor differences in the contour or size of vulvar structures are not unusual. Often, there is considerable variation in the distance between the posterior fourchette and the anus or between the urethra and the clitoris, giving the vulva different appearances.[58] There is also considerable variation in the size and shape of the labia minora. One labium may be considerably larger than the other, or both labia may be unusually large (Fig. 19–15). Labial enlargement and asymmetry have been wrongly assumed by some to be the result of masturbation. The physician should reassure the patient that these differences are simple minor variations that require no treatment. If the asymmetry is significant or the labia are pulled into the vagina during intercourse, the hypertrophied labia may be trimmed surgically.[58]

Anomalies of the Clitoris, Epispadias, and Bladder Exstrophy

Clitoral agenesis is a rare condition.[76] Clitoral enlargement almost invariably suggests that the infant had been exposed in utero to elevated levels of androgens. Such enlargement of the clitoris is often associated with fusion of the labioscrotal folds and is discussed under the section on abnormal sexual differentiation. Enlargement of the clitoris caused by a benign neoplasm has been observed in a few infants. For example, Von Recklinghausen's neurofibromatosis, lymphangiomas, and fibromas may involve the clitoris and cause enlargement.[77] Progressive idiopathic clitoral enlargement also has been described. When an isolated neoplasm causes enlargement of the clitoris, therapy consists of excision of the neoplasm and thereby reduction of the clitoris to normal size.

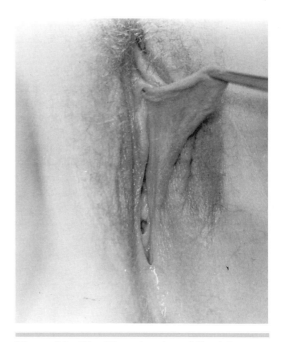

Figure 19–15. Hypertrophy of the labia minora in a 10-year-old girl.

Splitting or duplication of the clitoris is caused by the failure of the corpora to fuse in the midline. Bifid clitoris usually occurs in conjunction with bladder exstrophy, epispadias, and absence or cleavage of the symphysis pubis. The labia majora are widely separated, and the labia minora are separated anteriorly but can be traced posteriorly around the vaginal orifice. The vaginal orifice is narrow, and the vagina is shortened and rotated anteriorly.[78] The pelvic floor is incomplete, and uterine prolapse is often observed in these patients (Fig. 19–16). Other congenital anomalies may be present (e.g., spina bifida). At puberty, pubic hair growth is absent over the midline. Major urologic reconstruction is required immediately, but the gynecologic defects can be repaired later during the adolescent years.[78]

Anomalies of the Hymen

Variations in the appearance of the hymen are extremely common. The orifice may vary in diameter from small to large.[79] There may be one or more small orifices. A thick median ridge separating two lateral hymenal orifices may suggest

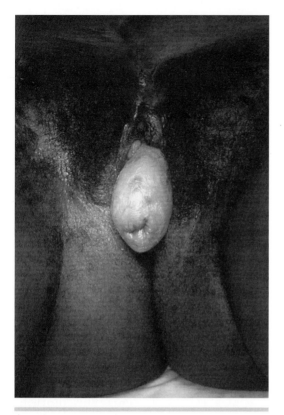

Figure 19–16. Uterine prolapse in a 15-year-old girl with bladder exstrophy.

ing a mucocolpos or hydrocolpos. When this occurs, the thin hymenal membrane is stretched out and forms a bulging, shiny, thin protuberance. Unless a mucocolpos is diagnosed and the fluid drained, the distended vagina forms a large mass, which may interfere with urination and at times may be mistaken for an abdominal tumor.[58]

Anomalies of the Vagina

Failure of Vertical Fusion

Transverse vaginal septa are the result of faulty canalization of the embryonic vagina. These septa may be without an opening (complete or obstructive) or may have a small central aperture (incomplete or nonobstructive). They are usually found in the midvagina but may occur at any level.[78] When the septum is located in the upper vagina, it is more likely to be patent (incomplete), whereas those located in the lower part of the vagina more often are complete.

An incomplete septum is usually asymp-

a septate vagina. The hymenal diaphragm may be a thin membrane or a thickened and fibrous one, forming a firm partition. Occasionally, what initially appears to be an imperforate hymen is found to have one or more tiny openings and is called a microperforate hymen.[58]

Although most of these variants are of no clinical significance, hymenal anomalies require surgical correction if they block the escape of vaginal secretions or menstrual fluid, interfere with intercourse, or prevent an indicated vaginoscopy and treatment of a vaginal disorder.[58] An imperforate hymen occurs when the hymen forms a solid membrane without an aperture (Fig. 19–17). It is assumed that an imperforate hymen represents a persistent portion of the urogenital membrane and occurs when the mesoderm of the primitive streak abnormally invades the urogenital portion of the cloacal membrane. When the vagina is obstructed, accumulation of vaginal secretions may distend the vagina, form-

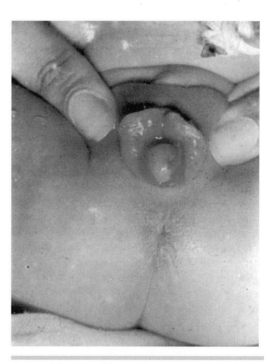

Figure 19–17. Mucocolpos secondary to an imperforate hymen.

tomatic and therefore does not require correction during childhood or early adolescence. The central aperture allows for vaginal secretions and menstrual flow to egress from the vagina. A complete septum, however, results in signs and symptoms similar to those of an imperforate hymen.[73,78,80] Unfortunately the diagnosis of a transverse vaginal septum is often delayed until after menarche when menstrual blood is trapped behind an obstructing membrane. If the diagnosis of a complete septum is established before menarche, it should be incised, creating an aperture to allow drainage. Incision of a complete septum should be done only when the upper vagina is distended and the membrane is bulging. The distention confirms the presence of an upper vaginal segment and facilitates the procedure and reduces the risk of injury to adjacent structures.[73,80]

Failure of Longitudinal Fusion

When the distal ends of the müllerian ducts fail to fuse properly, the mesenchymal tissue between the ducts forms a longitudinal septum that divides the vagina lengthwise. If asymptomatic, longitudinal septa require no treatment. Division of the septum is indicated when dyspareunia is present, when obstruction of drainage from one half of the vagina is noted, or when the physician suspects that a septum would interfere with a vaginal delivery.[73,80]

Vaginal Agenesis

Individuals with the Rokitansky syndrome are genetic females. They develop normally in adolescence and have all of the usual feminine attributes, but because the müllerian ducts fail to develop, the uterus and vagina do not form. The external genitalia, however, are normal. A ruffled ridge of tissue represents the hymen, inside which there is an indentation marking the spot where the introitus would normally be found.

In many patients, other developmental defects are present as well, affecting the urinary tract (45% to 50%), the spine (10%), and less frequently the middle ear and other mesodermal structures.[81] Therefore, at some time during childhood, in any child with vaginal agenesis, there should be an evaluation of the urinary tract, the spine, and hearing. In addition, a chromosome analysis may be required in some patients with vaginal agenesis to rule out the rare instances in which vaginal agenesis represents the effects of testicular activity. An exploratory laparotomy is not indicated in these patients, and the absence of the uterus can be confirmed by a pelvic sonogram.

Creation of a functional vagina is the objective in treatment of vaginal agenesis, and this should be deferred until the young woman is contemplating an active sexual life. Several techniques have been used. The nonoperative creation of a vagina using graduated vaginal dilators has been described by Frank[82] and Ingram.[83] It is relatively risk-free but requires motivation and patient cooperation. The area that the vagina should occupy is a potential space filled with comparatively loose connective tissue that is capable of considerable indentation. The patient is given a series of dilators of graduated sizes and lengths and is taught how to place them against the vaginal dimple and apply constant pressure. This maneuver is repeated daily for 20 to 30 minutes using wider and longer dilators. The procedure takes a few months to complete and requires persistence and patience.

If it fails, the vaginal space can be developed surgically, between the urethra and bladder anteriorly and the perineal body and rectum posteriorly. This cavity is then lined by a split-thickness skin graft overlying a plastic or soft silicone mold (McIndoe procedure).[84] Although the use of an amnion may prevent pain and scarring at the site from which the skin graft was taken, fears regarding acquired immunodeficiency syndrome (AIDS) have rendered this method unsafe.

An alternative procedure is the Williams vulvovaginoplasty, which uses the labia majora to construct a coital pouch.[85] The labia are placed under tension. A U-shaped incision is carried from the level of the urethra along the margins of the labia majora to the midpoint between the posterior fourchette and the anus.

The vulvar skin is dissected from the subcutaneous fat to allow approximation without tension. Closure is in three layers. First-layer closure of the incision begins posteriorly and proceeds anteriorly, approximating the inner layer of skin. Interrupted sutures are then used to approximate the subcutaneous tissues, then the outer layer of skin is closed over the midline.

PUBERTY

Puberty is the period of life during which secondary sexual development occurs, the sex organs mature, and the reproductive capacity is attained. Puberty in the female begins with the first sign of secondary sexual development and continues until ovulation occurs. These changes occur largely as a result of the maturation of the hypothalamic-pituitary-ovarian (HPO) axis. The HPO axis begins to function early in the second trimester with the synthesis of gonadotropin-releasing hormone (GnRH). GnRH is then transported to the anterior pituitary gland and stimulates production of both pituitary gonadotropins, follicle-stimulating hormone (FSH) and luteinizing hormone (LH).

In early infancy, gonadotropins, and in particular FSH, are secreted in large amounts, and their level remains relatively high throughout the first 2 years of life. Afterwards, a higher central nervous system center begins to suppress the HPO axis, thereby limiting the production of GnRH. Subsequently the serum levels of FSH and LH fall to the low, prepubertal levels. At approximately 10 years of age, there is an increase in the amplitude and frequency of pulsatile GnRH secretion. This sets off a cascade of hormonal and physical changes that constitutes the pubertal development. The mechanism that initiates this increase in GnRH production is unknown, although the timing of puberty correlates better with skeletal maturity than with chronologic age.[86]

Increased GnRH secretion first occurs at night and stimulates nocturnal pulsatile secretion of LH, usually associated with sleep. This elevation of LH is the first measurable hormonal change of puberty.

As puberty progresses, LH pulses become more frequent, until at late puberty, they occur every 90 minutes. Basal levels of FSH also increase in early puberty, but then they plateau, and the FSH response to GnRH becomes less pronounced.

FSH and LH, in turn, stimulate the ovary to produce sex steroids. LH promotes the production of androgen precursors in the theca cells, and FSH activates the aromatase enzyme that converts these precursors to estrogen in the granulosa cells. Sex steroids, in addition to the physical changes, increase the basal levels of prolactin and growth hormone (GH).[87] The rise in GH secretion leads to increased serum concentrations of insulin-like growth factor 1 (IGF-1). The pubertal growth spurt is related to the increased secretion of sex steroids, GH and IGF-1.[88]

The visible physical changes of puberty generally proceed in the following manner: breast development (thelarche), growth acceleration, appearance of pubic hair (pubarche or adrenarche) and later axillary hair, and onset of menstruation (menarche). The onset of both thelarche and pubarche for North American girls are variable, with a mean of 10.9 and 11.2 years. Although the onset of the *adolescent growth spurt* at a mean age of 9.6 precedes breast development, this acceleration of growth is seldom documented and often goes unnoticed. Peak growth velocity occurs almost 2.5 years later and precedes the onset of menses (mean age 12.7 years). Regular ovulation, 20 months later, marks the completion of the pubertal cycle. The interval between the onset of thelarche and menarche is 2.3 ± 1.0 years and is independent of the age at which thelarche occurs. Marshall and Tanner[89] recorded the progression of pubertal development of 192 English girls. This classification (Table 19–1) is useful in following pubertal development in adolescents.

The chronologic span of puberty is wide but not infinite. The normal range for thelarche is 8.0 to 13 years. Sexual precocity is the onset of sexual maturation at any age that is 2.5 SD earlier than the norm. At present, the appearance of any secondary sexual characteristics before 8 years of age or onset of menarche

Table 19–1.   Sexual Development—Girls

Breast Development

Stage 1	Preadolescent. Elevation of papilla only
Stage 2	Breast bud stage. Elevation of breast and papilla as small mound. Enlargement of areolar diameter
Stage 3	Further enlargement and elevation of breast and areola with no separation of their contours
Stage 4	Projection of areola and papilla to form a secondary mound above the level of the breast
Stage 5	Mature stage. Projection of papilla only caused by recession of the areola to the general contour of the breast

Pubic Hair

Stage 1	Preadolescent. The vellus hair over the pubes is similar to that over the abdominal wall; that is, no visible pubic hair
Stage 2	Sparse growth of long, slightly pigmented downy hair, straight or curled, primarily along labia
Stage 3	Considerably darker, coarser, and more curled. The hair spreads sparsely over the junction of the pubes
Stage 4	Hair now adult in type, but area covered is still considerably smaller than in the adult. No spread to the medial surface of the thighs
Stage 5	Adult appearance in quantity and type with distribution of the horizontal (or classically feminine) pattern. Spread to medial surface of thighs but not up linea alba or elsewhere above the base of the inverse triangle (spread up linea alba occurs late and is rated stage 6)

before age 10 is considered precocious. Similarly, puberty is delayed when no signs of sexual development have begun by age 13 or absence of menarche by age 15.

Delayed Puberty

Delayed sexual development is defined as the absence of normal pubertal events at an age greater than 2.5 SD from the mean. The physician need not always delay evaluation until these criteria are met. The concern of the patient, her family, or the referring physician are reasons enough for initiating an evaluation. Because some degree of sexual maturation occurs in greater than 30% of patients with gonadal dysgenesis, an investigation is necessary when a girl presents following thelarche with delay in progression of pubertal development.[90]

Patients presenting with abnormal puberty may be classified according to gonadal function. Thus, patients are divided into three major clinical groups according to secondary sexual development:

1. Delayed menarche with adequate secondary sexual development (i.e., primary amenorrhea). These disorders have been collectively referred to as *eugonadism.*
2. Delayed puberty with inadequate or absent secondary sexual development. These disorders have been collectively referred to as *hypogonadism.* When FSH levels are high, the condition is called *hypergonadotropic hypogonadism,* and when FSH levels are low, the condition is called *hypogonadotropic hypogonadism.*
3. Delayed puberty and heterosexual secondary sexual development (i.e., *virilization*).

Patients with Adequate Secondary Sexual Development

Patients with functioning ovaries and delayed sexual maturation usually consult a physician in their midteens for primary amenorrhea. They have a well-formed female configuration with appropriately developed breasts. Most of these patients (approximately 80%) suffer from inappropriate LH feedback, anovulatory cycles, unopposed estrogens, and, in some patients, an excess of androgenic hormone production. Primary amenorrhea may persist until the patient is challenged with a progestin. Following a withdrawal bleeding, patients should be monitored for continued menstrual function because in some anovulation persists. Continued amenorrhea is treated with cyclic progestins, administered monthly or every other month, to ensure endometrial shedding and to prevent potentially heavy menstrual bleeding. Obviously, if the patient is sexually active, birth control pills are preferable to cyclic progestins.

Anovulation and the resulting endocrine disturbance—distortion of the estrogen-to-androgen ratio—are also encountered in adolescents with postnatal adrenogenital syndrome and patients with polycystic ovarian disease. The signs and symptoms are similar in these conditions, and when hyperandrogenism is present, evaluation of adrenal function should be performed.

The possibility that an adolescent may become pregnant before she menstruates is highly unlikely but must be borne in mind when considering the causes of delayed menarche in these patients.

Congenital anomalies of the paramesonephric (müllerian) structures are sometimes seen in patients (approximately 20%) with amenorrhea.[20,91] The most frequent defect is congenital absence of the uterus and vagina. Other anatomic causes of amenorrhea include imperforate hymen, transverse vaginal septa, agenesis of the cervix, and partial or complete agenesis of the vagina. These anomalies have been described elsewhere in this chapter. Gynecologic examination supplemented by sonography establishes the diagnosis of these congenital anomalies.

Adolescents with complete androgen insensitivity may also present with primary amenorrhea. This condition is relatively rare and accounts for only 1% of patients presenting with primary amenorrhea. These patients are genetic males in whom the testes developed normally and produce adequate amounts of androgens. End organ tissues (e.g., sexual hair, genitalia) are not responsive to androgens, and as a result, the patients do not virilize in utero or at puberty. In utero, the fetus develops along female lines, but the müllerian ducts regress under the influence of the müllerian inhibiting hormone. The newborn infant appears to be a normal female because the external genitalia appear normal. The vagina is absent, but the diagnosis is rarely

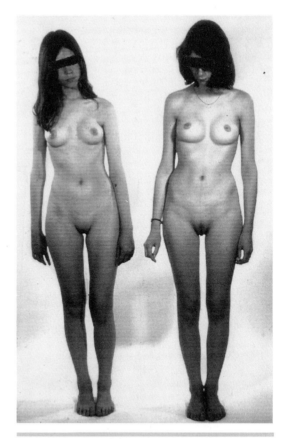

Figure 19–18. XY sisters with androgen insensitivity syndrome. (Courtesy of Professor Sir John Dewhurst. From Huffman JW, Dewhurst CJ, Capraro VJ: The Gynecology of Childhood and Adolescence, 2nd ed. Philadelphia, WB Saunders, 1981, p 187.)

made during childhood. During puberty, adequate breast development is often present, secondary to the small amounts of unopposed estrogen produced by the testis. Pubic and axillary hair are scant and often missing (Fig. 19–18). Only a short or blind vaginal pouch is present, and the patient presents with complaints of primary amenorrhea. The testes are often palpable in the inguinal canals. Once pubertal development has been completed, surgical extirpation of the gonads and reconstruction of the vagina are necessary.

Patients with Inadequate Secondary Sexual Development

The most common cause of pubertal delay is a normal variation in the timing or

---

Table 19-2. Delayed Sexual Maturation

Delayed menarche with adequate secondary sexual development
  Inappropriate hypothalamic-pituitary-
    ovarian axis feedback mechanism
  Anatomic defect
    Obstructed outflow tract
    Vaginal agenesis
  Complete androgen insensitivity syndrome
Delayed puberty (no signs of secondary sexual development)
  Gonadal failure (hypergonadotropic hypo-
    gonadism)
  Constitutional delay
    Chronic illness
    Weight loss
    Gymnasts
  Hypothalamic (hypogonadotrophic hypo-
    gonadism) pituitary failure
Delayed puberty with virilization
  XY female
  Virilizing tumors
  Congenital adrenal hyperplasia

---

tempo of the pubertal development, a condition known as *constitutional delayal puberty*. The statistical limits of normal variation of a defined population group indicate that by definition, 2.5% of all normal adolescents develop later than what is defined as normal. This group has been commonly labeled *late bloomers.* In addition, maturation is determined in part by genetic factors and also dependent on environmental factors. The lack of signs of puberty (including the pubertal growth spurt) often concerns the patient when her adolescent friends have secondary sexual features and the characteristic increase in height.

The various causes of delayed puberty are listed in Table 19-2. The diagnosis of constitutional delay is made by excluding other causes of delayed sexual maturation. The GnRH challenge test may differentiate constitutional delay from similar conditions associated with a deficiency of gonadotropin-releasing factor. Reassurance is the only necessary treatment, but the patient must be kept under observation until she begins normal menstrual cycles. Occasionally an adolescent requires temporary hormonal replacement therapy because of the emotional distress caused by the delay and the associated immature appearance.

Isolated deficiency of gonadotropin-releasing factor, often associated with intracranial anomalies and anosmia (Kallmann's syndrome), is uncommon. Every patient suspected of having the syndrome should be tested for sense of smell because many have only a minor degree of anosmia. These patients fail to develop secondary sexual features, and blood levels of gonadotropins are low. A rise in gonadotropin levels is normally expected following a GnRH challenge test. Estrogen therapy is used to initiate and later sustain sexual development. Induction of ovulation with menotropins (Pergonal) or GnRH should be given when fertility is desired.

A pituitary or parasellar tumor, particularly craniopharyngioma or pituitary adenoma, must be considered in the evaluation of a patient with delayed sexual maturation. Craniopharyngiomas are rapidly growing tumors that often develop in late childhood, whereas pituitary adenomas, although slow growing, may become symptomatic during puberty and interfere with sexual maturation.

An occult pituitary prolactinoma in adolescents with unexplained delayed sexual maturation must also be ruled out. Serum prolactin levels should be measured yearly in patients with unexplained delayed sexual maturation.

Weight loss because of severe dieting, marked protein deficiency, and fat loss without notable loss of muscle (often seen in athletes) may also delay or suppress hypothalamic pituitary maturation. Additionally, heroin addiction may cause amenorrhea, but its effect on sexual maturation has not been documented.

A large number of patients with delayed sexual development suffer from gonadal failure.[92] Lack of gonadal function most frequently occurs as a result of primary ovarian failure and is associated with a marked elevation of serum FSH. Most of these patients with ovarian failure suffer from a loss of X chromosome material and important ovarian determinant genes.

Two intact X chromosomes are usually necessary for normal ovarian structure and function. Chromosomal abnormalities that may be associated with failure of ovarian development include loss of all of one X chromosome, deletion of part of one, or transverse division at the centromere rather than longitudinal division leading to isochromosome formation. Mosaicism with two or more cell lines, one containing an abnormal X chromosome, is probably more common than nonmosaic abnormalities.[92] Somatic abnormalities with gonadal dysgenesis may be the result of the deletion of genetic material carried with the lost portion of the X chromosome. As a result, some with gonadal dysgenesis have only failure of sexual maturation, whereas others exhibit the complete phenotype of Turner's syndrome.

Adolescents with ovarian failure present with undeveloped breasts, little or no pubic hair, an atrophic vaginal smear, and elevated FSH levels. When X chromosome material is missing, somatic anomalies may also be present. The classic features of Turner's syndrome are well recognized: short stature, absent or minimal secondary sexual development, neck webbing, and coarctation of the aorta.[92] In all patients with gonadal failure, chromosomal analysis should be undertaken to help define its nature. Replacement hormonal therapy given in a cyclic manner is the treatment of choice. When a Y chromosome complement or derivative is discovered, gonadectomy is indicated because of the possibility of neoplastic changes in the retained gonad.[93,94]

Some patients may have ovarian failure with normal sex chromosomes (46,XX). In these patients, ovarian failure may be secondary to causes other than privation of X chromosome material. An autosomal recessive form of ovarian failure has been determined in some families.[95] Other causes of follicular depletion include chemotherapy, irradiation, infections (mumps), infiltrative disease processes of the ovary (tuberculosis), autoimmune diseases, and other known environmental agents. Submicroscopic X chromosome deletions in ovarian determinant region, however, may result in ovarian failure, similar to that found in patients with Turner's syndrome.

The resistant ovary syndrome is characterized by delayed menarche or primary amenorrhea, a 46,XX karyotype, high FSH levels, and ovaries that despite apparently normal follicle apparatus do not respond to endogenous gonadotropins. It is assumed the absence of follicular receptors for gonadotropins is responsible for ovarian failure in these patients. These individuals have normally developed secondary sexual characteristics, which contrasts with other adolescents having delayed sexual maturation, high FSH levels, and a normal chromosome constitution. Estrogen replacement therapy should be initiated to prevent long-term complications (e.g., vaginal dryness and osteoporosis). Pregnancies have been reported in some patients treated with Pergonal or following discontinuation of estrogen therapy.[96]

Virilization at puberty is the result of elevated androgens from adrenal or gonadal sources. These may be the result of an enzyme deficiency (e.g., late-onset congenital adrenal hyperplasia) or a neoplasm (e.g., Leydig cell tumor). A small group of these patients are male pseudohermaphrodites, that is, adolescents who are being reared as girls, have female external genitalia, intra-abdominal or ectopic malfunctioning testes, and a normal 46,XY chromosomal constitution. This may be the result of mutation within the testis-determining region found in the Y chromosome.

Evaluation of the Patient with Delayed Sexual Development

Determination of gonadal function for categorization into hypogonadal or eugonadal groups can be accomplished by obtaining a medical history and performing a physical examination. Historical information should center around previous growth and pubertal development. Linear and velocity growth charts as well as a pubertal development chart clarify previous growth patterns and are useful in subsequent follow-up. Knowledge of previous medical disorders may help identify the cause of aberrant puberty.

Physical examination must include height, weight, and a search for somatic anomalies. Staging of pubertal development by Tanner classification is most important in determination of gonadal function. Presence of breast development signifies prior gonadal function. A vaginal smear for cytohormonal evaluation can determine whether the gonad is continuing to produce estrogen. Pelvic and rectal examination identifies patients with an obstructed outflow tract as well as patients with congenital absence of the vagina and uterus. Further confirmation of patients with Rokitansky sequence is dependent on a karyotype to identify normal 46,XX complement and a pelvic sonogram to confirm uterine absence and ovarian presence.

Absence of pubic hair is suggestive of the androgen insensitivity syndrome. Karyotype analysis identifies 46,XY individuals with testicular feminization syndrome. Patients with complete pubertal development, evidence of continued estrogen production, and normal müllerian systems probably have inappropriate positive feedback and, hence, chronic anovulation. Progesterone challenge in such patients is helpful; a withdrawal bleed signifies a normal müllerian system and continued estrogen production.

When breast development is minimal, the usual diagnosis is hypogonadism. Serum gonadotropin assays are performed for further elucidation; elevated FSH levels suggest gonadal failure. Other endocrine profiles should be obtained if hypothyroidism, congenital adrenal hyperplasia, or Cushing's syndrome is suspected. Karyotype is necessary in patients with gonadal failure. Gonadal extirpation is required when Y chromosome material is identified.

Low FSH levels suggest an interference with hypothalamic pituitary maturation and gonadotropin release. Skull films and prolactin assays must be obtained for all patients to rule out the more serious irreversible causes, such as pituitary tumors. Appropriate endocrine evaluation identifies the occasional patient with hypothyroidism or congenital adrenal hyperplasia and the rare patient with Cushing's syndrome. Diagnosis of Kallmann's syndrome is suspected in hypogonadotropic patients who have associated anosmia but is confirmed only after GnRH challenge tests are performed. The presumed diagnosis of physiologic delay is made by exclusion of all other causes and by the typical gonadotropin release patterns after GnRH challenge.

Early Pubertal Development

Isosexual precocious puberty is defined as the onset of secondary sexual development before age 8 or menarche before age 10. The signs of puberty may result from endogenous sex steroids produced by the ovaries or the adrenal glands or may derive from exogenous, environmental sex steroid exposure or drugs. In the case of endogenous steroids, sexual precocity may result from premature activation of the HPO axis and is referred to as *true precocious puberty* or GnRH-dependent precocious puberty. When mechanisms other than the normal activation of the HPO axis are responsible for the sexual development, the condition is labeled as *pseudoprecocious puberty* or GnRH-independent precocious puberty. Occasionally, for reasons that remain unclear, only one sign of pubertal development is present: breast development, pubic hair, or menstruation (Table 19–3).

True precocious puberty affects both sexes but is four to eight times more common in girls. The peak incidence of true precocious puberty occurs between the ages of 4 and 5 years. These patients

Table 19–3. Early Sexual Maturation

Complete Forms
Immature HPO axis (GnRH independent)
  Exposure to estrogens
    In the food chain
    Medications
  Endogenous estrogen production
    Functional ovarian cysts
    Ovarian neoplasms
    Other hormone-producing neoplasms
  McCune-Albright syndrome
Mature HPO axis (GnRH dependent)
  Constitutional precocious puberty
  Central nervous system lesions

Incomplete Forms
Premature thelarche
Premature adrenarche
Premature menarche

HPO = Hypothalamic-pituitary ovarian; GnRH = gonadotropin-releasing hormone.

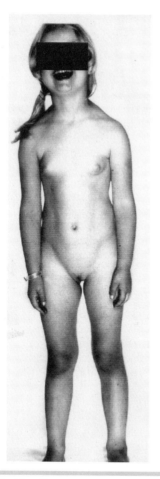

Figure 19–19. Precocious puberty in a 4-year-old child.

have no abnormality except for the early development of pubertal changes that progress in an orderly sequence (Fig. 19–19). In some of these girls, a CT scan of the brain occasionally demonstrates the presence of small hypothalamic hamartomas. The ovaries, stimulated by the mature HPO axis, produce sex steroids and, subsequently, the physical changes of puberty. Follicular development occurs, and pregnancies have been reported. Girls with idiopathic precocious puberty have some loss of adult height because of an accelerated bone maturation. In other respects, however, prognosis is favorable, and future menstrual pattern and fertility in this group of patients are expected to be normal.[97]

Central Nervous System Lesions

Patients with central nervous system lesions such as tumors, severe head injuries, meningitis, and encephalitis occasionally have early sexual development, possibly as a result of an irritative phenomenon on the hypothalamus resulting in an earlier than normal activation of the HPO axis. Usually pubertal development is slower than normal and progresses gradually over many years. The clinical findings (apart from the early pubertal development) are related to the nature of the primary central nervous system lesion. When such lesions are large, concurrent neurologic deficit may be present. Treatment is directed toward the primary disorder, and precocious puberty is treated symptomatically. Prognosis is determined by the nature of the primary central nervous system lesion. Primary pituitary tumors secreting gonadotropins are unusual and rare causes of precocious puberty.

Lastly, primary hypothyroidism may present as isosexual precocity with growth retardation. Precocious puberty in these girls may be the result of an overlapping production of FSH and LH in response to thyroid-stimulating hormone (TSH). It is also possible that the reduced metabolic rate in patients with hypothyroidism results in reduced catabolism of gonadotropins thereby prolonging their biologic activity.

Gonadotropin-Releasing Hormone–Independent Precocious Puberty

In these disorders, the increase in sex steroid production is independent of GnRH production or secretion of gonadotropins. In other words, these disorders are not an expression of early maturation of the HPO axis. Accidental ingestion of estrogens (e.g., estrogen-containing food) or the prolonged use of creams containing estrogens is a possible (yet uncommon) cause of early feminization. If such exposure is documented, prompt discontinuation is the proper treatment. Gonadotropin-independent precocious puberty may also occur in girls with functional ovarian cysts, adrenal neoplasms, and ovarian neoplasms (e.g., granulosa cell tumor). The ovary of a newborn contains 1 to 2 million primordial follicles, most of which undergo atresia during childhood without producing significant quantities of estrogen. Large follicular cysts capable of estrogen production may occur, however, and lead to early feminization. In addition, other benign tumors of the ovary (i.e., teratoma, cystadenoma) are capable of either producing estrogens or inducing the surrounding ovarian tissue to produce sex steroids. Finally, granulosa cell tumors capable of estrogen production are a rare cause of feminization of a prepubertal child. Other tumors of extragonadal origin may produce estrogens, and these include adrenal adenomas and hepatomas but are extremely rare.

McCune-Albright Syndrome

The diagnosis of McCune-Albright syndrome is established by the presence of the typical clinical triad of polyosthotic fibrous dysplasia, irregular cutaneous pigmentation, and precocious puberty. McCune-Albright syndrome has been attributed to defects in the LH receptor, interfering with the synthesis of cyclic adenosine monophosphate, which is the intracellular messenger required for estrogen production.[98] In these girls, estrogen secretion is episodic, although it corresponds to ovarian follicular development and regression. These children usually present at a younger age than those with idiopathic precocious puberty. Vaginal bleeding occurs early and in most is the first sign of puberty. The diagnosis is made on the basis of the skin pigmentation (Fig. 19–20) and the presence of the typical bone lesions or pathologic fractures.

The prognosis is unfavorable. Adult height is significantly reduced, not only because of the early epiphyseal closure, but also because of skeletal abnormalities and pathologic fractures of the long bones. In addition, most adults with this disorder suffer from severe menstrual abnormalities and infertility.[97]

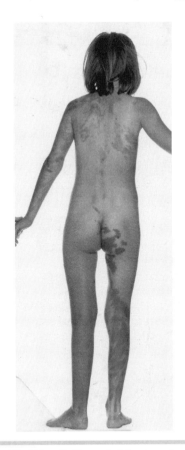

Figure 19–20.   Café-au-lait lesions in a child with McCune-Albright syndrome.

Pseudoprecocious Puberty (Incomplete Puberty)

Occasionally, for reasons that remain unclear, only one sign of pubertal development is present (breast development, pubic hair, or menstruation). It is possibly the result of transient elevations in the levels of circulating steroid hormones produced by small follicular ovarian cysts or, alternatively, may be caused by extreme sensitivity of the end organ to the low, prepubertal levels of sex hormones. Such isolated development, however, may also be the first sign of true precocious puberty, and reevaluation at regular intervals is indicated.

Premature Thelarche

Premature thelarche is the isolated development of breast tissue before age 8. It may occur at an earlier age but is most common between 1 and 3 years. It may affect one or both breasts. On examination, somatic growth pattern is not accelerated; bone age is not advanced; and estrogen levels are within the normal, low, prepubertal range. The diagnosis is made by exclusion of other disorders, such as hypothyroidism. Surgical biopsy of the breast is contraindicated because a relatively large portion of breast tissue may be unwittingly excised, causing permanent damage to the breast. Follow-up is necessary to identify those patients in whom such breast development heralds the onset of true precocious puberty. The prognosis is favorable: In 32% of patients, there is spontaneous regression; in 54%, there is no change; and in only 11%, breast size increases.[99] Pubertal development is unaffected, and menstrual pattern and fertility are reported to be normal.[97]

Premature Pubarche

Premature pubarche is the isolated development of pubic or axillary hair before age 8 without other signs of precocious puberty. Such hair growth may be idiopathic and of no clinical significance. In some series, these individuals tend to be slightly taller, bone age tends to be marginally advanced, and DHEAS levels in the blood tend to be slightly elevated.[100]

Early pubarche may also be a sign of excess androgen production because of an enzyme deficiency (e.g., congenital adrenal hyperplasia) or tumor (e.g., Leydig cell tumor). Thorough evaluation of adrenal and gonadal function as well as assessment of androgen production is necessary to exclude such abnormalities. Thus, the diagnosis of idiopathic premature pubarche is made only after such an evaluation fails to detect a hormonal abnormality.

Premature Menarche

Premature menarche denotes the appearance of cyclic vaginal bleeding in girls under age 10 in the absence of other signs of secondary sexual development. Examination of these children is usually normal, and the genital appearance as well as cytologic vaginal smears shows lack of constant estrogenic stimulation. Growth and development are appropriate for age, and the bone age is not advanced. When these girls are given GnRH challenge, the response of the pituitary gland is similar to that seen in prepubertal children.

The diagnosis is formulated by exclusion of other causes of vaginal bleeding. With time, the diagnosis is confirmed when the cyclic nature of the bleeding becomes apparent. Prognosis for these girls is excellent; adult height is uncompromised, future menstrual pattern is normal, and fertility potential remains unimpaired.[101]

Evaluation of the Patient with Accelerated Sexual Development

The evaluation of a child presenting with early sexual maturation requires a detailed history, in particular, onset and progression of growth and secondary sexual features, use of medications, history of head injury or central nervous system lesions, and family history of early sexual maturation. A complete physical examination should include height, weight, and Tanner staging of breast and pubic hair development. Growth should be plotted on standard growth charts as well as on growth velocity charts. Careful inspection of the skin should be performed in search of pigmented nevi or neurofibromas. Inspection of the genitalia is required to determine the degree of estrogenic stimulation. A rectoabdominal palpation is required to delineate large ovarian lesions.

Initial laboratory evaluation in patients with isolated breast development consists of plasma estrogen levels, prolactin, and, when clinically indicated, thyroid function tests. A left hand and wrist x-ray is obtained to determine bone age. If all these tests are normal, the diagnosis of premature thelarche is highly likely. These patients require follow-up to determine whether progression occurs. Absence of further development confirms the diagnosis.

Initial laboratory evaluation in patients with isolated pubic hair development consists of plasma androgen levels, 17α-hydroxyprogesterone, and, when clinically indicated, ACTH stimulation and suppression tests. A left hand and wrist x-ray is obtained to determine bone age. If all these tests are normal, the diagnosis of premature adrenarche is highly likely. These patients require follow-up to determine whether progression occurs. Absence of further development confirms the diagnosis.

Initial laboratory evaluation in patients with suspected true precocious puberty consists of plasma estrogen levels (or an evaluation of vaginal smear for estrogen effects), a left hand and wrist x-ray to determine bone age, a pelvic sonogram, and CT or MRI of the skull. Diagnosis is confirmed by a pubertal response to a GnRH challenge test.

Therapy

Treatment of early sexual development depends on the exact cause. Patients with incomplete puberty (e.g., premature thelarche, premature adrenarche) require only observation and serial follow-up visits. In patients with gonadal or adrenal neoplasms, the treatment consists of surgical excision of the neoplasm. Patients with congenital adrenal hyperplasia require steroid replacement therapy. Patients with central nervous system lesions may require surgery or irradiation depending on the histologic features and the location of the lesion.

Treatment of patients with true precocious puberty is aimed at suppression of gonadotropin secretion. The most common treatment today is the administration of GnRH agonists. These drugs lower the production rate and secretion of gonadotropins by the pituitary gland. If GnRH agonists are not available, 100 to 200 mg of medroxyprogesterone acetate may be given intramuscularly weekly or twice monthly.

ABNORMAL UTERINE BLEEDING IN THE ADOLESCENT

Excessive or irregular bleeding from the vagina is a common disorder of menstru-

Table 19–4. Differential Diagnosis of Dysfunctional Uterine Bleeding

Pregnancy complications
  Abortion
  Ectopic pregnancy
  Trophoblastic disease
Benign and malignant neoplasms of the
    genital tract
  Endometrial polyp
  Cervical polyp
  Vaginal adenosis
  Vaginal carcinoma
  Cervical carcinoma
  Granulosa-theca cell tumors
  Endometriosis
  Leiomyoma
Genital tract infection
  Vaginitis
  Cervicitis
  Vaginal foreign body
  Intrauterine contraceptive device
  Salpingo-oophoritis
Endocrinopathies
  Polycystic ovarian disease
  Hyperprolactinemia
  Hypothyroidism
  Hyperthyroidism
Administration of drugs or hormones
Trauma
Coagulation disorders
  Idiopathic thrombocytopenic purpura
  von Willebrand's disease
Chronic systemic illness
  Liver cirrhosis
  Renal failure

al function. Although few adolescents do have an organic lesion that causes the bleeding, most of these patients suffer from dysfunctional uterine bleeding (DUB), a condition defined as abnormal bleeding from the uterine endometrium that is unrelated to anatomic lesions of the genital tract. Almost all cases in the adolescent age group are caused by anovulation resulting in a total lack of progesterone. DUB is only a symptom; before therapy can be instituted, the more serious causes of genital bleeding in the adolescent age group should be ruled out (Table 19–4).

Anovulatory uterine bleeding tends to follow one of several patterns, and the specific pattern encountered depends on the duration and intensity of estrogen stimulation of the endometrium. In the presence of continual high levels of estrogen, continued endometrial proliferation occurs. When estrogen levels become insufficient to support further endometrial growth or to maintain endometrial integrity, desquamation and bleeding occur. The menstrual cycles are usually longer than the average span for ovulatory cycles, and the bleeding is often heavy. In the presence of continual low circulating levels of estrogen, endometrial growth extends for a longer period, with a greater interval of amenorrhea between successive menstrual periods. The bleeding may be heavy and prolonged. In the presence of fluctuating levels of estrogens, there is an increase in the frequency of bleeding episodes. The patient often has more than one bleeding episode each month. With each decline in circulating estrogen levels, endometrial integrity is compromised and bleeding ensues.[102]

The diagnosis of DUB is based on history, general physical examination, pelvic examination, and (rarely) selected laboratory tests. It requires the exclusion of all organic causes of abnormal vaginal bleeding. In a typical teenager with DUB, the history reveals irregular periods since menarche with a heavy flow that lasts several days or even weeks. Generally the physical examination is normal. A Papanicolaou smear is obtained at the time of the pelvic examination. It is often useful to obtain a simple vaginal smear for cytology (maturation index). Although there is no typical anovulatory pattern, a progesterone-dominated maturation index is consistent with an ovulatory cycle and might therefore suggest a diagnosis other than dysfunctional bleeding (e.g., pregnancy). To complete the evaluation of a patient with presumed DUB, the following tests should be included: a pregnancy test, urinalysis, complete blood count, serum prolactin level, and, in selected cases, thyroid function tests. Although an endometrial biopsy is often performed in adult patients, it is seldom necessary in a teenager.

The possibility of an underlying coagulation disorder in the adolescent patient with perimenarchal menorrhagia needs to be considered. Idiopathic thrombocytopenia purpura and von Willebrand's disease are the most common. A careful medical history with specific questioning as to episodes of easy bruising, epistaxis, gingival bleeding, and family history is recommended. A thorough physical examination, blood smear, and coagulation screen should be performed routinely in any patient with severe menorrhagia or prolonged episodes of DUB.[103] The coagulation screen should include prothrombin time, partial thromboplastin time, phase platelet count, and bleeding time. This relatively simple screen effectively rules out all but the rare hematologic disorders. These tests should be performed before transfusion and administration of hormones.[103]

A simple classification based on hemoglobin concentration is required for effective clinical management (Table 19–5). Those who have hemoglobin levels greater than 12 g/dL are considered to have a mild disturbance (group I); those with hemoglobin levels between 10 and 12 g/dL have a moderate abnormality (group II); and those with hemoglobin levels less than 10 g/dL have a severe problem

---

Table 19–5.   Management of Dysfunctional Uterine Bleeding

Hgb >12 g/dL
Reassurance
Menstrual calendar
Iron supplement
Periodic reevaluation

Hgb 10–12 g/dL
Reassurance and explanation
Menstrual calendar
Iron supplement
Cyclic progestin therapy or OCP
Reevaluation in 6 mo

Hgb <10 g/dL: No Active Bleeding
Explanation
Transfusion/iron supplement
OCP
Reevaluation in 6–12 mo

Hgb <10 g/dL: Acute Hemorrhage
Transfusion
Fluid replacement therapy
Hormonal hemostasis (intravenous conjugated estrogens [Premarin])
Intensive progestin therapy
Dilation and curettage when hormonal hemostasis fails
OCP for 6–12 mo
Periodic reevaluation

OCP = Oral contraceptive pill.

(group III). In group I, reassurance and explanation are necessary, with an ongoing review of the patient's progress at regular intervals. The patient is given a menstrual calendar and encouraged to take a daily dietary iron supplement.[104] The majority of patients spontaneously convert to normal menstrual cycles within 1 or 2 years. In group II, the bleeding is severe enough to warrant action. One may choose to use oral contraceptive pills (OCPs) for a short period of time. The pill reverses the effects of estrogens and prevents further endometrial proliferation. The use of OCPs should be considered in all sexually active girls. The other alternative, to be considered for girls who are not sexually active, is to institute intermittent progestin therapy using medroxyprogesterone acetate (Provera), 10 mg daily for 5 to 7 days every 35 to 40 days. This is an excellent cycle regulator because it allows spontaneous menses to occur between treatment cycles, and it prevents chronic unopposed estrogen stimulation of the endometrium. In group III, the bleeding episodes are severe, and some patients require emergency hospital management. Patients who are bleeding heavily or become hypotensive require transfusions and fluid replacement. Associated pathology, specifically complications of pregnancy and coagulopathy, must be excluded. In one series, 20% of all adolescent patients requiring hospitalization for DUB were found to suffer from a coagulation disorder.[103] Regardless of the cause, the bleeding may be controlled in most patients by the administration of estrogens or, sometimes, progestins. In a few rare instances, when primary medical management has failed, dilatation and curettage may be required. Initial hormonal hemostasis may be achieved by the administration of Premarin 20 to 25 mg intravenously every 4 hours for a maximum of six doses. It is usually unnecessary to continue the parenteral estrogen therapy beyond 24 hours.[103,105] Continued bleeding beyond this time is an indication for diagnostic dilatation and curettage. Concurrently a highly progestational OCP (i.e., Ovral) is given. An initial loading dose of two tablets is followed by one tablet four times daily, and the dosage is tapered gradually over the succeeding month. Despite the dosage, this regimen is well tolerated, and antiemetics are seldom required.

Following this intense hormonal therapy, 6 months of cyclic therapy with conventional combined OCPs is undertaken. It is expected that the withdrawal flow will be reasonable and regular and that each successive cycle will be accompanied by a progressive reduction in endometrial height. After 6 months, the patient is reassessed. If she is sexually active, continued treatment with OCPs is recommended. Otherwise, the patient may be allowed to menstruate without medication. Careful follow-up is undertaken to assess the timing and duration of menses with the aid of a menstrual calendar and to treat any relapses that may occur. If the anovulatory pattern recurs, Provera is used as described for group II patients. By adhering to this medical protocol of initial hormonal hemostasis followed by cyclic regulation of menses and continuous long-term observation, unnecessary dilatation and curettage can be avoided, and surgical management may be reserved for the small percentage of patients who fail to respond to conservative measures.

In general, adolescent menstrual problems are viewed with optimism, and 50% of adolescents with DUB return to a regular menstrual pattern within 4 years following menarche.[106] If anovulation persists longer than 4 years, however, the chance of recovery is low. The risks of exposure to continued unopposed estrogen stimulation must then be considered.

DYSMENORRHEA

Dysmenorrhea affects almost half of all female adolescents today and is probably the most frequently encountered gynecologic disorder. The term *dysmenorrhea* is derived from the Greek, and although it means difficult monthly flow, it is commonly used to refer to painful menstruation. Dysmenorrhea is classified as primary or secondary. Primary dysmenorrhea has no detectable pelvic pathology, whereas in secondary dysmenorrhea, the pain is the result of an existing pelvic disease.

Adolescent dysmenorrhea often begins shortly after menarche (within 6 to 12 months) and coincides with the onset of ovulatory cycles. The patient complains of colicky pain that begins several hours before or just at the onset of menstrual flow. The pain usually begins in the mid-pelvis and radiates to the back and sometimes to the legs. The pain is most severe during the first day of menstruation but may last for 2 or 3 days. In more than half the patients, the pain is accompanied by other systemic signs, including nausea and vomiting, fatigue, diarrhea, headaches, and irritability. In rare instances, syncopal attacks have been reported. Patients with primary dysmenorrhea have reported diminishing symptoms with increasing age. In some, the pain may disappear after the first childbirth.

The diagnosis of primary dysmenorrhea is made on the basis of its clinical features and the onset of pain at or shortly after menarche. The pain begins shortly before or immediately following menstruation and disappears completely within 2 or 3 days. The pain is crampy in nature, and pelvic examination is normal.

It is now well accepted that in many adolescents with primary dysmenorrhea the production and release of endometrial prostaglandins give rise to abnormal uterine activity and that this abnormal activity is perceived by the patient as discomfort or pain. It has been shown that the intensity of abnormal uterine activity is related to the amount of prostaglandins released into the menstrual flow from the degenerating decidua. Prostaglandin levels are highest during the first 48 hours of menstruation. In addition to uterine hyperactivity, prostaglandins may give rise to pain by directly affecting nerve endings.[107]

Both OCPs and prostaglandin inhibitors were found to be highly effective in the treatment of dysmenorrhea. The use of OCPs was found to be effective in at least 90% of women with primary dysmenorrhea. OCPs suppress endometrial proliferation, resulting in an endocrine environment similar to that of the early proliferative phase of the menstrual cycle, when prostaglandin levels are lowest. OCPs are the drug of choice for sexually active teens, who need contraception as well.[107]

Prostaglandin inhibitors are used mainly in young patients who do not need con-

traception. It is the drug of choice for the treatment of primary dysmenorrhea because the pills are taken only during the first 2 or 3 days of the menstrual cycle. The medication either inhibits cyclic endoperoxide synthesis or acts through the cyclic endoperoxide cleavage enzyme system. As a result, endometrial prostaglandin synthesis is suppressed, restoring normal uterine activity and providing relief from menstrual cramps.[107]

SECONDARY DYSMENORRHEA

In patients with secondary dysmenorrhea, the pain is the result of an existing pelvic pathology. Endometriosis has been reported in adolescents with obstructive genital malformations. At times, there is a history of previous pelvic inflammatory disease. Although the presence of dysmenorrhea in an adolescent often suggests that the patient has primary dysmenorrhea, it is now well accepted that in some patients endometriosis may occur soon after the onset of menarche.[108,109] If the patient fails to respond to medical therapy, she should be further evaluated to exclude pelvic pathology. Diagnostic laparoscopy is indicated to establish the diagnosis of endometriosis. The treatment for secondary dysmenorrhea is directed toward the underlying pelvic disorder.

REFERENCES

1. Hammerschlag MR, Alpert S, Rosner I, et al: Microbiology of the vagina in children: Normal and potentially pathogenic organisms. Pediatrics 1978; 62:57–62.
2. Muram D: Vaginoscopy. In Stovall T, Ling F, eds: Atlas of Benign Gynecologic Surgery. London, Mosby-Wolf 1994; pp 191–205.
3. Muram D, Jones CE: The use of video-colposcopy in the gynecologic examination of children and adolescents. Adolesc Pediatr Gynecol 1993; 6:154–156.
4. Grunberger W, Fisch LF: Pediatric gynecological outpatient department: A report on 600 patients. Wien Klin Wochenschr 1982; 94:614–618.
5. Muram D: Pediatric and adolescent gynecology. In DeCherney A, Pernol M,

eds: Current Gynecologic and Obstetric Diagnosis and Treatment. Norwalk, CT, Appleton & Lange, 1994; pp 633–661.

6. Ingram DL, White S, Durfee M: The association of gonorrhea (GC) in children and sexual contact. *In* Ambulatory Pediatric Association Program and Abstracts, 1982.

7. Ingram DL: The gonococcus and the toilet seat revisited. Pediatr Infect Dis 1989; 8:191.

8. Lewis LS, Glauser TA, Joffe MD: Gonococcal conjunctivitis in prepubertal children. Am J Dis Child 1990; 144:546–548.

9. Farrell MK, Billmire E, Shamroy JA, et al: Prepubertal gonorrhea: A multidisciplinary approach. Pediatrics 1981; 67:151–153.

10. Lipsitt HJ, Parmet AJ: Nonsexual transmission of gonorrhea to a child. N Engl J Med 1984; 311:470.

11. White ST, Loda FA, Ingram DL, et al: Sexually transmitted diseases in sexually abused children. Pediatrics 1983; 72:16–21.

12. DeJong AR: Sexually transmitted diseases in sexually abused children. Sex Transm Dis 1986; 13:123–126.

13. Nelson JD, Mohs E, Dajani AS, et al: Gonorrhea in preschool and school-aged children: Report of the prepubertal gonorrhea cooperative study group. JAMA 1976; 236:1359–1364.

14. Silber TJ, Controni G: Clinical spectrum of pharyngeal gonorrhea in children and adolescents. J Adolesc Health Care 1983; 4:51–54.

15. Whittington WL, Rice RJ, Biddle JW, et al: Incorrect identification of *Neisseria gonorrhoeae* from infants and children. Pediatr Infect Dis J 1988; 7:3–10.

16. Hammerschlag M: Pitfalls in the diagnosis of sexually transmitted diseases in children. *In* The Advisor, American Professional Society on the Abuse of Children (APSAC). 1989, pp 4–5.

17. Centers for Disease Control: Sexually transmitted diseases treatment guidelines. MMWR 1993; 42(RR-14):1–102.

18. Rettig PJ, Nelson JD: Genital tract infection with *Chlamydia trachomatis* in prepubertal children. J Pediatr 1981; 99:206–210.

19. Harrison HR, Alexander ER: Chlamydial infections in infants and children. *In* Holmes KK, eds: Sexually Transmitted Diseases. New York, McGraw-Hill, 1990; pp 811–820.

20. Alexander ER: Maternal and infant sexually transmitted diseases. Urol Clin North Am 1984; 11:131–139.

21. Frau LM, Alexander ER: Public health implications of sexually transmitted diseases in pediatric practice. Pediatr Infect Dis 1985; 4:453–467.

22. Hammerschlag MR, Chandler JW, Alexander ER, et al: Longitudinal studies on chlamydial infections in the first year of life. Pediatr Infect Dis 1982; 1:395–401.

23. Schachter J, Grossman M, Sweet RL: Prospective study of perinatal transmission of *C. trachomatis*. JAMA 1986; 255:3374–3377.

24. Bell TA, Stamm WE, Kuo CC, et al: Delayed appearance of *Chlamydia trachomatis* infections acquired at birth. Pediatr Infect Dis J 1987; 6:928–931.

25. Schachter J, Grossman M, Holt J: Infection with *Chlamydia trachomatis:* Involvement of multiple anatomic sites in neonates. J Infect Dis 1979; 139:232.

26. Bell TA, Stamm WE, Kuo CC: Chlamydial Infections. Cambridge, Cambridge University Press, 1986, pp 305–308.

27. Bell TA, Stamm WE, Wang SP, et al: Chronic *Chlamydia trachomatis* infections in infants. JAMA 1992; 267:400–402.

28. Paradise JE, Campos JM, Friedman HM, et al: Vulvovaginitis in premenarcheal girls: Clinical features and diagnostic evaluation. Pediatrics 1982; 70:193–198.

29. Hammerschlag MR, Rettig PJ, Shields ME: False positive results with the use of chlamydial antigen detection tests in the evaluation of suspected sexual abuse in children. Pediatr Infect Dis J 1988; 7:11–14.

30. Ginsburg CM: Acquired syphilis in prepubertal children. Pediatr Infect Dis 1983; 2:232–234.

31. Neinstein LS, Goldenring J, Carpenter S: Nonsexual transmission of sexually transmitted diseases: An infrequent occurrence. Pediatrics 1984; 74:67–76.

32. Dorfman DH, Glaser JH: Congenital syphilis presenting in infants after the newborn period. N Engl J Med 1990; 323:1299–1302.

33. Sanchez P, Wendal G, Norgard MV: Congenital syphilis associated with negative results of maternal serologic tests at delivery. Am J Dis Child 1991; 145:967–969.

34. Corey L: Genital herpes. *In* Holmes KK,

ed: Sexually Transmitted Diseases. New York, McGraw-Hill, 1990, pp 391–413.

35. Hibbard RA: Herpetic vulvovaginitis and child abuse. Am J Dis Child 1985; 139:542.

36. Gushurst CA: The problem of genital herpes in prepubertal children. Am J Dis Child 1985; 139:542–545.

37. Kaplan KM, Fleisher GR, Paradise JE, et al: Social relevance of genital herpes simplex in children. Am J Dis Child 1984; 138:872–874.

38. Nahmias AJ, Dowdle WR, Naib ZM, et al: Genital infection with herpesvirus hominis types 1 and 2 in children. Pediatrics 1968; 42:659–666.

39. Gardner M, Jones J: Genital herpes acquired by sexual abuse of children. J Pediatr 1984; 104:243–244.

40. Miller RG, Whittington WL, Coleman RM, et al: Acquisition of concomitant oral and genital infection with herpes simplex virus type 2. Sex Transm Dis 1987; 14:41–43.

41. Douglas JM, Corey L: Fomites and herpes simplex viruses: A case of non-venereal transmission? JAMA 1983; 250:3093.

42. Sweet RL, Gibbs RS: Perinatal infections. *In* Sweet RL, Gibbs RS, eds: Infectious Diseases of the Female Genital Tract. Baltimore, Williams & Wilkins, 1990, pp 290–319.

43. Sweet RL, Gibbs RS: Herpes simplex virus infection. *In* Sweet RL, Gibbs RS, eds: Infectious Diseases of the Female Genital Tract. Baltimore, Williams & Wilkins, 1990, pp 144–157.

44. Bender ME: New concepts of condyloma acuminata in children. Arch Dermatol 1986; 122:1121–1123.

45. Obalek S, Jablonska S, Favre M, et al: Condylomata acuminata in children: Frequent association with human papillomaviruses responsible for cutaneous warts. J Am Acad Dermatol 1990; 23:205–213.

46. Hanson RM, Glasson M, McCrossin I, et al: Anogenital warts in childhood. Child Abuse Negl 1989; 13:225–233.

47. DeJong AR, Weiss JC, Brent RL: Condyloma acuminata in children. Am J Dis Child 1982; 136:704–706.

48. Herman-Giddens ME, Gutman LT, Berson NL: Association of coexisting vaginal infections and multiple abusers in female children with genital warts. Sex Transm Dis 1988; 6:63–67.

49. Boyd AS: Condylomata acuminata in the pediatric population. Am J Dis Child 1990; 144:817–824.

50. Goldenring JM: Condylomata acuminata: Still usually a sexually transmitted disease in children (letter). Am J Dis Child 1991; 145:600–601.

51. Fleming KA: DNA typing of genital warts and a diagnosis of sexual abuse in children. Lancet 1987; 2:454.

52. Friedman-Kien AE, Eron LJ, Conant M, et al: Natural interferon alfa for treatment of condylomata acuminata. JAMA 1988; 259:533–538.

53. Healy GB, Gelber RD, Trowbridge AL, et al: Treatment of recurrent respiratory papillomatosis with human leukocyte interferon. N Engl J Med 1988; 319:401–407.

54. Gale C, Muram D: The surgical treatment of condyloma acuminata in children. Adolesc Pediatr Gynecol 1990; 3:189–192.

55. Dewhurst J: Lichen sclerosus of the vulva in childhood. Pediatr Adolesc Gynecol 1983; 1:149–162.

56. Jenny C, Kirby P, Fuquay D: Genital lichen sclerosus mistaken for child sexual abuse. Pediatrics 1989; 83:597.

57. Redmond CA, Cowell CA, Krafchik BR: Genital lichen sclerosus in prepubertal girls. Adolesc Pediatr Gynecol 1988; 1:177–180.

58. Huffman JW, Dewhurst CJ, Capraro VJ: The Gynecology of Childhood and Adolescence, 2nd ed. Philadelphia, WB Saunders, 1981.

59. Ben-Ami T, Boichis H, Hertz M: Fused labia: Clinical and radiological findings. Pediatr Radiol 1978; 7:33–35.

60. Muram D: Labial adhesions: A possible marker of sexual abuse. JAMA 1988; 259:352–353.

61. Berkowitz CD, Elvik SL, Logan MK: Labial fusion in prepubescent girls: A marker for sexual abuse? Am J Obstet Gynecol 1987; 156:16–20.

62. Stovall TG, Muram D: Urinary retention secondary to labial adhesions. Adolesc Pediatr Gynecol 1988; 1:203–204.

63. Muram D, Elias S: The treatment of labial adhesions in prepubertal girls. Surg Forum 1988; 34:464–466.

64. Capraro VJ, Bayonet-Rivera NP, Magosas I: Vulvar tumor in children due to prolapse of urethral mucosa. Am J Obstet Gynecol 1970; 108:572.

65. Velcek FT, Kugaczewski JT, Klotz DH, et al: Surgical therapy for urethral prolapse in young girls. Adolesc Pediatr Gynecol 1989; 2:230–233.

66. Mercer LJ, Mueller CM, Hajj SN: Medical treatment of urethral prolapse. Ad-

olesc Pediatr Gynecol 1988; 1:182–184.

67. Muram D: Vaginal bleeding in children and adolescents. Obstet Gynecol Clin North Am 1990; 17:389–408.

68. Dewhurst J: Botryoid sarcoma of the cervix and vagina in children. *In* Studd J, ed: Progress in Obstetrics and Gynecology. Edinburgh, Churchill Livingstone, 1983, pp 151–157.

69. Crist WM, Garnsey L, Beltangady MS, et al: Prognosis in children with rhabdomyosarcoma: A report of the Intergroup Rhabdomyosarcoma Studies I and II. J Clin Oncol 1990; 8:443–452.

70. Newton AWJ, Soule EH, Hamoudi AB: Histopathology of childhood sarcomas, Intergroup Rhabdomyosarcoma Studies I and II: Clinicopathologic correlation. J Clin Oncol 1988; 6:67–75.

71. Muram D: Genital tract injuries in the prepubertal child. Pediatr Ann 1986; 15:616–620.

72. Hostetler BR, Jones CE, Muram D: Sharp penetrating injuries of the hymen. Adolesc Pediatr Gynecol 1994; 7:94–96.

73. Jones HW Jr, Rock JA: Reparative and Constrictive Surgery of the Female Genital Tract. Baltimore, Williams & Wilkins, 1983.

74. Muram D: Congenital malformations. *In* Copeland LJ, ed: Textbook of Gynecology. Philadelphia, WB Saunders, 1993, pp 121–141.

75. Rock JA: Surgery for anomalies of the Müllerian ducts. *In* Thompson J, Rock J, eds: Te Linde's Operative Gynecology. Philadelphia, JB Lippincott, 1992, pp 603–646.

76. Falk HC, Hyman AB: Congenital absence of the clitoris: A case report. Obstet Gynecol 1971; 38:269.

77. Kaneti J, Leiberman E, Moshe P, et al: A case of ambiguous genitalia owing to neurofibromatosis: Review of the literature. J Urol 1988; 140:584.

78. Dewhurst CJ: Congenital malformations of the lower genital tract. Clin Obstet Gynecol 1978; 5:250.

79. Pokorny SF: Configuration of the prepubertal hymen. Am J Obstet Gynecol 1987; 157:950–956.

80. Rock JA, Azziz R: Genital anomalies in childhood. Clin Obstet Gynecol 1987; 30:682–696.

81. Griffin JE, Edwards C, Madden JD, et al: Congenital absence of the vagina: The Mayer-Rokitansky-Kuster-Hauser syndrome. Ann Intern Med 1976; 85:224–236.

82. Frank R: Formation of artificial vagina without operation. Am J Obstet Gynecol 1938; 35:1053.

83. Ingram JM: The bicycle seat stool in the treatment of vaginal agenesis and stenosis: A preliminary report. Am J Obstet Gynecol 1981; 140:867.

84. McIndoe AH, Banister JB: An operation for the cure of congenital absence of the vagina. J Obstet Gynaecol Br Emp 1938; 45:490.

85. Williams EA: Congenital absence of the vagina: A simple operation for its relief. J Obstet Gynaecol Br Commonw 1964; 71:511.

86. Sizonenko PC, Burr IM, Kaplan SL, et al: Hormonal changes in puberty: II. Correlation of serum luteinizing hormone and follicle-stimulating hormone with stages of puberty and bone age in normal girls. Pediatr Res 1970; 4:36.

87. Wennink JMB, Delemarre-van de Wall HA, Shoemaker R, et al: Growth hormone secretion patterns in relation to LH and estradiol secretion throughout normal female puberty. Acta Endocrinol (Copenh) 1991; 124:129.

88. Rosenfield RL, Furlanetto R: Physiologic testosterone or estradiol induction of puberty increases plasma somatomedin-C. J Pediatr 1985; 107:415.

89. Marshall WA, Tanner JM: Variations in the pattern of pubertal changes in girls. Arch Dis Child 1969; 44:291.

90. Simpson JL, Golbs MS, Martin AO, et al: Genetics in Obstetrics and Gynecology. Orlando, Grune & Stratton, 1982.

91. Shulman LP, Elias S: Developmental abnormalities of the female reproductive tract: Pathogenesis and nosology. Adolesc Pediatr Gynecol 1988; 1:230–238.

92. Simpson JL: Disorders of Sexual Differentiation: Etiology and Clinical Delineation. New York, Academic Press, 1976.

93. Simpson JL, Photopulos G: The relationship of neoplasia to disorders of abnormal sexual differentiation. Birth Defects 1976; 12:15–50.

94. Talerman A: Germ cell tumors of the ovary. *In* Blaustein A, ed: Pathology of the Female Genital Tract. Springer Verlag, New York, 1977.

95. Dewhurst SJ: Female Puberty and Its Abnormalities. Edinburgh, Churchill Livingstone, 1984.

96. Muram D, Jolly EE: Pregnancy and gonadal dysgenesis. J Obstet Gynecol 1982; 3:87–88.

97. Muram D, Grant DB, Dewhurst SJ: Precocious puberty: A follow-up study. Arch Dis Child 1984; 59:77–78.

98. Shenker A, Weinstein LS, Moran A, et al: Severe endocrine and non-endocrine manifestations of the McCune Albright syndrome associated with activating mutations of stimulatory G protein Gs. J Pediatr 1993; 123:509.

99. Milles JL, Stolley PD, Davies J, et al: Premature thelarche: Natural history and etiologic investigation. Am J Dis Child 1981; 135:743.

100. Kaplowitz PB, Cockrell JL, Young RB: Premature adrenarche: Clinical and diagnostic features. Clin Pediatr 1986; 25:28.

101. Muram D, Dewhurst SJ, Grant DB: Premature menarche: A follow-up study. Arch Dis Child 1983; 58:142–143.

102. Yen SSC, Jaffe RB: Reproductive Endocrinology, 2nd ed. Philadelphia, WB Saunders, 1986.

103. Claessens EA, Cowell CA: Acute adolescent menorrhagia. Am J Obstet Gynecol 1981; 139:277.

104. Arvidsson B, Ekenved G, Rybo G, et al: Iron prophylaxis in menorrhagia. Acta Obstet Gynaecol Scand 1981; 60:157.

105. DeVore GR, Owens O, Kase N: Use of intravenous Premarin in the treatment of dysfunctional bleeding—a double-blind randomized control study. Obstet Gynecol 1982; 59:285.

106. Southam AL, Richart RM: The prognosis for adolescents with menstrual abnormality. Am J Obstet Gynecol 1966; 94:637.

107. Smith RP: Primary dysmenorrhea and the adolescent patient. Adolesc Pediatr Gynecol 1988; 1:23–30.

108. Goldstein DP, deCholnoky C, Emans SJ: Adolescent endometriosis. J Adolesc Health Care 1980; 1:37.

109. Chatman DL, Ward AB: Endometriosis in adolescents. J Reprod Med 1982; 27:156–160.

Index

Note: Page numbers in *italics* indicate figures; those with a t indicate tables.

W

Warts, genital, 53–54
  children with, *255*, 255–256
  treatment of, 54
Weight loss, amenorrhea with, 148
  delayed puberty with, 269
Wernicke's encephalopathy, 242
Williams vulvovaginoplasty, 265–266

Wilms' tumor, 114t
World Health Organization (WHO), menopause
  defined by, 184
  Pap smear terminology of, 68, 69t

Y

Yeast infections, 49–50, 50t

ISBN 0-7216-6433-4

90038

9 780721 664330